Management Decision Making for Nurses

124 Case Studies

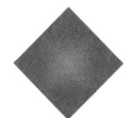

Third Edition

Bessie L. Marquis, RN, CNAA, MSN

Professor of Nursing
California State University
Chico, California

Carol J. Huston, RN, CNAA, MSN, DPA

Professor of Nursing
California State University
Chico, California

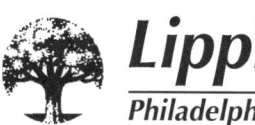
Lipp
Philadelph

D1044380

Sponsoring Editor: Jennifer E. Brogan
Coordinating Editorial Assistant: Susan V. Barta
Project Editors: Susan Deitch, Roberta Spivek
Production Manager: Helen Ewan
Production Coordinator: Patricia McCloskey
Design Coordinator: Kathy Kelley-Luedtke
Indexer: Ellen Murray

Third Edition

9 8 7 6 5 4 3 2 1

Library of Congress Cataloging in Publications Data

Marquis, Bessie L.
   Management decision making for nurses: 124 case studies / Bessie L. Marquis,
Carol J. Huston. —3rd ed.
     p. cm.
   Includes bibliographical references and index.
   ISBN 0-397-55429-X (alk. paper)
   1. Nursing services—Administration—Case studies. 2. Nursing—Decision making—
Case studies. I. Huston, Carol Jorgensen. II. Title.
   [DNLM: 1. Nursing, Supervisory. 2. Nursing Services—organization & administration.
3. Decision Making. WY 105 M357m 1998]
RT89.M388 1998
362.1′73′068—DC21
DNLM/DLC
for Library of Congress   97-24663
                                             CIP

Care has been taken to confirm the accuracy of the information presented and to describe generally accepted practices. However, the authors, editors, and publisher are not responsible for errors or omissions or for any consequences from application of the information in this book and make no warranty, express or implied, with respect to the contents of the publication.

The authors, editors and publisher have exerted every effort to ensure that drug selection and dosage set forth in this text are in accordance with current recommendations and practice at the time of publication. However, in view of ongoing research, changes in government regulations, and the constant flow of information relating to drug therapy and drug reactions, the reader is urged to check the package insert for each drug for any change in indications and dosage and for added warnings and precautions. This is particularly important when the recommended agent is a new or infrequently employed drug.

Some drugs and medical devices presented in this publication have Food and Drug Administration (FDA) clearance for limited use in restricted research settings. It is the responsibility of the health care provider to ascertain the FDA status of each drug or device planned for use in their clinical practice.

Dedication

*We dedicate this book
to the future leaders of the nursing profession:
those individuals who are willing to take risks
by challenging what is,
in hopes of what can be.*

Bessie L. Marquis
Carol Jorgensen Huston

Preface

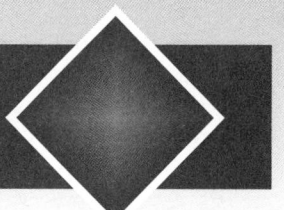

The first edition of this book developed as a result of several events that occurred more or less simultaneously. The first event dealt with our growing conviction that, although our students enjoyed and performed well in our nursing management course, they appeared to have some difficulty applying management theory to the workplace following their graduation.

The next event occurred as we became involved with the "teaching to think" movement, which developed as a result of criticism leveled against academia by numerous investigative bodies examining the status of education in America. Among those criticisms were reports that there was a serious decline in the ability of young adults to problem solve, and many were incapable of inferential reasoning. Organizations were formed by educators to address this problem and to identify and develop teaching strategies that would do more than merely give learners information—strategies providing learners with opportunities to use information in a manner that would result in improved decision-making skills.

After becoming involved in the teaching to think movement, we were convinced that a primary reason for student difficulty in transferring theory to practice and drawing inferences occurred because students of management theory had less opportunity to practice their new skills than did students of other nursing theory courses. Thus, we began to examine modes of teaching management theory that provided opportunities for practice simulation.

The next step was our growing interest in the case method approach, as a result of the Harvard Business School's use of the case method in their M.B.A. program. We began a search for an appropriate casebook for teaching new managers. Being unable to locate a text that would serve our needs, we undertook the task of writing our own casebook. After using the casebook for several years we added a theory component and published the first edition of *Management Decision Making for Nurses*. This is now the third edition of that text.

Since first publishing this textook, we have authored two editions of another text, *Leadership Roles and Management Functions: Theory and Application*. This second text uses a complete experiential approach to learning, with a dual emphasis on leadership and management. It also has an expanded theory base and a more sophisticated writing style.

However, there continues to be a need for a concise textbook with a strong management focus that uses a case approach for teaching management. Thus, we have written the third edition of *Management Decision Making for Nurses*. In writing the third edition we have made every effort to maintain the strengths of earlier editions and to correct shortcomings. We continue to respond to users' and reviewers' comments and have also included contemporary theory and new cases that illustrate the changing times in health care.

Because we believe that management problems are universal but that management science changes rapidly as our knowledge increases and the needs of society change, we have included a current bibliography at the end of each chapter to help readers solve the cases. In addition, we have updated content and references so the text remains contemporary. Some cases have been rewritten to make them more effective, new cases have been added, and ineffective or outdated cases were deleted. We have also somewhat reorganized the book's format, moving some theory to what we believe are more appropriate units, and although we have added a unit, we have not increased the book's size. We have eliminated outdated material, but for the most part the format remains the same. Per reviewer feedback, the *concise* theory component and writing style have been retained.

We continue to believe that the ability to transfer management theory will not occur unless the learner has an opportunity to apply management concepts over and over again in real life situations. Therefore, major concepts and theories are repeated throughout the book as each chapter builds upon information presented in prior chapters. In this way, learners develop skills in solving complex problems through the use of inferential reasoning.

We believe the abundance of cases in this text contributes greatly to its value and its potential for learning. The third edition contains 124 cases. Of these cases, approximately 20% are solved, and the rest are left for the learner to solve.

Many of the cases are straightforward and use traditional management theory as the rationale for decision making. Other cases are complex, requiring a greater degree of analysis and the need to synthesize a larger amount of didactic theory. The variation in complexity allows the book to be used with a wide range of learners, who have varying maturity levels and theoretical knowledge. The instructor therefore has a variety of choices in selecting case studies to best meet the needs of a particular group. We have made an effort to include case studies representing problems beyond the traditional hospital setting. All cases use current terminology and concepts, and most cases are derived from situations the authors or their nursing management colleagues actually experienced.

In this edition, we incorporated additional assignments requiring group problem solving. Regardless of the audience or the cases selected, we urge that the group process be used in some manner to facilitate problem solving. We believe group problem solving expands alternatives for decision making.

In order to assist individuals who have not previously used this mode of teaching/learning, there is a teacher's/learner's guide in the front of the text. In addition, the first chapters of the text are devoted to decision making and the management process. Those experienced in these aspects may not need to use all of this material.

We have found that management principles are just as applicable for managing one's personal life as for managing a nursing unit or department. Indeed, we have found that when learners begin to apply management principles to managing their personal lives, it not only makes their lives function better, it also makes learning management theory fun. Therefore, we have again included a personal notebook section at the end of each set of cases. We strongly encourage students and instructors or facilitators to use this unique part of our text, for we believe that the personalization of learning adds another valuable dimension to vicarious learning.

We have created this book in an effort to promote critical thinking in management. This will not occur if only past approaches to learning, such as lecture and discussion, are used. We therefore urge users of this book to incorporate experiential teaching techniques in order to facilitate analysis, synthesis, and communication—three elements of critical thinking most important in nursing management.

Reader and Instructor Guidelines for Using Case Studies

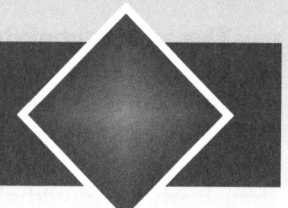

There is little question that vicarious learning, or learning through "simulated experience" has tremendous value and application to nurses. Examples of experiential or vicarious learning methods include group discussions, role playing, simulations, games, guided fantasy, psychodrama, and problem-solving exercises (Marquis, 1994). In all these methods, learning occurs *through* or *with* experience. In learning *through* experience, a situation is designed to allow participants to gain insight through participation. In learning *from* experience, participants look back at past experiences in their lives in order to glean new meanings from them or to compare them with their present situation.

Using case studies is one form of vicarious learning that allows participants to learn both through and from experiences. The case study approach allows learners to ask the "what, they, and how" questions to instill a habit of inquiry, gain a sense of how securely a conclusion is held, learn to discriminate clearly when evidence is available or not, discover implicit and explicit assumptions, analyze the reasoning of others, draw inferences, test their own line of reasoning, draw conclusions, and learn to transfer knowledge from familiar to unfamiliar concepts.

The case study provides a means for new learning for both students and teachers. Teachers can use case studies to demonstrate critical conditions in concrete situations rather than using abstract generalizations. Students derive additional significance from the information gathered about a problem when they have the opportunity to take action on the problem.

Because experiential learning provides the unique opportunity of gaining and sharing experiences without actually having to undergo the experience, case studies provide an opportunity for learners to vicariously live and learn how to make difficult decisions in a systematic and analytical manner. This allows for immediate application of learning and translating theory and principles into practice. This results in a reduction of risk, as novice managers are allowed to make simulated decisions before they occur in a management setting.

Use of case studies provides the opportunity for teachers/facilitators to recognize students or group members as mature, responsible human beings. Students gain confidence in their ability to problem solve and be risk takers.

5. Who is affected by the problem?
6. What is happening?
7. Why is it happening? What are the causes of the problem? Can the causes be prioritized?
8. What are the basic underlying issues? Areas of conflict?
9. What are the consequences of the problem? Which of these is most serious?

ANALYSIS OF SOLUTIONS

In analyzing possible solutions for a case study, individuals may want to look at the following questions:

1. What factors can be influenced? How can the positive factors be enhanced and the negative factors minimized?
2. What are the financial and political consequences of each possible solution? What are the departmental and interdepartmental consequences and time constraints? Is adequate support available?
3. What are the criteria for action?
4. What are the alternative plans of action?
5. What are the influencing factors?
6. What should be done?
7. What is the "best" solution?
8. Will a less than optimum solution be satisfactory?
9. What is the means for evaluation?

PRESENTATION OF FINDINGS

When assigned or called on to present a case and its solution, the presentation usually includes:

Introduction of self
Identification of the situation or problem
Analysis of key alternatives
Recommendations for specific action
Means of evaluation

If case presentations are to be graded, how factors are weighted should be determined in advance and shared with group members prior to case presentations. The evaluation of the presentation by facilitators and group members should consider the following factors:

1. Poise, clarity, dynamism, articulation, accuracy, nonverbal communication (appropriate and inappropriate), and use of audiovisual aids
2. Soundness of rationale used to support decision making and problem solving, and the quality of the problem solving
3. Evidence of preparation to address the questions posed in the case, and whether the objectives and questions were addressed completely

CRITIQUE OF THE PRESENTATION

Case studies provide an opportunity for critique by either the instructor/ facilitator or peers. Those critiquing should present feedback in a manner that is neither aggressive nor passive, but assertive. They must contribute information to the case presentation — for example, why the presentation was an example of effective problem solving or wise decision making, or what was faulty, illogical, or omitted. As with case presentations, it is possible to measure an individual's ability to objectively and assertively critique a presentation. The critique should be evaluated in terms of:

1. Poise, clarity, articulation, and concision
2. Soundness of rationale used
3. Fairness and assertiveness

Individuals selected to critique a case presentation may be assigned in advance or may be chosen at random immediately following the case presentation or critique. A case presentation and solution may be done on a volunteer basis.

◆ Strategies for Implementing the Case Study Approach

The preparation, presentation, and analysis of a case study requires a systematic approach if it is to be beneficial. However, there is no single, specific system for case preparation, as several principles are necessary for its successful use.

1. There must be a sufficient number of cases for participants to begin to draw conclusions. The case study approach is inappropriate if a spectrum of cases cannot be offered. Individual cases will often reveal variances from the norm but do not allow the participant to draw generalizations or to recognize patterns.
2. There is no absolute right or wrong solution to a case presentation, although some solutions will have a much greater possibility of successful implementation. Divergence, rather than convergence, of ideas and problem solving must be the goal. Perhaps the greatest value in using case studies is the number of solutions that are generated in response to every problem and the subsequent increase in the experiential and knowledge base of all the individuals involved in making that decision.
3. The particular organizational setting in which the case takes place is not of critical importance. Management concepts are transferable from one type of organization to another. Likewise, participants should not be concerned about the decision maker's position within the nursing administration hierarchy. Incidents should be analyzed using the best judgment possible, even if the participant never has occupied the particular role reflected in the incident.

4. It is critical to look for underlying problems in each case study as opposed to simply treating the symptoms of the problem, as this will only allow the problem to recur.

5. Experiential learning is frequently used in conjunction with, but is not synonymous with, group work. However, if the desired outcome for teaching critical thinking is an interaction between the participants that results in the ability to critically examine issues, then the group process must be employed in some manner (Marquis, 1994).

◆ Group Work Using the Case Study Approach

When the case study approach is used in a group, certain responsibilities must be recognized by group members.

THE FACILITATOR

There is little agreement about how active or passive the teacher's or the facilitator's role should be in learning. However, because experiential learning is still relatively new, the following proposals may assist educators in facilitating the application of theory.

1. An essential prerequisite for a successful case study is planning. The teacher or facilitator must try to imagine him- or herself as a participant and ask: What would I learn from this case? How would I go about solving the problem? If I found myself faced with these problems, would I miss the real problem? What parts of the case would help me toward an understanding of the real problem?

2. The facilitator must understand the cases and be able to identify their learning objectives. When alternatives are not formulated or issues not clarified, it may be difficult for group members to see what is involved in the case. The facilitator must try to identify the "universality" or primary focus of the case without squelching creativity in identifying solutions.

3. The group should be assisted past the point of dependence on the leader as solver of the problem. The facilitator should be the "enabler" of the group.

4. With increased experience in managerial and leadership problem solving, it is very easy for the facilitator to unconsciously direct group members toward a particular solution and to consider other solutions inappropriate. Flexibility and objectivity, therefore, are essential. The facilitator must also be willing to relinquish some control.

5. Discussion questions should be correlated to the participant's level of theoretical knowledge and practical experience. These questions should promote discussion rather than single-word responses, elicit a variety of appropriate problem solutions, highlight important concepts or principles, and build to generate increasingly complex responses.

6. Time can be a constraint in any type of experiential learning. The facilitator should predetermine how much time should be devoted to each case study or how many case studies the allotted period of time allows. Factors to consider include the learning objectives and the maturity of group members.

GROUP MEMBERS

Group members must assume the following responsibilities:

1. A willingness to listen to what is being said by other group members and the facilitator, rather than focusing on their own rebuttal.
2. A responsibility to share ideas to allow mutual learning. Consistent participation in group discussions will strengthen verbal skills.
3. Advance case preparation. This includes careful reading of the cases and completion of assigned didactic material before attempting to problem solve.
4. A willingness to subject themselves to open debate and criticism, as little can be gained when nothing is risked. The ultimate goal of criticism is to assist other group members in making good decisions. Criticism received must be viewed as an opportunity to learn with the risks being small and the potential for gain great.

◆ Modes for Case Study Presentation

Case studies traditionally have been used in group work for group problem solving. The case studies in this book can be used individually, or by a large or small group. The primary factors determining appropriate modes are the learning objectives for class and the maturity of group members. This book has been written for use by senior generic nursing students, the new first- and middle-level manager, and LVN/LPNs and RNs returning to school.

◆ Use of This Book with Senior Generic Nursing Students

With senior generic nursing students, the cases may be assigned to individuals or solved by the class as a whole. Many nursing students have limited knowledge regarding management theory and have had even less exposure to management in a clinical setting. The instructor or facilitator must recognize that outside preparation and reading will be necessary before group members can attempt to solve the cases. Assigning students specific cases in advance allows them to fully prepare for their specific case presentation. Calling on students spontaneously encourages advance preparation by all class members, but probably not to the extent as when cases are assigned in advance. The instructor must scrutinize the academic workload of the students in determining how many cases students will have adequate time to prepare for each class session, as well as how many cases can be solved during the academic quarter or semester. The instructor should seek case studies that provide many significant factors related to the problem, as the students will bring limited prior management experience from which to draw in their problem solving. As the book progresses the complexity of the case studies increases, and students may want to creatively embellish details of the situation.

The instructor may prefer group problem solving over selecting individuals to present cases. Using group problem solving presents both advantages and disadvantages. In a formal academic setting, time constraints often limit the use of group problem solving, as a knowledgeable instructor can often deliver the same content in much less time. In addition, digressions should be expected in groups that are not accustomed to the case method, as students frequently find that their listening skills are not as well developed as their verbal skills.

Evaluation of individual group members is also more difficult when group case study preparation and presentation are used. Instructors must be careful in grading individual group members based on the group product. The input into the case study analysis most likely will not be equal, as the abilities of individual group members usually differ. When using group case study analysis, the instructor must decide in advance if and how individual students will be evaluated. The instructor must also decide how problem solving will be weighted versus the appropriateness of group process. Although most instructors weigh quality more heavily than quantity of contributions, the assertive, articulate student will probably do best in evaluation.

Solving cases by the group process enhances both verbal and listening skills as well as group dynamics. Students learn to become better listeners. They learn to give and receive constructive criticism. Group process also encourages risk taking. As individual verbal and listening skills improve, the group learns how to improve its collective performance.

Perhaps the best approach for the use of case studies is for the problem solving to occur outside of actual class time. Use of small study groups prior to class allows learners to use small group process in solving cases. This method is advantageous because it does not consume needed class time and one member from the group can be randomly selected for the presentation.

There is much to be said for an individual rather than a group making the presentation of the case solutions. The individual making an unassisted presentation practices the art of communication, a critical thinking skill (Marquis and Huston, 1996).

◆ Use of the Text with Returning Students

All returning students, both vocational/practical nurses and ADN or diploma RNs, generally have a wide range of management/leadership backgrounds. They may have been managers in other fields, or held positions of management in nursing. Many returning students have held management positions and functioned in a variety of leadership roles. Even those who have not held management positions will have had the personal experience of being managed by someone in health administration.

It is important that the previous experience of these students be acknowledged. However, the instructor must also see that their practical experience be supplemented with concrete didactic information. Some may have had a short course in management theory, but many will not have. Occasionally, returning students have histories of being exposed to poor management and leadership styles. Such student exchanges will add personal meaning to the case studies.

Because there is a wide variety of life experiences in these groups, group process works very well and members tend to learn from each other. However, for this same reason there is still a need to add some structure. The text itself may serve adequately as the structure for the class, or the instructor may find that some class time needs to devoted to short organized lectures. Returning students also respond well to teacher-led discussion and if the class is not too large this often serves as an excellent alternative to the lecture.

◆ Use of This Book with New Managers

New managers may use this book within small seminar groups and workshops, or on an individual basis should adequate resources be available or should the new manager have a sound management theory base. If the case studies are used in the seminar/workshop setting, the instructor/facilitator must recognize that group members most likely have varying levels of knowledge and expertise. Applying an awareness of adult learner concepts, the facilitator should attempt to include the work experiences of group members, and should focus on case studies that examine problems relevant to group members at the time. Case studies selected for this group may be less specific or complete than those used for senior generic nursing students, as participants should have the benefit of life experience from which to draw or relate.

Seminars/workshops will probably not allow for advance preparation by group members and therefore, individual problem solving and case presentation is not a viable option. The facilitator should also recognize that because of the varying levels of expertise, some group participants will contribute more to the problem solving than others. The new manager with little experience will probably find the seminar the most helpful, whereas more experienced nurses may define their role as being that of a teacher and mentor.

Because there is rarely a need to evaluate individual performance in the seminar/workshop setting, the instructor/facilitator does not have the same concerns as with nursing students in differentiating between individual and group performance.

The relatively new manager with a sound management theory base may find value in reviewing the cases on an individual basis. With adequate resources, the new manager can search for the various alternatives to the case study solution and recommend solutions. Certainly, the lack of feedback or cor-

DECISION MAKING IN MANAGEMENT

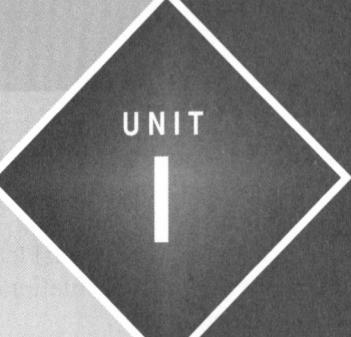

. . . An executive decision is a moment in the process.

—*Mary Parker Follett*

The foundation of this book rests on the premise that professional judgment, critical thinking, and wise decision making can be taught. In order to accomplish this task the reader (both learner and teacher) needs to have an understanding of the theories and processes of learning and teaching critical thinking. When individuals learn, they acquire new information that should assist them in problem solving. Unfortunately, many individuals have difficulty with the transference of information. Although able to demonstrate the acquisition of new knowledge they are frequently unable to make appropriate inferences in a real situation requiring the use of the new information. This inability to appropriately transfer learning leads to unwise decision making.

Carnevali and Thomas (1993) maintain that real learning occurs only by applying knowledge and practicing skills. In nursing education, clinical experiences accompany most learning; thus, the learner has the opportunity to apply new knowledge as it is learned, thereby assisting in knowledge transfer. A frequent exception to this normal occurrence of simultaneous theory and clinical application is nursing management. Because many learners are never able to fully experience this role or apply management theory, there has been poor transference of management theory into practice.

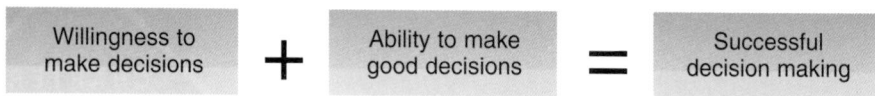

FIGURE 1-1.
A model of the successful decision maker.

sion making is both the pivotal leadership activity and the core of management. How do managers become successful decision makers? Successful decision making can be learned through life experience, but not everyone learns to make appropriate decisions by this trial and error method. Additionally, using one's life experiences as a method to learn decision making leaves much to chance. Learning decision making using a systematic, scientific approach eliminates trial and error and focuses the learning on a proven process. A systematic, scientific approach to decision making always involves the application of theoretical systems for decision making (Marquis and Huston, 1995).

◆ Theoretical Systems for Decision Making

Decision making is a critical task, possibly the most critical of the thinking skills. In the past, it was felt that some people were unable to be successful decision makers because the *process* of decision making was not taught in schools. Today, decision-making autonomy is often equated with professional nursing practice and nurses are taught to gain control over decisions that affect them and their patients (Huston and Marquis, 1995). The best method to improve decision-making skills is to use an adequate process model as the theoretical base for learning and practicing decision making.

There are many problem-solving and decision-making models in the literature. Although many people use the terms problem solving and decision making synonymously, there is a small but significant difference. *Problem solving* is a systematic process that focuses on analyzing a difficult situation and always includes a decision-making step (Marquis and Huston, 1996). In problem solving, much time and energy are spent in pursuit of the underlying problem identification.

Decision making, on the other hand, is usually triggered by a problem, but is often dealt with in a manner that does not eliminate the problem. An example is a conflict situation in which you decide to handle the conflict crisis in some manner at that time, but do not make an effort to get at the real problem causing the conflict. You might decide to address the real cause of the conflict at a later time. It is even possible for a decision maker to do nothing about a problem. The decision is not to problem solve. The decision maker may select this alternative because of a lack of energy, time, or resources to problem solve. For some situations, this is an appropriate decision. For example, if a nursing supervisor has information that a staff nurse who has begun calling in sick frequently is retiring within the next three months, the supervisor may decide not to take action on the problem. This conscious decision reflects the supervisor's determination that the problem will soon no longer exist and that the time and energy needed to correct the problem now is not warranted.

Of the many problem-solving and decision-making models that have been identified, only four are discussed in this chapter. The model each individual selects should be determined in part by what is comfortable for him or her; however, quality and self-confidence in decision making tend to increase when one model is used consistently (Marquis and Huston, 1996).

TRADITIONAL PROBLEM-SOLVING PROCESS

This problem-solving model uses seven steps, with the actual decision making occurring at step five (see Display 1-1). One of the reasons the traditional problem-solving model continues to be widely used is that it is well known and has been proved effective. However, it remains a problem-solving model, not a decision-making model, and therefore has several weaknesses when used for certain types of decision making.

One such weakness is that the setting of objectives is often omitted. If no objective or overall goal for the problem solving is identified, the identification of alternatives may become endless and the problem-solving efforts may become unfocused.

HARRISON'S MANAGERIAL DECISION-MAKING PROCESS

Harrison's (1981) managerial decision-making process is a modification of the traditional problem-solving model and eliminates the weakness of the traditional model by the addition of the goal-setting step (see Display 1-2).

NURSING PROCESS

The nursing process is the systematic approach the professional nurse uses to diagnose and treat human responses to actual or potential health problems. It

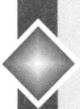

DISPLAY 1-1
Traditional Problem-Solving Process

1. Identify the problem.
2. Gather data to identify the causes and consequences of the problem.
3. Explore alternative solutions.
4. Evaluate the alternatives.
5. Select the appropriate solution.
6. Implement the solution.
7. Evaluate the results.

DISPLAY 1-2
Harrison's Managerial Decision-Making Process (1981)

1. Set objectives.
2. Search for alternatives.
3. Evaluate alternatives.
4. Choose.
5. Implement.
6. Follow up and control.

is also a theoretical system for decision making. The strength of the nursing process as a decision-making model is its feedback mechanism. This feedback mechanism allows for reevaluation throughout decision making.

The nursing process has been identified as an effective decision-making tool and as a problem-solving model because of the constant information flow (Morrison, 1995). The initial decision making occurs when the decision point has been identified, but there continues to be decision making throughout the process (see Fig. 1-2). Although the nursing process was designed for nursing

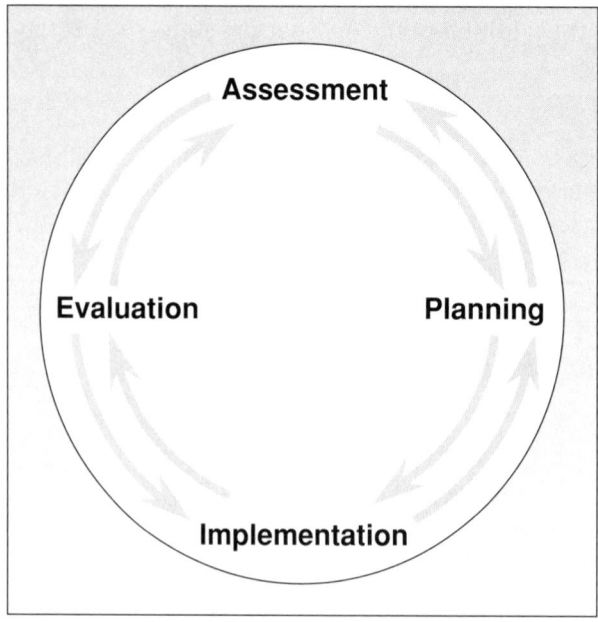

FIGURE 1-2.
Feedback mechanism of the nursing process.

practice with regard to client care and nursing accountability, it can be adapted easily as a theoretical model for use in management and organizational decision making. Table 1-1 shows how closely the nursing process parallels the decision-making process.

The weakness of the nursing process is a lack of clearly stated objectives. The planning phase of the nursing process is where goals should be clearly defined, but in reality this step is frequently omitted or obscured. However, because nurses are familiar with the nursing process and because of its proven effectiveness, it is one of the recommended theoretical systems for adaptation to managerial decision making.

INTUITIVE DECISION-MAKING MODEL

Romiszowski (1981) built on the nursing process in creating the Intuitive Decision-Making Model (see Fig. 1-3). In this model, the decision maker consciously incorporates recall or cumulative nursing knowledge that has come from education, both formal and informal, as well as experience, in planning the decision. Inexperienced or novice decision makers spend more time in the assessment, recall, and planning phases, whereas experienced decision makers gather information, recall, and often leap directly to implementation, because planning has become automatic (Casebeer, 1991). That novice nurses and experienced nurses process information differently has been supported by the work of Carnevali and Thomas (1993) and Benner (1994). Ironically, this "leap" from information gathering to implementation may be the greatest weakness of this model.

◇ **TABLE 1-1**
Comparison of the Decision-Making Process to the Simplified Nursing Process

Decision-Making Process	Simplified Nursing Process
Identify the decision.	Assess.
Collect data.	
Identify criteria for decision.	Plan.
Identify alternatives.	
Compare alternatives with criteria.	
Choose alternative.	Implement.
Implement alternative.	
Evaluate steps in decision.	Evaluate.

lead to poor-quality decisions. There are three primary ways in which individuals think illogically.

1. *Over-generalization.* This type of "crooked" thinking assumes that if "A" has a characteristic, then every "A" has the same characteristic. An example is the assumption that if one manager has excellent interpersonal skills, then all managers must have excellent interpersonal skills.
2. *Affirming the Consequences.* In this type of illogical thinking we decide that if "B" is good and we are doing "A," then "A" must not be good. If a new method of performing a nursing procedure is heralded as the best way to execute the procedure and the nurses in your facility are not using that technique, this does not necessarily mean that the technique used in your facility is wrong or bad. For example, if your nursing unit is using a total patient care structure for nursing care delivery and primary nursing is currently the most commonly used nursing care delivery system nationwide, total patient care may still be totally acceptable and may, in fact, be the best care delivery system for your unit at this time. In this example, affirming the consequences is avoided.
3. *Argument from Analogy.* This is a manner of applying a component that is present in two separate concepts and stating that because "A" is present in "B," then "A" and "B" are alike in all respects. An example here would be stating that since intuition plays a part in clinical and managerial nursing, then any characteristic present in a good clinician should also be present in a good manager. However, we know this is not necessarily true and that a good manager does not necessarily possess all the skills of a good clinician.

INABILITY TO CHOOSE AND ACT

It is not enough to gather adequate information, think logically, select from several alternatives, and be aware of the influence of one's values. In the final analysis, one must act. It is at this last point in the decision-making process that many individuals become vulnerable. They often choose to delay taking action because of personal risk. In every decision there lies some element of risk, some set of consequences, as well as accountability. If we choose to wear a wool suit and the weather turns very hot, we pay the consequences of our poor decision by being uncomfortable all day.

It may help the reluctant decision maker to remember that decisions, although often having long-term consequences and far-reaching effects, are frequently not cast in stone. Decisions found to be ineffective or inappropriate often can be changed. Evaluation of the decisions made will assist the decision maker in learning more about his or her decision-making ability and how it is faulty. However, we must continue to make decisions even though they are sometimes of questionable quality, because the only way individuals can become successful decision makers is to make decisions and make decisions and make decisions.

◆ Characteristics of the Successful Decision Maker

Various experts on decision making have attempted to characterize what attributes successful decision makers have. Although all experts do not agree, Huston (1990) notes the following qualities of successful decision makers.

1. *Courage.* Courage is of particular importance and involves the willingness to take risks.
2. *Sensitivity.* Good decision makers seem to have an antenna that makes them particularly sensitive to situations and others.
3. *Energy.* People must have the energy and desire to make things happen.
4. *Creativity.* Successful decision makers tend to be creative thinkers, developing new ways to solve problems.

◆ Summary

The successful decision maker is an individual who has a great deal of self-awareness and possesses courage, sensitivity, energy, and creativity. He or she is someone who has developed a systematic, scientific approach to problem solving, an approach that begins with a fixed goal and ends with an evaluation process. The successful decision maker understands the significance that each individual's values, life experiences, preferences, and ways of thinking have on selected alternatives. The critical thinker pondering a decision is aware of the areas of vulnerability that hinder successful decision making and will expend effort to avoid the pitfalls of faulty logic and data gathering. Finally, the successful decision maker is cognizant that the very act of deciding and evaluating decisions increases his or her expertise.

◆ References

Agor WH (1986). The logic of intuition: how top executives make important decisions. Organizational Dynamics Winter, 5–18

Benner P (1994, July 17). Engaged reasoning: critical evaluation of critical thinking. Paper Presented at Improving the Quality of Thinking in a Changing World. Massachusetts Institute of Technology, Cambridge, MA

Boughn S (1988). A lack of autonomy in the contemporary nursing student: a comparative study. J Nurs Educ 27(4):150–155

Bradham CU, Dalme FC, and Thompson PJ (1990). Personality traits valued by practicing nurses and measured in nursing students. J Nurs Educ 29(5):225–232

Carnevali DL and Thomas MD (1993). Diagnostic Reasoning and Treatment Decision Making in Nursing. Philadelphia: JB Lippincott

Casebeer L (1991). Fostering decision making in nursing. J Nurs Staff Dev Nov/Dec, 271–274

Corcoran S (1986). Task complexity and nursing expertise as factors in decision making. Nurs Res 35:107–112 process. Authors also disagree about the middle portion, or the "doing" part of the management process. These differences concern both the nomenclature used and the inclusion or omission of staffing as a step in the management process. Staffing as a phase of the management process is rarely found in texts outside of nursing. However, because staffing is an important element, many nursing management authors include this as a phase in the process.

For the purposes of organizing this text the management process of plan, organize, staff, direct, and control will be used as shown in Display 2-1. Regardless of how the steps of the management process are labeled, it is important to understand that the principles used are identical. In addition, the process, concepts, and principles that assist nursing managers in making wise decisions are the same for managers in other industries. Briefly described, the functions for each phase of the management process are as follows.

1. *Planning.* Planning functions include determining philosophy, goals and objectives, policies, procedures, and rules; carrying out long-range, intermediate, and short-range planning; fiscal planning; and managing planned change.

2. *Organizing.* Organizing includes establishing the structure to carry out plans, determining the most appropriate type of patient care delivery, and grouping activities to meet unit goals. Other functions include working within the structure of the organization as well as understanding and using power and authority appropriately.

3. *Staffing.* Staffing functions include recruitment, interviewing, hiring, and orientation. Scheduling and staff development are additional staffing functions. Socialization of employees is also frequently included as a staffing function.

4. *Directing.* Some management experts place several staffing functions under the directing phase of the management process. However, the usual functions listed in this phase are the human resource management functions; that is, motivating, managing conflict, delegating, communicating, and facilitating collaboration.

5. *Controlling.* Controlling functions include performance appraisals, fiscal accountability, quality control, legal and ethical control, and professional and collegial control.

Because of the cyclical nature of the management process, many different phases occur simultaneously. To illustrate, let us suppose a manager spent part

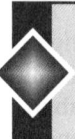

DISPLAY 2-1
The Management Process

Planning → Organizing → Staffing → Directing → Controlling

of the day working on a budget for next year (Planning); had a meeting about reorganizing patient care management from team nursing to primary care nursing (Organizing); altered the staffing pattern to include 12-hour shifts (Staffing); held a meeting to resolve a conflict between physicians and nurses (Directing); and conducted an employee job performance appraisal (Controlling). Not only would the manager have been performing all parts of the management process, but each one of these activities would have had a planning, implementing, and controlling phase. Each duty and every decision of a manager should begin with a plan and includes some sort of evaluation or control.

◆ The Effect of Organizational Power on Decision Making

There is an important additional component in organizational decision making that varies from individual decision making. This additional component is organizational power and a discussion of managerial decision making is incomplete without examining the influence of power on organizational decision making.

In the previous chapter, there was a discussion of the effect of the individual's values and preferences on the decision. Because organizations are made up of people with differing values and preferences, there are often conflicts in decision dynamics within organizations (Glendon and Ulrich, 1992). Powerful individuals within organizations are more apt to have decisions made (by themselves or their subordinates) that are congruent with their preferences and values. On the other hand, people wielding little power in organizations must always consider the preference of the powerful when they make management decisions (Marquis and Huston, 1996).

The influence of organizational politics on decision making is a reality in management decision making. Power interacts as a decision factor, since the preference of the powerful influences the decisions of others and inhibits the preferences of the less powerful.

Bennis (1989) maintains that individuals who remain and advance in organizations are those who feel and express values and beliefs congruent with those of the organization. Thus the potential for autonomous decision making and creativity in problem solving within the organization becomes limited. A balance must be found between the limitations posed by the organizational power structure and totally independent thinking that can lead to organizational chaos.

This ability of the powerful to influence individual decision making in an organization often results in the development of two types of personality— the *private* personality and the *organizational* personality. For example, a person may believe that he or she would have made a different decision if acting individually, but went along with the organization's decision. This "going along" in itself constitutes a decision: a decision that we can or cannot accept an organizational decision that differs from our own individual preferences and values.

◆ Rational and Administrative Decision Making

For many years it was widely believed that most managerial decisions were based on a careful, scientific, and objective thought process. Not until the work of Simon (1947) was it recognized that most managers made a great many decisions that could not be categorized as fitting the objective rationality theory. Simon suggested there were two types of decision makers. The rational decision maker was referred to as the economic man, whereas the second type was labeled the administrative man. The outcome desired for the decisions made by the administrative man is that they be effective, whereas the goal of decisions made by the economic man is that they be the best possible alternative. A comparison of these two types of decision making is shown in Display 2-2.

Managers who are successful decision makers attempt to make rational decisions. That is, they gather as much information as possible and generate many alternatives, since a restricted knowledge base and few alternatives directly affect the quality of the decision. They then attempt to select the best alternative. This approach, however, is often unsuitable for various reasons. The problems may not have been encountered previously and therefore, the consequences are unknown. Additionally, in this day of complex information acquisition and information overload, it becomes impossible for the human brain to store and retain the amount of information available for each decision.

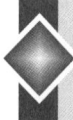

DISPLAY 2-2
Comparison of the Economic and Administrative Man

Economic Man
1. Makes decisions in a very rational manner.
2. Has complete knowledge of the problem or decision situation.
3. Has a complete list of possible alternatives.
4. Has a rational system of ordering preference of alternatives.
5. Selects the decision that will maximize utility function.

Administrative Man
1. Makes decisions that are good enough.
2. Because complete knowledge is not possible, knowledge is always fragmented.
3. Because consequences of alternatives occur in the future, they are impossible to accurately predict.
4. Usually chooses from among a few alternatives, not all possible ones.
5. Selects a final choice that is "satisficing" rather than maximizing.

(Adapted from Simon, 1974.)

Last, the need for rapid decision making and the lack of the time necessary for rational decision making results in many management decisions with an outcome that is "satisficing" or good enough. The decision must "work," that is, the outcome of the decision should be successful, but the alternative selected need not have been the optimal alternative. The "best" choice for many decisions is often found to be too costly in terms of time or resources, so another less costly, but workable, solution is found.

◆ Management Decision-Making Technology

Morrison (1995) maintains that nurses must be taught decision making skills because decision-making is such a vital component of management. In order to assist the manager in making decisions, management analysts have developed tools that provide order and direction in obtaining and using information, or that are helpful in selecting who should be involved in making the decision. Because there is such a wide selection of these decision aids, only a few have been included in this text. An attempt has been made to select decision technology that would be the most helpful to the novice manager.

A. QUANTITATIVE DECISION-MAKING TOOLS

Various management authors label management decision-making aids as "models"; others use the term "tools." It is only important to remember that the end result of any decision-making aid requires the need for the individual to make the final decision and that all aids are subject to human error.

1. Decision Grids—A decision grid allows the decision maker to visually examine the alternatives and compare each against the same criteria. Any criteria may be selected, but the same criteria are used to analyze each alternative. When many alternatives have been generated or when a group or committee is working on making a decision, this is an easy and helpful assistance method. An example of a decision grid is depicted in Figure 2-1.

A decision grid could be appropriately used in evaluating different methods of managing care on a unit. The unit manager and the nursing staff would evaluate all the alternatives available using the same criteria.

2. Pay-off Tables—The decision aids that fall in this category have a cost–profit–volume relationship, and are very helpful in decisions where some quantitative information is available, such as the cost of the item or predicted usage of the item. In order to use pay-off tables, it is necessary to determine probabilities and to use historical data, such as a previous hospital census, numbers of procedures performed, or other available quantitative data.

One might use a pay-off table to determine how many participants it would take to make an in-service program break even. If the instructor for the class cost $400, the in-service director would need to charge each of 20 participants

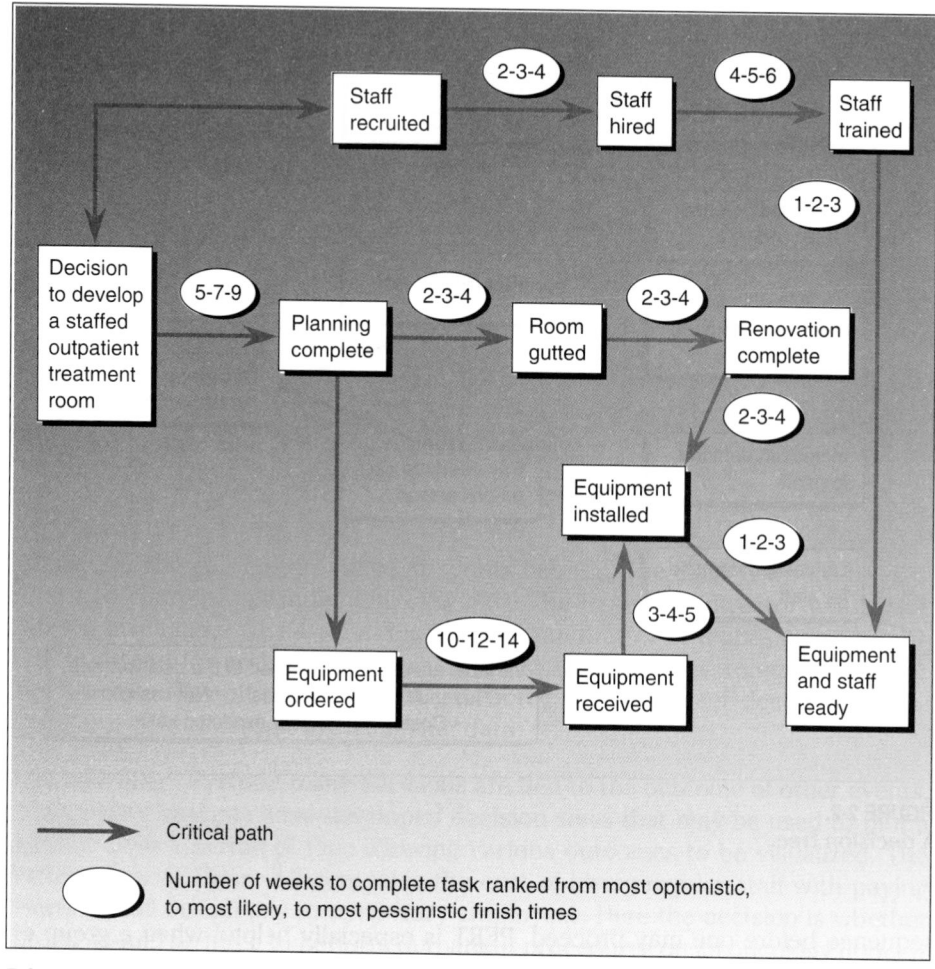

FIGURE 2-3.
An example of a PERT flow diagram.

Seven situation variables have also been identified by Vroom (1973). These situation variables become decision rules that determine which of the five decision-making styles is appropriate in a given situation. The seven rules identified by Vroom are listed in the following:

1. *The Information Rule.* If the quality of the decision is important and if the leader does not possess enough information or expertise to solve the problem by himself, AI is eliminated from the feasible set. (Its use risks a low-quality decision.)
2. *The Goal Congruence Rule.* If the quality of the decision is important and if the subordinates do not share the organizational goals to be obtained in solving the problem, GII is eliminated from the feasible set.

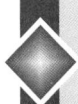

DISPLAY 2-3
Types of Management Decision Styles

AI   You solve the problem or make the decision yourself, using information available to you at that time.

AII   You obtain the necessary information from your subordinate(s), then decide on the solution to the problem yourself. You may or may not tell your subordinates what the problem is in getting the information from them. The role played by your subordinates in making the decision is clearly one of providing the necessary information to you, rather than generating or evaluating alternative solutions.

CI   You share the problem with relevant subordinates individually, getting their ideas and suggestions without bringing them together as a group. Then *you* make the decision that may or may not reflect your subordinates' influence.

CII   You share the problem with your subordinates as a group, collectively obtaining their ideas and suggestions. Then *you* make the decision that may or may not reflect your subordinates' influence.

GII   You share a problem with your subordinates as a group. Together you generate and evaluate alternatives and attempt to reach agreement (consensus) on a solution. Your role is much like that of chairman. You do not try to influence the group to adopt "your" solution and you are willing to accept and implement any solution that has the support of the entire group.

(Reprinted, by permission of publisher, from *Organizational Dynamics.* Spring 1973. © American Management Association, New York p. 67. All rights reserved.)

(Alternatives that eliminate the leader's final control over the decision reached may jeopardize the quality of the decision.)

3. *The Unstructured Problem Rule.* In decisions in which the quality of the decision is important, if the leader lacks the necessary information or expertise to solve the problem by him or herself, and if the problem is unstructured, that is, he or she does not know exactly what information is needed and where it is located, the method used must provide not only for the leader to collect the information, but to do so in an efficient and effective manner. Methods that involve interaction among all subordinates with full knowledge of the problem are likely to be both more efficient and more certain to generate a high-quality solution to the problem. Under these conditions, AI, AII, and CI are eliminated from the feasible set. (AI does not provide for the leader to collect the necessary information, AII and CI represent more cumbersome, less effective, and less efficient means of bringing the necessary information to bear on the solution of the problem than methods that do permit those with necessary information to interact.)

4. *The Acceptance Rule.* If the acceptance of the decision by subordinates is critical to effective implementation, and if it is not certain that an auto-

cratic decision made by the leader would receive that acceptance, AI and AII are eliminated from the feasible set. (Neither provides an opportunity for subordinates to participate in the decision and both risk the necessary acceptance.)

5. *The Conflict Rule.* If the acceptance of the decision is critical, and an autocratic decision is not certain to be accepted, and subordinates are likely to be in conflict or disagreement over the appropriate solution, AI, AII, and CI are eliminated from the feasible set. (The method used in solving the problem should enable those in disagreement to resolve their differences with full knowledge of the problem. Accordingly, under these conditions, AI, AII, and CI, which involve no interaction or only "one-on-one" relationships and therefore provide no opportunity for those in conflict to resolve their differences, are eliminated from the feasible set. Their use runs the risk of leaving some of the subordinates with less than the necessary commitment to the final decision.)

6. *The Fairness Rule.* If the quality of the decision is unimportant and if acceptance is critical and not certain to result from an autocratic decision, AI, AII, CI, and CII are eliminated from the feasible set. (The method used should maximize the probability of acceptance as this is the only relevant consideration in determining the effectiveness of the decision. Under these circumstances, AI, AII, CI, and CII, which create less acceptance or commitment than GII, are eliminated from the feasible set. To use them is to run the risk of getting less than the needed acceptance of the decision.)

7. *The Acceptance Priority Rule.* If acceptance is critical, not assured by an autocratic decision, and if subordinates can be trusted, AI, AII, CI, and CII are eliminated from the feasible set. (Methods that provide equal partnership in the decision-making process can provide greater acceptance without risking decision quality. Use of any method other than GII results in an unnecessary risk that the decision will not be fully accepted or receive the necessary commitment on the part of subordinates.)*

The following are examples of management problems requiring a decision. Attempt to solve these problems in groups or individually using the Vroom and Yetton decision styles. Follow the decision rules outlined by Vroom in selecting your decision style.

PROBLEM 1**

You are the head nurse of a 30-bed medical unit. At your request, after consultation, you recently put into effect a system for incorporating nursing diagnosis within the patient care plans. This was expected to reduce reporting time between shifts and to improve the quality of patient care. To everyone's surprise, including your own, you find that the system is not working.

---

*Reprinted, by permission of publisher, from *Organizational Dynamics,* Spring 1973. © American Management Association, New York, p. 71. All rights reserved.

**From Marquis and Huston, 1996

You do not think there is anything wrong with your idea; many other hospitals in the area are using nursing diagnosis with success. You had a consultant come from another hospital and give an update to your nurses on the use of the system. The consultant reported that your staff seemed very knowledgeable and appeared to understand their responsibilities in implementing the system.

You suspect that a few nurses might be sabotaging your efforts for planned change, but your charge nurses do not agree; they feel the failure may be owing to a lack of proper incentives or poor morale among the staff.

Your nursing director is anxious to implement the system on other patient care units, but wants it to be working well on your unit first. You have just come from a head nurse meeting where your nursing director advised you to solve the problem and report back within a week regarding the steps you had taken to solve your problem. You share your director's concern; how should you solve this problem?

Decision Style Selected _____

PROBLEM 2*

You are one of two supervisors in a Home Health Agency. The director of the agency has offered to send four nurses to a Home Health Care Conference in a nearby city. The Director wants each supervisor to submit two names of the selected nurses in 2 weeks.

All the nurses you supervise would like to go, and from a staffing standpoint there is no reason why any one of them could not go. All the nurses are active in the local home health care organization. You would like to send them all, but financial resources limit the selection to only two. You supervise eight full-time nurses.

Decision Style Selected _____

PROBLEM 3

You are the day charge nurse on a surgical unit. Your supervisor has made you responsible for selecting a new type of blood warming unit. As you are recognized as having expertise in this area, you want to be sure that you select the right unit. Although several salespeople have made samples available to the staff for trial use, you have not received much feedback regarding their preference.

Today your supervisor requested the price and the name of the manufacturer of the unit you had selected to submit with her budget, which is due in 2 days.

Decision Style Selected _____

◆ Summary

The management process guides organizations and managers in a systematic manner. Although steps in the process may have various names, there is always a planning and an evaluation step.

---

*Adapted from Managerial Decision Making, La Monica and Finch, 1977

There are several areas of organizational decision making that differ between personal and professional decision making. Two major considerations in organizational decision making are how power affects decision making, and the assumption that management decision making need only be "satisficing." Management science has produced a great many tools and techniques used for analyzing decisions to be made. There are also models available to assist new managers in determining which decision style to use. Although these management tools can be very useful for the novice manager, they are not foolproof and often do not allow for the human element in management.

◆ References

Bennis W (1989). Why Leaders Can't Lead: The Unconscious Conspiracy Continues. San Francisco: Jossey-Bass

Gillies DA (1994). Nursing Management, 3rd ed. Philadelphia: WB Saunders

Glendon K and Ulrich D (1992). Using cooperative decision-making strategies in nursing practice. Nurs Adm Quart 17(1):69–71

Johnson LJ (1990). The influence of assumptions on effective decision-making. J Nurs Admin 20(4):35

La Monica E and Finch FE (1977). Managerial decision making. J Nurs Admin May–June (7):18–26

Marquis BL and Huston J (1996). Leadership Roles and Management Functions in Nursing, 2nd ed. Philadelphia: JB Lippincott

Morrison RS (1995). Validation of nursing management diagnoses. Image 27(4): 267–271

Simon HA (1947). Administrative Behavior. New York: Harper Textbooks

Vroom VH (1973). A new look at managerial decision-making: organizational decision-making. Org Dynam 1(4):66–80

Vroom V and Yetton PW (1973). Leadership and Decision-Making. Pittsburgh: Univ Pittsburgh Press

◆ Bibliography

Baggs JG (1993). Collaborative interdisciplinary bioethical decision making in intensive care units. Nursing Outlook 41(3):108–112

Dwyer D, Schwartz R, and Fox M (1992). Decision making autonomy in nursing. JONA 22(2):17–23

Felman C, Olberding L, Shorridge L, and Zappin P (1993). Decision making in case management of home healthcare clients. J Nurs Admin 23(1):33–38

Grobe S, Drew J, and Fonteyn M (1991). A descriptive analysis of experienced nurses' clinical reasoning during a planning task. Res Nurs Health 14:305–314

Huston CJ and Marquis BL (1995). Seven steps to successful decision-making. AJN 95(5):65–68

Huston CJ and Marquis BL (1989). Retention and Productivity Strategies for Nurse Managers. Philadelphia: JB Lippincott

Marquis BL and Huston CJ (1994). Decisions, decisions. Adv Prac Nurse 1, March

Nagelkerk JM and Henery BM (1990). Strategic decision making. J Nurs Admin 20(7/8):21–24

Sarazen S (1990). The tools of quality: Part II: Cause and effects diagram. Qual Prog July 59–62

Yates JF (1990). Judgment and Decision Making. Englewood Cliffs, NJ: Prentice-Hall

Chris Argyris (1964) supported McGregor and Mayo by stating that managerial domination causes workers to become discouraged and passive, and if employee self-esteem and independence needs are not met, they will become discouraged, troublesome, or may leave the organization. Argyris stressed the need for employee participation in decision making and flexibility within the organization.

By the late 1960s, there was growing concern that the human relations approach to management was not without its own problems. Most people continued to function in a bureaucratic environment, making it difficult to always apply a participatory approach to management. The human relations approach was time-consuming and did not always result in organizational goals being met. In addition, not every employee liked working in a less structured environment. Table 3-1 summarizes the development of management theory up to 1970.

Until the late 1960s, leadership theory developed separately from management science, but by 1960 management researchers began to examine how both concepts were intertwined. As a result there is a better understanding of the complexity of both management and leadership.

◆ The Relationship Between Leadership and Management

Although the literature clearly demonstrates the need for effective leaders *and* managers, the relationship between leadership and management is less clear. Tranbarger (1988) states that leadership is but one of many functions of management, whereas Gardner (1990) proclaims that leadership requires more complex skills than management and that management is only one role of leadership. Manthey (1990) delineates the two, stating that a manager guides, directs, and motivates, whereas a leader empowers others. Therefore, she states, every manager should be a leader. Farley (1990) implies that manage-

◇ **TABLE 3-1**
Management Theory Development

Theorists	Theory
Taylor	Scientific Management
Weber	Bureaucratic Organizations
Fayol	Management Functions
Mayo	Hawthorne Effect
McGregor	Theory X and Theory Y
Argyris	Employee Participation

ment preparation occurs before leadership, when she states that young nursing managers must be developed as leaders.

In an effort to better understand the relationship between leadership and management, it may be helpful to look at how they are different.

Managers:

1. are always assigned a position within an organization.
2. have a legitimate source of power owing to the delegated authority that accompanies their position.
3. are expected to carry out specific functions.
4. emphasize control, decision making, decision analysis, and results.

Leaders:

1. may or may not have delegated authority, but are capable of obtaining their power through means other than delegated authority.
2. have a wider variety of roles than do managers.
3. are frequently not part of a formal organization.
4. focus on the group process, information gathering, feedback, and empowering others.

Holloman (1986) uses the term *headship* to define the manager, and makes a distinction between headship and leadership. Holloman maintains that it is a mistake to refer to the dean of a school of nursing, a nursing supervisor, or a head nurse as a leader. A job title does not make a person a leader; these individuals are in a headship position, rather than a leadership position. Only a person's behavior determines whether a person occupies a leadership position.

What then is the relationship between leadership and management? Most scholars now agree that a good manager must also have leadership abilities. The authors feel that *every* nurse is a leader and manager at some level and that the nursing role requires *both* leadership and management skills. Gardner (1986) asserts that leader/managers distinguish themselves from the more traditional manager in six ways.

1. They think longer term. They are visionary and futuristic. They consider what effect their decisions will have years from now, as well as the immediate consequences.
2. They look outward toward the larger organization, and maintain a broad focus. They are able to understand how their unit or department fits into the bigger picture.
3. They influence others beyond their own group. Effective leader/managers in an organization rise above bureaucratic boundaries.
4. They emphasize vision, values, and motivation. They understand intuitively the unconscious and often nonrational aspects that are present in interactions with others. They are very sensitive to others and to differences unique to each situation.
5. They are politically astute and are capable of coping with conflicting requirements and expectations from among their many constituencies.

6. They think in terms of change and renewal. The traditional manager accepts the structure and processes of the organization, but the leader/manager examines the ever-changing reality of the world and seeks to make revisions in the organization in order to keep pace with that changing world.

There is less agreement among scholars regarding a definition of leadership than there is about the definition of management (Marquis and Huston, 1996). Gardner (1990) defines leadership as "the process of persuasion and example by which an individual (or team) induces a group to take action that is in accord with the leader's purposes or the shared purposes of all." Robbins (1991) concurs that leadership is a process that empowers other social transaction in which one person influences another. Kotter (1988) and Bernhard and Walsh (1990) also believe that leadership is a process that moves groups toward goals in a noncoercive manner. Yura, Ozimek, and Walsh (1981) maintain that it is the behaviors an individual exhibits that makes them a leader, and have condensed the behaviors of leadership into four components: 1) deciding, 2) relating, 3) influencing, and 4) facilitating.

◆ Historical Development of Leadership Theory

Much of the early work on leadership centered on the behaviors or characteristics of the leader, rather than looking at others involved in the interactive leadership process.

TRAIT THEORIES

Early theories were based on the assumption that some individuals are natural leaders (i.e., leaders are born not made), and that they have certain characteristics or personality traits that make them better leaders than others. One such trait theory is called the *Great Man Theory*. Researchers studied the lives of great men throughout history to determine what traits they had in common that made them great leaders. Contemporary theorists argue that leadership skills can be developed not just inherited and that trait theorists ignored other historical events, such as the impact followers had, or the impact of the situation itself on that moment in time (Gardner, 1990; Senge, 1990).

Later theories focused on identifying common characteristics researchers found in most good leaders. Although such theories also have obvious shortcomings they are worth examining. Many of these characteristics (see Table 3-2) can still be used to describe successful leaders in our contemporary world.

BEHAVIORAL THEORIES

During the human relations era many behavioral and social scientists studying management science also studied leadership. For example, McGregor's theo-

◆ **TABLE 3-2**
Characteristics of a Leader

Intelligence	Personality	Abilities
Knowledge	Adaptability	Able to enlist cooperation
Judgment	Creativity	Interpersonal skills
Decisiveness	Cooperativeness	Tact, diplomacy
Oral fluency	Alertness	Prestige
	Self-confidence	Social participation
	Personal integrity	
	Emotional balance and control	
	Nonconformity	
	Independence	

Adapted from Bass, 1982; Huston, 1990; and Swansburg, 1990.

ries had as much influence on leadership research as they did on management science. As research developed in this era, there was a move away from studying what traits the leader possessed and a greater emphasis placed on what the leader did and their leadership style.

A major breakthrough occurred when both Lewin (1951) and White and Lippitt (1960) isolated commonly occurring leadership styles. Later, these styles came to be referred to as authoritarian, democratic, and laissez-faire.

The *authoritarian* leader is characterized by the following leadership behaviors.

1. Maintains strong control over the work group.
2. Motivates others by coercion.
3. Gives directions as commands.
4. Communication flows downward.
5. Makes decisions without involving others.
6. Emphasis is placed on differences in status ("I" and "you").
7. Criticism is punitive.

Authoritarian leadership results in well-defined group actions that are usually predictable. This reduces frustration in the work group and gives members a feeling of security. Productivity is usually high, but creativity, self-motivation, and autonomy are reduced. Authoritarian leadership is useful in crisis situations and is frequently found in very large bureaucracies, such as the armed forces.

◆ **TABLE 3-3**
Transactional and Transformational Leaders

Transactional Leader	Transformational Leader
Focuses on management tasks	Identifies common values
Caretaker	Committed
Uses trade-offs to meet goals	Inspires others with vision
Shared values not identified	Has long-term vision
Examines causes	Explores effects
Uses contingency reward	Empowers others

◆ Summary

There is a need to understand how management science has evolved histori-cally. Our perceptions of the "best" way to operate an organization or manage employees within that organization are rooted within management theory and have changed as we have gained a better understanding of the complexity of organizations and individuals within those organizations.

Being well-grounded in management science will assist novice managers in selecting an approach to decision making that is more apt to be effective in handling contemporary organizational problems. Every effort should be made to incorporate a leadership approach in management decision making and for integrating leadership components into all management functions.

◆ References

Argyris C (1964). Integrating the Individual and the Organization. New York: Wiley

Bass BM, Avoliio BJ, and Goodheim L (1987). Biography and the assessment of trans-formational leadership at the world-class level. J Manage Jan, 7–19

Bass BM (1982). Stogdill's Handbook of Leadership. New York: Free Press

Bennis W, Nanus B (1985). Leaders: The Strategies for Taking Change. New York: Harper & Row

Berhard LA and Walsh M (1990). Leadership. St. Louis: CV Mosby.

Blake RR and Mouton JS (1964). The Managerial Grid. Houston: Gulf Publishing

Burns JM (1978). Leadership. New York: Harper & Row

Cottingham C (1990). Transformational leadership. In Hein EC and Nicholson MJ (eds): Contemporary Leadership Behavior, 3rd ed. Glenview, IL: Scott, Foresman

Dunham J, and Klafehn KA (1990). Transformational Leadership and the Nurse Executive. J Nurs Admin 20(40):28–34

Farley S (1990). Leadership. In Swansburg RC (ed): Management and Leadership for Nurse Managers. Boston: Jones and Bartlett

Fayol H (1925). General and Industrial Management. London: Pittman and Sons

Fiedler F (1967). A Theory of Leadership Effectiveness. New York: McGraw-Hill

Gardner JW (1986). The Nature of Leadership: Introductory Considerations. Washington, DC: The Independent Sector, 6

Gardner JW (1990). On Leadership. New York: Free Press

Hersey P and Blanchard K (1977). Management of Organizational Behavior: Utilizing Human Resources, 3rd ed. Englewood Cliffs, NJ: Prentice-Hall

Herzberg F (1977). One More Time: How Do You Motivate Employees? In Carroll L, Paine R, and Miner A (eds): The Management Process, 2nd ed. New York: Macmillan

Hollander EP (1978). Leadership Dynamics: A Practical Guide to Effective Relationships. New York: Free Press

Holloman CR (1986). Headship leadership: there is a difference. Notes Quotes 365:4

Huston CJ (1990). What makes the difference? Attributes of the exceptional nurse. Nursing 90(5):20

Huston CJ and Marquis BL (1989). Retention and Productivity Strategies for Nurse Managers. Philadelphia: JB Lippincott

Kotter JP (1988). The Leadership Factor. New York: The Free Press

Lewin K (1951). Field Theory in Social Sciences. New York: Harper & Row

Manthey M (1900). The nurse manager as leader. Nurs Manage 21(6)

Marquis BL and Huston CJ (1996). Leadership Roles and Management Functions in Nursing, 2nd ed. Philadelphia: JB Lippincott

Maslow A (1970). Motivation and Personality, 2nd ed. New York: Harper & Row

Mayo E (1953). The Human Problems of an Industrialized Civilization. New York: Macmillan

McGregor D (1960). The Human Side of Enterprise. New York: McGraw-Hill

Ouchi WG (1981). Theory Z: How American Business Can Meet the Japanese Challenge. Reading, MA: Addison-Wesley

Robbins A (1991). Awaken the Giant Within. New York: Fireside Books

Schein EH (1970). Organizational Psychology, 2nd ed. Englewood Cliffs, NJ: Prentice-Hall

Senge PM (1990). The Fifth Discipline. New York: Doubleday Books

Stogdill RM (1974). Handbook of Leadership: A Survey of Theory and Research. New York: Free Press

Stout-Shaffer S and Larrabee J (1992). Everyone can be a visionary leader. Nurs Manage 23(12):54–58

Strader MK (1987). Adapting theory Z to nursing management. Nurs Manage 18(4)

Swansburg RC (1990). Management and Leadership for Nurse Managers. Boston: Jones and Bartlett

Tannenbaum R and Schmidt W (1983). How to choose a leadership pattern. Harvard Bus Rev, May/June

Tappen RM (1995). Nursing Leadership and Management: Concepts and Practices, 3rd ed. Philadelphia: FA Davis

Taylor FW (1911). The Principles of Scientific Management. New York: Harper & Row

Tranbarger R (1988). The nurse executive in a community hospital. In Johnson M (ed): Series on Nursing Administration, vol. 1. Menlo Park, CA: Addison-Wesley

Tyrrell RA (1994) Visioning: An important management tool. Nurs Econ 12(2):93–95

White RK and Lippitt R (1960). Autocracy and Democracy: An Experimental Inquiry. New York: Harper & Row

Wolf GA, Boland S, and Aukerman M (1994). A transformational model for the practice of professional nursing. Part II. Nurs Admin 24(5):38-40

Yura H, Ozimek D, and Walsh M (1981). Nursing Leadership: Theory and Process. New York: Appleton-Century-Crofts

◆ Bibliography

Achenbach R and Shepard J (1989). The study of management styles. Nurs Manage 20:60–76

Barker AM (1991). An emerging leadership paradigm: transformational leadership. Nurs Health Care 12(4):204

Beck JDW and Yeager NM (1994). The Leader's Window: Mastering the Four Styles of Leadership to Build High Performing Teams. New York: Wiley

Boston C and Forman H (1994). A time to listen: staff and manager views on education, practice and management. J Nurs Admin 24(2):16–18

Curtin LL (1991). Leaders: the organization's pacemakers. Nurs Manage 22(3):6–8

Frieswick G (1990). Theory Z: what can it do for nursing? Nurs Manage 21(7):104

Heifetz RA (1994). Leadership without Easy Answers. Cambridge, MA: Harvard University Press

Keenan MJ, Hurst JB, and Dennis RS (1990). Situational leadership for collaboration in health care settings. Health Care Super 8(3):19–25

Lucas MD (1991). Management style and staff nurse job satisfaction. J Prof Nurs 22(4):216–228

Mark BA (1994). The emerging role of the nurse manager. J Nurs Admin 24(5):38–39

Steven DL (1991). Profile of a good manager. Nurs Manage 22(1):60–61

Viau JJ (1990). Theory Z: "magic potion" for decentralized management. Nurs Manage 21(12):34–36

PERSONAL NOTEBOOK

1. Recall the periods during which you have been a manager, not necessarily a nursing manager. Perhaps you were the head lifeguard or an evening-shift manager at a fast food restaurant. During those times do you believe you displayed more management skills or leadership skills?

2. Think of all the supervisors that you have had. Which ones were the best? What made them better than others? Which were better developed, their management or leadership skills?

3. Make a list of your greatest strengths as a leader, followed by a list of your management strengths.

PLANNING: AN OVERVIEW

Plans are worthless, planning is essential.
—Dwight David Eisenhower

Planning is the first phase of the management process. The planning phase is the most critical phase and precedes all other management functions. Without adequate planning the management process fails.

Planning may be defined as deciding in advance what to do; who is to do it; and how, when, and where it is to be done. Therefore, all planning involves choice: a necessity to choose from among alternatives. Therefore, planning can be considered a decision-making process.

Planning is important because it offsets uncertainty and chance by linking good intentions and action. It also focuses attention on the objectives of the organization. Good planning makes an economical operation possible and establishes a means of control. It also allows the manager to maxmize the utilization of scarce resources.

Planning may be long-term, intermediate, or short-term in nature. It may also be proactive or reactive. Some types of plans that will be discussed in Unit 2 include:

- the planning hierarchy including mission, philosophy, goals, objectives, policies, procedures, and rules
- strategic, intermediate, and operational planning
- planned change, and
- fiscal planning.

Regardless of which of these types of plans the manager is engaged in, the following principles and guidelines apply.

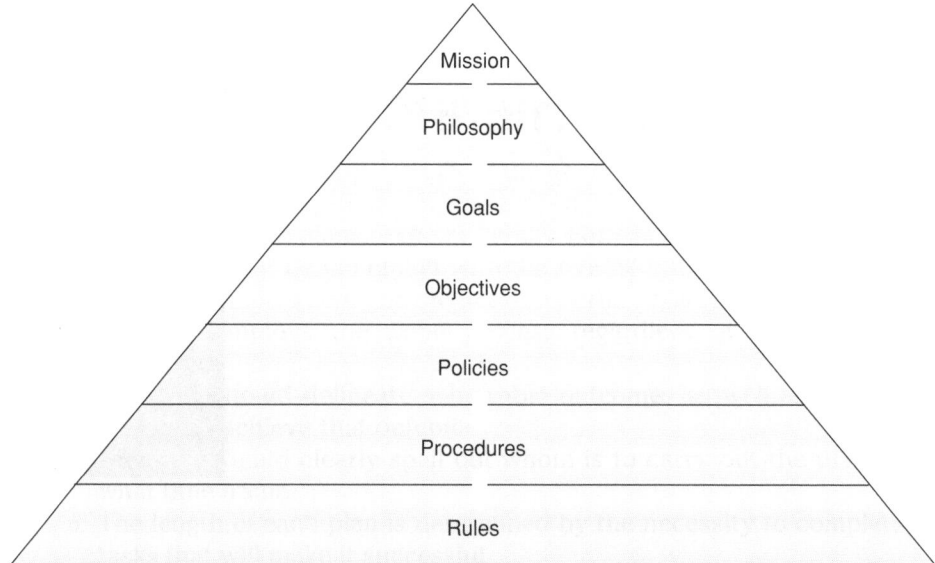

FIGURE 4-1.
The planning hierarchy.

aim and function. It may also address the organization's vision for the future. A sample mission statement for a teaching hospital is shown in Display 4-1.

The mission statement is the highest priority in the planning hierarchy. It influences the development of an organization's philosophy and goals, from which the objectives, policies, and procedures giving direction to employees are derived.

◆ Philosophy

A philosophy is defined as a set of values or beliefs that guides the actions of an organization and is developed from its purpose. Statements of philosophy can only be helpful if they truly direct the work of the organization (Marquis and Huston, 1996).

Every department and unit in an organization must use the larger organization's philosophy in developing its own philosophy. There must be congruence in formulating beliefs within an organization.

Individuals also have a personal philosophy or set of values. *Values* are beliefs, ideas, objects, and behaviors that are important to us. McNally (1980) identified the following four characteristics of a *true value*.

1. It must be freely chosen from among alternatives only after due reflection.
2. It must be prized and cherished.
3. It must be positively affirmed and acted on.
4. Evidence of it must be consciously and consistently repeated, becoming part of a pattern.

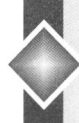

DISPLAY 4-1
Sample Mission Statement

Hospital X is a tertiary care facility and provides comprehensive, holistic care to all state residents who seek treatment. The purpose of Hospital X is to combine high-quality, holistic health care with the opportunity for learning for students in medicine, nursing, and the allied health sciences. Research is encouraged as a means of identifying new treatment regimens and for the promotion of high-quality health care for generations to come.

If a value does not meet all four criteria, it is a *value indicator.* Most individuals have many value indicators, but few true values.

Robbins (1991) suggests that the only way people can ever feel happy and fulfilled in the long term is to live in accordance with their true values. If they do not, they are likely to experience intense pain and to have significant difficulty making important decisions. Therefore, all individuals should consciously examine their values system and recognize its role in how they make decisions, resolve conflicts, and perceive the world. This is called *values clarification.* Catalano (1996) suggests that values clarification is an important element in critical thinking. Values clarification involves examining values, assigning them priorities, and determining how they influence behavior so that lifestyle is consistent with prioritized values. Values clarification is invaluable for all individuals and should be performed periodically, as values are frequently changed as a result of life experience or newly acquired knowledge.

Most of the values we have as children are a reflection of the values we have been taught by our parents. Later, these are modified as we are exposed to peers and role models who have differing values systems. Although learned, they cannot be forced on an individual, since one must internalize values. However, limited exposure to other viewpoints also limits the alternatives available to an individual. Therefore, learning more about the world in which we live increases our awareness of available options.

The values of the individual may or may not coincide with that of the organization. Since the philosophy of an organization determines its priorities, goals selection, and distribution of resources, it is important to understand the organizational philosophy in the agency where one is employed. The philosophy should speak for the primary mission of the organization, the level of responsiveness to the community, any special approaches to care, and any particular beliefs regarding patients and/or employees (Huston and Marquis, 1989).

Unfortunately, individuals are often employed in agencies where their philosophy differs or is in direct conflict with that of the organization. For example, nurses employed by large teaching hospitals, where teaching is clearly the primary purpose, should not be surprised to find that opportunities for learning take a priority over other actions. It is feasible that such a philosophy would result in most deaths in that hospital being handled as "code" situations, thus, enabling physicians to obtain adequate practice in code procedures. If, in this situation, the beliefs of a nurse differed from those of the organization, great personal conflict could occur.

The greatest safeguard for individuals to avoid this type of situation is to request a copy of the philosophy or mission of the institution *prior* to seeking employment. Sometimes, however, an organization's philosophy is not reflected in its actions.

Therefore, in addition to obtaining a copy of the philosophy of the institution, prospective employees need to talk with other employees to determine whether they feel the organization's philosophy is actually implemented, and to observe the priorities of the organization. Mallison (1989) emphasizes the need for the philosophy to direct the actions, priorities, and behaviors of an organization. An individual should also review budgetary priorities and talk to patients.

Although it is important for all individuals to have a philosophy congruent with that of the employing agency, it is especially important for the new manager to have a values system compatible with that of the organization. Requests by the organization that are not in conflict with the manager's personal values system will receive greater effort and higher priority than those requests that create personal values conflicts for the manager. As the discussion of organizational preferences in decision making in Chapter 2 suggests, managers frequently making decisions that conflict with their personal values may experience confusion and anxiety. This intrapersonal conflict will ultimately lead to job stress and job dissatisfaction.

It is generally unrealistic for a manager to accept a position under the assumption that he or she can work to change the organizational philosophy to be more closely aligned with his or her personal philosophy. Such a change would require extraordinary energy and inevitable conflict. The philosophy of the organization reflects the historical development of the organization as well as the philosophy of those individuals who play a vital role in its management. Therefore, changing an organization philosophy is often very difficult.

◆ Goals and Objectives

All philosophies must be translated into specific goals and objectives if they are to result in action. A goal may be defined as the aim of a philosophy. Institutional goals are primarily determined by the highest administrative levels, although there is increasing emphasis on including workers in setting organizational goals. Organizations usually set long- and short-term goals regarding services rendered, economics, use of resource people, funds and facilities, innovations, and social responsibilities (Marriner-Tomey, 1996). Goals, much like philosophies and values, change over time and require periodic reevaluation and prioritization.

Objectives are more specific than goals and usually include how the goal is to be accomplished. There are normally multiple objectives aimed at meeting a single goal. Objectives can be written focusing on the desired process or the desired end result.

It is important to ensure that both goals and objectives be explicit, measurable, observable or retrievable, obtainable (realistic), and that they be communicated to all those in the organization responsible for their attainment. Objectives should also be accompanied by the target date on which they are expected to be accomplished. The more specific a goal can be outlined in an objective, the easier it is for all individuals involved in goal attainment to understand and carry out their specific role behaviors. This is especially important to remember when writing job descriptions; if there is limited ambiguity in the job description there will be little role confusion or distortion. Clearly written and communicated goals and objectives are one of the most important tools of effective management.

◆ Policies and Procedures

Policies are comprehensive statements, derived from the organization's philosophy, goals, and objectives that explain how goals will be achieved and serve as guides for the general course and scope of activities permissible for goal accomplishment (Marriner-Tomey, 1996). Policies direct individual behavior toward the mission of the organization and define broad limits and desired outcomes of commonly recurring situations, while leaving some discretion and initiative to those individuals who must carry out that policy.

Policies can be implied or expressed. Implied policies are neither written or expressed verbally. They are those that have usually developed over time and that follow a precedent. Expressed policies are delineated either verbally or in writing. Expressed policies have the advantage of being readily available to all individuals in the organization and promote consistency of action.

Procedures identify the process or steps to be taken to implement a policy. Since procedural instructions involve elements of organizing, some textbooks place the development of procedures in the organizing phase of the management process. Regardless of where procedural development is formulated, there must be a close relationship with planning; planning is the foundation for all procedures.

Procedures establish customary or acceptable ways of accomplishing a specific task by outlining a set of steps to be followed with the rationale for each set of activities. Established procedures save staff time, reduce cost, and increase productivity.

◆ Rules

Rules and regulations are plans that define specific action or nonaction. Generally included as part of policy and procedure statements, rules describe situations that allow only one course of action (Marquis and Huston, 1996).

CASE 3 (CONTINUED)

the "cancer" patients concentrated in one area. Nurse Bell was well liked by most of her subordinates and will be missed. Her appointment to another unit has just been approved. Several of the nurses applied for her former position on your unit, but you received the appointment.

You have now just come from your first planning session with the director of Nursing Service and find your head is spinning. She has given you several assignments, leaving you overwhelmed. The nursing director has given you a copy of Memorial Hospital's Nursing Service philosophy. (See Display 4-2, Memorial Hospital—Nursing Service Philosophy.) She has requested that you use this philosophy as a guide in preparing a philosophy for the new oncology unit.

● ●

Assignment

1. Outline your plan for designing the philosophy (it need not be new) for the new oncology unit. Would you involve anyone else? If so, who and why? What would you do first, second, and so on? What is the rationale for your plan?

2. What are some particularly important aspects of philosophy that need to be examined in this case? Why?

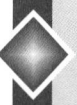

DISPLAY 4-2
Memorial Hospital—Nursing Service Philosophy

Our philosophy of nursing is based on respect for the dignity and worth of the individual. We believe each patient has the basic right to receive effective nursing care that is personal and based on his needs as they relate to him individually and to his clinical disease or condition.

Recognizing the obligation of nursing to help restore the patient to the best possible state of physical, mental, and emotional health and to maintain his sense of spiritual and social well-being, we pledge intelligent cooperation in coordinating nursing service with the medical and allied professional practitioners.

Understanding the importance of research and teaching for the improvement of patient care, the Nursing Department will support, promote, and participate in these activities.

Using knowledge of human behavior, we shall strive toward mutual trust and understanding between the nursing service and employees to provide an atmosphere for fully developing the potential of each individual member of the nursing team.

It is our belief that nursing personnel are individually accountable to the patient and his or her family for the quality and compassion of the patient care rendered and for upholding the standards of care as delineated by the nursing staff.

CASE 4 ◆

The director of nursing has also requested that *you* make a list of five goals that you wish to accomplish as head nurse on this unit in the next 3 years.

· ·

Assignment

1. List five goals for completion. Make sure that each goal states *who* will accomplish the goal, *what* the target or outcome of the goal is, and what the *timelines* are for goal completion. Explain your rationale for selecting these goals. Be sure that these goals are stated in measurable and behavioral terms.
2. The director has given you a list of broad goals and objectives that Sally Bell developed for the old medical-surgical unit. (See Display 4-3, Memorial Hospital Unit Goals and Objectives.) While the intent of the goals and objectives was appropriate, the director has decided that they lack specificity and measurability. Choose any four goals and restate them in specific measurable achievable terms with percentages (if necessary) and target dates.

CASE 5 ◆

Memorial Hospital is a medium-sized community hospital with a pulmonary care specialty unit (PCSU). Adjacent to the PCSU is a treatment room that the medical director of the PCSU, Dr. Smith, uses for both inpatient and outpatient bronchoscopies. Approximately two to three bronchoscopies are performed daily, usually before 10:00 A.M. and after 5:00 P.M. so as not to interfere with scheduled patient visits at his office, one block away.

A nurse from the PCSU is expected to assist during the bronchoscopies, although additional staffing to compensate for this is difficult to schedule. Many times the procedure is done on an emergency basis or the appointment is made at the physician's office during patient visits. This frequently leaves the PCSU understaffed.

The procedure for scheduling this room has always been on an informal first-come first-served basis and until the opening of the PCSU 1 year ago, was rarely used. In the past few months Dr. Smith has become increasingly more possessive of "his" treatment room and has told the PCSU charge nurse that other physicians wishing to do bronchoscopies must do them between 11:00 A.M. and 4:00 P.M.

Several new pulmonary medicine specialists (M.D.s) have joined the medical staff in the last 6 months. They also care for patients in the PCSU (although not as many as Dr. Smith) and do inpatient as well as outpatient bronchoscopies in addition to their routine office visits. They have approached you as the supervisor of the PCSU, complaining that these hours are very inconvenient and that they feel they have as much right to the treatment room as Dr. Smith. As a group, they plan to do two to three bronchoscopies per day.

· ·

Assignment

Devise a policy and procedure that will organize scheduling and will provide for the optimum use of the room and personnel.

CASE 6 (CONTINUED)

CASE 6

You are an obstetrical nurse in Jamestown Hospital, an acute care, for-profit hospital. The mission statement for Jamestown hospital states that the organization has two primary purposes: 1) to provide the highest possible quality of care for its clients and, 2) to maximize the efficiency and cost-effectiveness of resource utilization in recognition of its obligation to internal and external stakeholders.

Recently, you have become increasingly concerned regarding what you perceive to be the economically motivated, premature discharge of mothers and their babies, often less than 24 hours after delivery. Although you recognize that the majority of your patients do well at home following discharge, you are concerned that the short admission time does not allow for adequate assessment of potential complications that may arise for both the mother and baby within the first few days after delivery.

Assignment

In small groups, discuss whether you feel the dual-goal mission statement is in conflict. Why or why not? How will you handle the intrapersonal conflict you feel about the rapid discharge of patients from your unit? Is it realistic for you to attempt to change the organization's mission statement?

DISPLAY 4-3
Memorial Hospital—Unit Goals and Objectives

1. To maintain a safe environment for the patient by
   a. Utilizing the guidelines as outlined by the safety manual.
   b. Having an effective infection control by use of an infection control committee, and by using the guidelines of the isolation manual.
2. To coordinate both nursing and non-nursing services by
   a. Explaining and scheduling procedures.
   b. Interpreting services to the patient.
3. To carry out a therapeutic medical plan of care as ordered by the physician by
   a. Having an understanding and knowledge of acceptable medical practice.
   b. Noting and following through with the physicians plan of care.
4. To assess, plan, implement, and evaluate a nursing plan of care by
   a. Use of short- and long-term nursing goals.
   b. Ensuring the cooperation of all shifts in the use of nursing care plans.
   c. Evaluating the nursing care through the use of 1) a charting audit, 2) a patient questionnaire form, and 3) the use of team conferences.

DISPLAY 4-3 *(Continued)*
Memorial Hospital—Unit Goals and Objectives

5. To help the patient grow from his or her illness experience by
   a. Teaching aspects of health and illness.
   b. Assisting the patient with his or her own problem solving.
   c. Allowing the patient as much autonomy as possible in regard to his or her illness.
6. To do for the patient what he or she is unable to do for him- or herself by
   a. Using skilled bedside techniques in procedures and treatments.
7. To act as a family member surrogate and to relieve the anxiety of illness by
   a. Showing compassion and interest in the patient.
   b. Using therapeutic and listening techniques of communication.
   c. Answering questions and giving reassurance.
8. To think of the patient as a member of an open system by
   a. Including members of the family in aspects of teaching.
9. To provide for continuity of care by
   a. Use of nursing care plans.
   b. Utilizing referrals to other community agencies and resources.
   c. Coordinating a plan of care.
   d. The use of pertinent and accurate recording.
10. To provide a trained and knowledgeable nursing staff by
    a. Having an effective, meaningful, and well-attended program of in-service education.
    b. Encouraging the use of community educational resources.
    c. Having an employee educational reimbursement program.
    d. Encouraging staff to attend workshops and seminars.
    e. Having each member of the staff share knowledge and teach others.

◆ **Bibliography**

Butcher AH (1994). Supervisors matter more than you think: components of a mission-centered organizational climate. Hosp Health Serv Adm 39:505–520

Carroll AB (1993). Three types of management planning: making organizations work. Manag Quart 34; Spring:32–36

Connors R, Smith T, and Hickman C (1994). The Oz Principle: Getting Results Through Individual and Organizational Accountability. Englewood Cliffs, NJ: Prentice-Hall

Davis D and Salmen K (1991). Nursing, planning, and marketing: from theory to practice. Nurs Admin Quart 15(3):66–71

Demarzo DL (1993). Policies and procedures: protection or peril? RN 56(7):61–62

El-Namaki MSS (1992). Creating a corporate vision. Long Range Plan 25:25–29

Heenan ALJ (1994). A mission statement, Prof Nurse 10(2):72

Irurita VF (1994). Optimism, values, and commitment as forces in nursing leadership. J Nurs Admin 24(9):61–71

Martin LS and Hughes SR (1993). Using the mission statement to craft a least-restraint policy. Nurs Manag 24(3):65–66

Matejka K, Kurt L, and Gregory B (1993). Mission impossible? Designing a great mission statement to ignite your plans. Manag Dec 31:34–37

Paris LL (1995). Clarifying the team's work: writing a mission statement. Nurs Qual Connec 4(4):4,7

Peters J (1993). On vision and values. Manag Dec 31:14–17

Peters J (1993). On objectives. Manag Dec 31(6):28–30

Redman BK (1994). Nursing's agenda for health care reform: the profession's ability to create a health care system congruent with its philosophy. As found in Chapter 7 of Nursing Issues in the 90s. Strickland O and Fishman D (eds.) New York: Delmar

Steaban RL (1993). Value-based leadership: Using values clarification to change a unit culture. Aspen's Adv Nurse Exec 9(1):3–4

White CB (1990). Policies and procedures: a synergistic approach. Nurs Manag 21(10):82,84

PERSONAL NOTEBOOK

1. My basic beliefs about life are:
   (List 5–10)

2. My basic beliefs about nursing are:
   (List 5–10)

3. Are your beliefs about life and nursing consistent?

4. If you are presently employed in a health care institution, have you reviewed that organization's philosophy and compared it with your own?

5. Make a list of five personal goals and five professional goals you want to accomplish in the next 6 years.

nication between all levels of personnel, a cooperative spirit relative to solving problems, and a pervasive feeling that the departments are unified, goal-directed, and doing their part to help the organization accomplish its mission.

If there is one common fault among unit-level managers in planning, it is in not adequately developing long-range planning. Many managers operate in a crisis mode and do not use acknowledged historical patterns to assist them in planning for the future, nor do they examine present clues and projected statistics, called *forecasting*, to determine future needs. Forecasting takes advantage of the input from others, prescribes a sequence for activities, and protects an organization against undesirable changes. In an age of rapidly changing technology, payment structures, and resource availability, the manager who is unwilling or unable to predict with some degree of accuracy is a liability to the efficiency of the organization and the effectiveness of the unit in meeting organizational goals. Increased competition, governmental reimbursement, and decreasing hospital revenues have reduced intuitive managerial decision making. Nursing managers who lack knowledge regarding legal, political, economic, and social factors affecting health care can make planning errors that have disastrous implications for both their professional development and the financial viability of the organization (Marquis and Huston, 1996).

Because health care facilities are particularly vulnerable to external social, economic, and political forces, it is very difficult to accurately predict how these forces may change. Unlike the 20-year strategic plans of the 1960s and 1970s, most organizations find it difficult today to project even 5 or 10 years in the future. This means that long-range plans must be flexible, permitting change as these forces impact the health care facility.

Porter-O'Grady (1996) suggests that the realities emerging in today's rapidly changing health care system must be incorporated in planning for a healthcare organization's future. Such realities include:

- the rise of information as the new architecture for organizations, linking people and information in a way that allows people to function well, no matter where they are located
- the requirement to build different work relationships in light of the impact of information technology on the way we manage systems, people, processes, and outcomes
- the necessity to build on the "point of service" and construct organizational supports around the worker and customer to facilitate rather than impede that relationship
- the need for new, yet fewer leadership roles that require a higher level of competence and confidence than what was often considered acceptable before, and
- higher levels of expectations from those who do work; both competence and interdependence rank high as appropriate behaviors for workers in the future health care system.

Decker and Sullivan (1992) have identified eight major phases in the strategic planning process. Phase I incorporates a review of both the organization and the nursing mission, philosophy, goals, and objectives to clarify values and assumptions affecting current operation. In Phase II, the planning cycle is outlined, as well as the processes or structure to be used. In Phase III, an assessment is made of environmental variables, strengths, and weaknesses of the nursing department, as well as discrepancies between consumers, employees, and organizational expectations. Phase IV results in a revised mission statement, objectives, and goals, and an idealized design of a desired future. In Phase V, the organizational structure for strategic planning is developed with the clear identification of roles and role expectations. Employees are oriented to new roles and/or changes in currently existing roles. In Phase VI, measurable conclusions and evaluation criteria are designed as controls. The strategic plan becomes a written document in Phase VII and is implemented in Phase VIII.

Yoder-Wise (1995) suggests there are five phases in the strategic planning process. Phase I includes an assessment of the external and internal environments of the organization. Phase 2 includes a review of the organization's mission statement, philosophy, goals, and objectives. The third phase involves the identification of major issues, the establishment of goals, and the development of strategies to meet those goals. In the fourth phase of the strategic plan, specific plans for action are implemented. The last phase is evaluation at all levels to determine if the goals, objectives, and activities are on target.

Regardless of how many phases there are or what the phases are labeled, it is clear that the process of strategic planning in all organizations must be carefully thought out and appropriately implemented.

Intermediate planning, which works to achieve strategic planning goals, includes planning that covers a 1- to 5-year range. Intermediate planning involves program or project planning, which focuses on one event, such as developing a specific service, building a new facility, or projections for marketing and annual budgeting (Jernigan, 1988). In a study by Martinsons (1991), 83.7% of responding health care organizations stated they were planning major construction projects between 1991 and 1995. It is critical that managers participate in such facility planning to ensure that patient needs will be met and that the most effective use of nursing personnel is made (Munn and Saulsbery, 1992).

Most of the managers' plans, however, concern day-to-day *operational* planning, as well as procedural and policy planning. This day-to-day planning is more focused on achieving specific tasks and is often called *short-range planning.* Short-range plans may involve a time period of 1 hour to 1 year, and usually are much less complex than strategic plans or intermediate planning. Short-range planning may be done annually, bimonthly, weekly, or even daily as required.

A common mistake among novice managers lies in underestimating the importance of establishing a *daily* plan to organize the work or in not allowing adequate time for plan development. Managers may believe they are being unproductive if they sit at their desk designing the plan of care for the day, rather than accomplishing any specific task. Planning takes time as it requires the ability to think, analyze data, envision alternatives, and make decisions. Daily planning is essential if the manager is to manage efficiently rather than in response to crisis. Daily planning in the form of time management, is discussed more fully in Chapter 15.

Policy and procedural planning involves reviewing and revising policies and procedures that govern unit function. Because the unit is in a constant state of flux, the needs of the unit and the most appropriate means of meeting those needs constantly change. Therefore, the unit manager must periodically review and revise written policy and procedure statements to ensure they are current and applicable. For example, the unit manager is responsible for seeing that a clearly written policy exists regarding holiday and vacation time off and that this policy be clearly communicated to all those affected by it. In addition, the unit manager must assure that there is a clearly written procedural statement regarding requesting vacation or holiday time on that specific unit. If a long-term change in patient census or availability of human resources occurred, the unit manager would assess those changes and revise the policy and procedural statements accordingly.

◆ Management by Objectives

All managers are responsible for ensuring that the goals of the organization are met. The manager may do this by assisting employees in setting personal and organizational objectives intended to satisfy organizational goals. This planning by objectives is known as Management by Objectives (MBO) and was developed by Peter Drucker in the mid-1950s. In MBO, each nurse sets personal objectives to meet organizational goals. These goals are reviewed with the appropriate department head for feedback on how to more clearly specify goals and to ensure that these goals are realistic. Intermittent periodic evaluation is then suggested in order to monitor and recognize employee progress. Display 5-1 identifies standard steps in the MBO process.

DISPLAY 5-1
The MBO Process (Management by Objectives)

1. Employees are informed of the intent to implement MBO.
2. Employees are asked to provide feedback and additional information is given in response to concerns and questions.
3. Organizational goals are reviewed with employees.
4. Employees prepare personal objectives that include a time limit.
5. Employees and managers meet to review employee objectives.
6. Employees work to meet personal objectives.
7. Managers provide ongoing feedback to evaluate progress made on employee objectives. Annual or semiannual conferences are held to review prior objectives and set new ones as necessary.

A basic belief underlying MBO is that if employees are allowed to participate in personal and organizational goal setting, they will be more inclined to
feel they have an investment in the organization itself. Why then don't all nurse
managers use MBO? Possibly because it takes time to implement correctly and
requires the cooperation and support from all levels of the administrative hierarchy. In addition, many nurses have not used MBO before and as in all change,
resistance of the unknown can and does occur. MBO does, however, offer managers an effective and consistent means of organizing the work of others to
meet organizational goals. A further discussion of MBO is found in Chapter 21,
Performance Appraisal.

◆ Planning Strategies

Because effective planning is essential for managers, barriers must be overcome. The benefits of good planning include the ability to accomplish a higher
quality of work on time and more effective use of capital and human resources.
The manager must remember several points if effective organizational planning
is to be achieved.

1. The organization can be more effective if movement within that organization is directed at prespecified goals and objectives. Unfortunately, a
   step frequently omitted by the novice planner is establishing a goal or
   objective prior to outlining plans. Establishing an end for the plan helps
   keep the individual focused on the "big picture" and prevents him or her
   from getting lost in the minute details. Just as nursing-care plans establish patient care goals prior to delineating problems and interventions,
   so must managers establish goals for their planning strategies.
2. Because a plan is a guide for action to reach a goal, it must be flexible
   and allow for readjustment as unexpected events occur.
3. The manager should include all individuals and organizational units that
   could be affected by the planning process. Although not everyone will
   want to contribute, they should be invited to do so. The manager also
   needs to communicate clearly to all those responsible for assisting in
   carrying out the plans, what the end goals are as well as the specific
   responsibilities of each participant to ensure a coordinated effort in
   meeting the goals.
4. Plans should be specific, simple, and realistic. A plan that is vague is impossible to implement. A plan that is too global or unrealistic will discourage
   employees rather than motivate them to meet organizational goals.
5. Know when to and when not to plan, as it is possible to over- as well as
   underplan. An example of over planning is devoting an excessive amount
   of time to concentrating on details that might be better left to the initiative of others involved. Underplanning occurs when the manager
   assumes that people and events will naturally fall into some desired and
   efficient method of production.

6. Effective plans have a time for evaluation built-in, so that there can be a midway correction if unexpected events occur. Another evaluation should always take place at the end of the plan time frame. If goals were not met the plan should be reexamined to determine the reason for failure. The evaluation process assists the manager in future planning.

◆ Summary

It is critical to remember that planning does not take place in a vacuum. As plans, goals, objectives, policies, rules, and procedures are established, there is inevitably an impact on organizational, controlling, and motivational issues. The proactive manager attempts to assess this impact and develops contingency plans as needed.

Short-range planning is a proactive and deliberate process that allows personal as well as organizational needs to be met. Most of the unit-level manager's planning time is spent in short-range planning and their performance is often measured by their ability to execute these plans effectively.

Likewise, today's managers must be proactive rather than reactive in their long-range planning strategy. The health care system is perpetually and chaotically changing at a frenzied pace, making it difficult for managers to identify forces that will influence their units on a short-, intermediate-, and long-term basis. Managers today must be able to accurately forecast unit needs with an understanding of the legal, political, economic, social, and legislative climate of the organization and unit or be left to pay the price in terms of fiscal, technological, and human resources.

◆ References

Bombard CF (1993). Strategic planning: a practical approach. J Nurs Admin 23(7/8):41–45

Decker PJ and Sullivan EJ (1992). Nursing Administration: A Micro/Macro Approach for Effective Nurse Executives. Norwalk, CT: Appleton and Lange

Douglass LM (1996). The Effective Nurse: Leader and Manager, 5th ed. St. Louis: Mosby

Jernigan DK (1988). Human Resource Management in Nursing. Norwalk, CT: Appleton and Lange

Marquis B and Huston C (1996). Leadership Roles and Management Functions: Theory and Application, 2nd ed. Philadelphia: JB Lippincott

Marriner-Tomey A (1996). Guide to Nursing Management, 5th ed. St. Louis: Mosby

Martinsons J (1991). Despite slump, health care construction still blooms. In Grayson MA, Hemmes M, and McLarney UJ (eds): Plant Technology and Safety Management Series (Health Facility Design and Construction). Oakbrook Terrace, IL: Joint Commission on Accreditation of Health Care Organizations, 44–46

Mintzberg H (1994). The Rise and Fall of Strategic Planning. New York: Free Press

Munn EM and Saulsbery PA (1992). Facility planning—a blueprint for nurse executives. J Nurs Admin 22(1):13–17

Porter-O'Grady (1994). The Nurse Manager's Problem Solver. St. Louis: Mosby

Porter-O'Grady T (1996). The seven basic rules for successful redesign. J Nurs Admin 26(1):46–53

Simms LM, Price SA, and Ervin NE (1994). The Professional Practice of Nursing Administration, 2nd ed. New York: Delmar

Swansburg RC (1990). Management and Leadership for Nurse Managers. Boston: Jones and Bartlett

Tappen RM (1996). Nursing Leadership and Management: Concepts and Practice, 3rd ed. Philadelphia: FA Davis

Yoder-Wise PS (1995). Leading and Managing in Nursing. St. Louis: Mosby

Young LC and Hayne AN (1988). Nursing Administration: From Concepts to Practice. Philadelphia: WB Saunders

SAMPLE CASE ANALYSIS

THE CASE ◆

You are a newly licensed graduate nurse from a baccalaureate nursing program. You completed your education in Arizona, although you hope to return to California (where your family lives) and find your first job. You especially enjoyed your critical care rotation in school and would like to find a job in critical care after completing 1 or 2 years of medical-surgical job experience.

Assignment

Devise your plan to make this happen. Your plan should include both long- and short-range goals, although most of your planning will be short-range. Identify what steps you propose to take to meet these goals.

Analysis

Although you have a general idea of what you would like to do in the future, it is important to identify specific long- and short-range goals.

Long-Range Goals
1. Become a competent critical care nurse with a critical care nursing certification.
2. Serve as a preceptor/mentor to other new graduate nurses in the critical care setting.

Short-Range Goals
1. Obtain employment in California to be closer to your family.
2. Be hired into a job that provides medical-surgical work experience.
3. Develop critical care expertise and knowledge.

Once you have identified your long- and short-term goals, it is important to break those goals down into more specific, workable steps. Your plan might look something like the following.

CASE 2 (CONTINUED)

- Discontinue the IV on a patient who is complaining of redness/tenderness at the insertion site.

CASE 3

You are a 25-year-old female in your senior year at a baccalaureate nursing school in the Midwest. One of your assignments for an issues class in nursing is to make a 10-year strategic plan for your career. Be sure you introduce flexibility within your plan.

Assignment

1. What is your overall career goal?
2. What are your strategic plans for reaching that goal? How did you overcome financial and family constraints?
3. What alternatives did you include in your plan?
4. Is marriage or parenthood part of your plan? Did you plan for aging parents?
5. What are your target dates? Are they feasible and realistic?

CASE 4

ASSIGNMENT

Strategic planning requires managerial expertise in health care economics, human resource management, political and legislative issues affecting health care and planning theory. It also requires the leadership skills of being sensitive to the environment, being able to appraise accurately the social and political climate, and being willing to take risks (Marquis and Huston, 1996). Write an essay identifying six forces affecting today's health care system. Prioritize these forces in terms of how they may affect you as a unit manager or staff nurse. You may include legal, political, economic, social, technological, or ethical forces.

◆ Bibliography

The following is a list of references to help you solve these cases:

Anvaripour PA (1990). A nursing department can and should plan for the future. Nurs Health Care 11(4):207–209

Berry FS (1994). Innovation in public management: the adoption of strategic planning. Public Admin Rev 54(4):322–329

Boyd BK (1991). Strategic planning and financial performance: a meta analytical review. J Manage Stud XXVIII, 4 (July):353–374

Buchana A (1992). Strategic planning for tomorrow's success. Caring 11(Nov):52–57

Buckhardt PJ and Reuss S (1993). Successful Strategic Planning: A Guide for Nonprofit Agencies. Newbury Park, CA: Sage

Curtin L (1991). Strategic planning: asking the right questions. Nurs Manage 22(1):7–8

Hardy K (1992). The three crimes of strategic planning. Bus Quart 57(spring):71–74

Howard LS, Mabon SA, and Piland NF (1993). Nursing department strategy, planning, and performance in rural hospitals. J Nurs Admin 23(4):23–24

Ives JR (1991). Articulating values and assumptions for strategic planning. Nurs Manage 22(1):38–39

MacDonald S, Beange J, and Blachford P (1992). Planning for strategic change? A participative planning approach for community hospitals. Healthcare Manage For 5(3):31–37

Naisbitt J and Aburdene P (1990). Megatrends 2000: Ten New Directions for the 1990s. New York: Morrow

Reeves PN (1993). Issues Management: The Other Side of Strategic Planning. Hosp Health Serv Admin 38(2)

Skafel J (1993). Change or business as usual. Healthcare Manage For 6(2):45–48

Smeltzer CH and Hinshaw AS (1993). Integrating research in a strategic plan. Nurs Manage 24(2):42–44

Thomas A (1993). Strategic planning: a practical approach. Nurs Manage 24(2):34–35, 38

Tuazon NC (1991). S-M-A-R-T planning for teaching sessions. Nursing 91 21(7):80–82

Wilson I (1992). Realizing the power of strategic vision. Long Range Plan 25(Oct):18–28

PERSONAL NOTEBOOK

My Professional Goals

My Personal Goals

1 year

1 year

1.

1.

2.

2.

3.

3.

5 years

5 years

1.

1.

2.

2.

3.

3.

10 years

10 years

1.

1.

2.

2.

3.

3.

Are your professional and personal goals congruent? Do they both reflect your overall philosophy? Is it possible to fulfill both your personal and professional goals?

Planned Change

CHAPTER

6

Most organizations today are undertaking a number of projects as part of a change effort. These projects are often directed at quality improvement, process and structure reengineering, and employee empowerment (Duck, 1993). The key to a successful change effort is not attending to each project in isolation, but instead, to connecting and balancing all the pieces. For when one piece of the organization is changed, the rest of the organization changes as well.

◆ Planned Change and the Change Agent

Planned change is a well-thought-out and deliberate effort to make something happen. Conversely, *accidental change,* also called *change by drift,* is unplanned change that occurs as a result of an imbalance in the system. Accidental change is always met with resistance and hostility as individuals being subjected to the change feel threatened and uninformed.

Planned change results because of an intended effort by a *change agent(s)* to deliberately move the system. Changes are implemented slowly and are carefully planned to increase the likelihood that the change will be successful. In planned change the manager often takes the role of change agent and assumes the responsibility for moving those affected by the change through its stages.

◆ Reasons for Change

Lewin (1951), perhaps the best known of the classical change theorists, identified several rules that should be followed in implementing change.

1. Change should only be implemented for good reason.
2. Change should always be gradual.
3. All change should be planned, and not be sporadic or sudden.
4. All individuals who may be affected should be involved in planning for the change.

Many change agents fail because they forget these four rules and often implement change without cause, too rapidly, or without adequately involving others. Sullivan and Decker (1988) maintain that there are only three good reasons for change that are applicable to a wide variety of situations.

1. Change in order to solve a problem.
2. Change to make work procedures more efficient.
3. Change to reduce unnecessary work.

◆ Resistance: The Natural Response to Organizational Change

Some of the processes used in planned change are the same as for long- and short-range planning, such as setting a goal and having flexibility as well as checkpoints built into the plans. However, since change implies movement from one point to another by those involved in the change, there are additional elements to examine. Consideration must be given to the feelings and frustrations of others involved in the change.

Because change disrupts the homeostasis or balance of the group, resistance is a natural response. The level of resistance generally depends on the type of change proposed. Technological changes encounter less resistance than changes that are perceived as social, or that are contrary to established customs or norms. Administrators must also recognize that subordinates' values, educational levels, cultural and social backgrounds, as well as past experiences with change (positive or negative) will have a tremendous impact on their degree of resistance.

Perhaps the greatest factor contributing to the resistance encountered with organizational change is a lack of trust between the employee and the manager or the employee and the organization. "One of the greatest paradoxes about change is that trust is hardest to establish at the times when you need it the most" (Duck, 1993; 114). Duck goes on to say that trust in a time of change is based on two things: *predictability* and *capability*. In any organization, workers want predictability; they want their work environment to be known and to be comfortable. They want security. That's why trust erodes when the ground rules change; as the assumed "contract" between the worker and the organization is altered. The public administrator must remember that people tend to consider the effects of change on their personal lives, status, and future, more than on the welfare of the organization.

The second factor in creating trust in the organization during change is capability. Both administrators and workers must accurately understand and believe in the capability of the other to successfully make the change. Roles and responsibilities of each person involved in the change must be negotiated and accepted before each will trust the situation. Thus, the change must be personalized before the risks can be accepted.

Because change is such a complex process, it requires a great deal of planning and intricate timing. Any change must allow adequate time for those involved to become fully assimilated to it. A change agent should not begin the process unless they have adequate time and a commitment to see it through. Marquis and Huston (1996) maintain that most planned change requires 3–6 months before the process is complete.

When a need for change is recognized by the system, the change agent has the responsibility to use appropriate strategies and techniques that will ensure that the change is effectively managed. Display 6-1 illustrates the responsibilities of the change agent during the various stages of the process.

DISPLAY 6-1
Stages of Change and Responsibility of the Change Agent

Step 1—Unfreezing
a. Gather data.
b. Accurately diagnose the problem.
c. Decide if change is necessary.
d. Make others aware of the need for change.

Do *not* proceed to step 2 until the status quo has been disrupted and there is a perceived and obvious need for change by others.

Step 2—Movement
a. Develop a plan.
b. Set goals and objectives.
c. Identify areas of support and resistance.
d. Include everyone in the planning that will be affected.
e. Establish target dates.
f. Develop appropriate strategies for alteration.
g. Implement the change.
h. Be available to support others through the process; offer encouragement as needed.
i. Employ tactics for overcoming resistance.
j. Evaluate the change.
k. Modify, if necessary.

Step 3—Refreezing
a. Support others so that the change remains in place.

DISPLAY 6-2 *(Continued)*
Ten Emotional Phases of Planned Change

Phase	Characteristics/Symptoms	Interventions
7. Resignation	Energy expended in passively accepting change. Lack of enthusiasm.	Expect employees to be accountable for reactions to behavior. Allow them to move at their own pace.
8. Openness	Availability to renewed energy. Willingness to expend energy on what has been assigned to individual.	Patiently explain again, in detail, the desired change.
9. Readiness	Willingness to expend energy in exploring new events. Reunification of intellect and emotions begins.	Assume a directive management style: assign tasks, monitor tasks and results so as to provide direction and guidelines.
10. Reemergence	Rechanneled energy produces feelings of empowerment and employees become more proactive. Rebirth of growth and commitment. Employee initiates projects and ideas. Career questions answered.	Mutual answering of questions. Redefinition of career, mission, and culture. Mutual understanding of role and identity. Employees will take action based on own decisions.

Source—Perlman D and Takacs GJ (1990). The ten stages of change. Nurs Manag 21(4):33–38; with permission.

This set of strategies is often referred to as the *rational empirical strategies.* The change agent using this set assumes man is a rational being who will change when he is given factual information supporting the reasons for the change.

Because peer pressure is often used to effect change, another collection of strategies that uses the group process to educate for change is called the *normative-reeducative* strategies. This set of tactics uses the group to socialize others and influence individuals, so change will occur. The change agent assumes man is a social animal who is more easily influenced by others than by facts.

The third group of methods often employed by change agents is called the *power-coercive strategies.* This group includes such things as influencing the enactment of new laws, or using the power of groups for strikes or sit-ins. Use of authority inherent in an individual position to effect change is another example of a power-coercive strategy. The change agent using this group of strategies assumes that individuals are often "set in their ways," resistant to change, and will only change when rewarded or forced by some other power-coercive method.

Often the change agent uses a variety of strategies from each group to assist in effecting the change. An example would be the one who wants his or

GOAL: RETURN TO SCHOOL

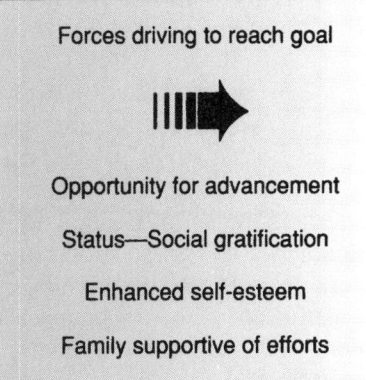

Forces driving to reach goal

Opportunity for advancement

Status—Social gratification

Enhanced self-esteem

Family supportive of efforts

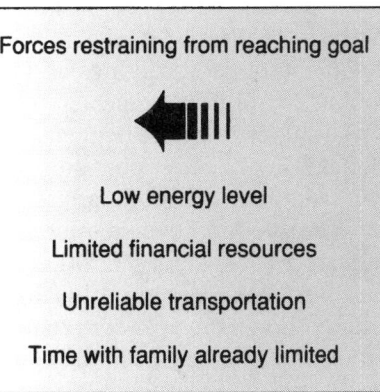

Forces restraining from reaching goal

Low energy level

Limited financial resources

Unreliable transportation

Time with family already limited

FIGURE 6-1.
Driving and restraining forces.

her spouse to stop smoking. The change agent would present the smoker with the latest research data on cancer and smoking (the rational approach); at the same time, an effort could be made to have friends and family educate the smoker socially as a means of influencing the change to occur (normative approach); and finally, the spouse might refuse to ride in the car of the smoker (coercive approach). By selecting an action from each set of strategies, the agent increases the chance of successful change.

Regardless of the strategies employed, the change agent needs to be supportive to those individuals affected by the change throughout the process. It is necessary that the support continue until refreezing occurs. Strong administrative support from higher levels of management is also necessary for change to occur. Adequate support includes mentoring those who are implementing the change, financial support for staff education and the allocation of necessary time to carry out the change process (Dumpe, 1996).

◆ The Role of the Nurse Manager in Fostering Appropriate Organizational Change

Because human beings are subjected to many unavoidable changes in their lives the change agent must remember that individuals function best when there is a workable balance between stability and change in the workplace (Perlman and Takacs, 1990). With the current widespread restructuring and reengineering that is occurring in health care organizations, many authors argue that such a balance has not been achieved.

Haveman (1992) argues that organizational change is generally disruptive and detrimental to organizational performance and survival chances, and that it can benefit organizational performance and survival chances only if it occurs in response to dramatic restructuring of environmental conditions and if it builds on established routines and competencies.

Amburgey (1993) suggests that organizational changes have two consequences: The first consequence is an immediate increase in the hazard of organizational failure. When change occurs, a "liability of newness" clock is reset and the risk of organization failure increases over what it would have been otherwise. The second consequence is an immediate increase in the likelihood of the same type of change at another time, particularly if it is organizational goals that are being changed. In other words, once the forces inhibiting change are overcome, the change process exhibits a momentum of its own. Organizations in motion tend to stay in motion, whereas aging organizations demonstrate a lower likelihood of change.

Amburgey concludes that the disruption produced by change can negate the benefits for a substantial period of time. Thus, proponents of organizational change should pay greater attention to determining both a desirable rate of change and the associated risk of organizational failure.

Despite the risks associated with major organizational change, the health care system of the 1990s is changing boldly and rapidly. This requires nurse managers with dramatically improved capacities to exercise relevant, reliable, and responsive leadership. Not only do nurse managers need to be visionary in identifying areas where organizational change is needed, they will have to be flexible in adapting to changes they have directly initiated or indirectly been affected by. Understanding when and how to initiate and coordinate organizational change are critical leadership skills required of the nurse manager. In addition, the nurse manager will need to learn to work with new employees early in their tenure to advise them of innovations that may help the organization be more effective and more responsive to the environment in which they function.

In an era of rapidly dwindling resources, exponential information technology growth, and virtually endless change, nurse managers must constantly strive to limit the disruptive effects of organizational change and bolster the adaptive effects. A failure to proactively do so may result in misdirected and poorly utilized fiscal and human resources.

◆ Summary

Planned change is a deliberate and well-thought-out process and a frequent part of a manager's planning. All change will elicit some resistance and it is up to the change agent to increase the driving forces toward change while decreasing the restraining forces, if the change is actually going to occur. Knowledge of the phases of planned change as well as the major change strategies will assist the manager in being a successful change agent.

◆ References

Amburgey TL, Kelly D, and Barnett WP (1993). Resetting the clock: the dynamics of organizational change and failure. Admin Sci Quart 38(1):51–73

Bennis W, Benne K, and Chinn R (1969). The Planning of Change, 2nd ed. New York: Holt, Rinehart, and Winston

Duck JD (1993). Managing change: the art of balancing. Harvard Bus Rev Nov/Dec 109–118

Dumpe ML (1996). Making a change: the importance of administrative support. Nurs Manage 27(5):61

Haveman HA (1992). Between a rock and hard place: organizational change and performance under conditions of fundamental transformation. Admin Sci Quart 37(1):48–75

Lewin K (1951). Field Theory in Social Sciences. New York: Harper & Row

Marquis BL and Huston CJ (1996). Leadership Roles and Management Functions for Nurses: Theory and Application, 2nd ed. Philadelphia: JB Lippincott

Perlman D and Takacs GJ (1990). The ten stages of change. Nurs Manag 21(4):33–38

Sullivan EJ and Decker PJ (1988). Effective Management in Nursing. Menlo Park, CA: Addison-Wesley

SAMPLE CASE ANALYSIS

THE CASE ◆

You are a 24-year-old, unmarried female RN and you have returned to your hometown to work in the local rural 55-bed hospital. Your only working experience has been on a general medical-surgical unit in the large city where you attended college. At that inner city hospital they had recently switched from a total patient care delivery model to team leading. At your present place of employment the nurses use task-oriented (functional) nursing-care management and you find this type of organization fragments patient care and, in addition, affords you little personal satisfaction. Your director of nurses seems open to new ideas and you decide that you would like to be the change agent, suggesting a newer method of patient care assignment. One evening after working the 3–11 P.M. shift you return to your parents' home and you sit down to spend the rest of the night working on your planned change.

Assignment

1. Is there a need for change?
2. What do you feel your approach should be in this case? Why?
3. Outline your plan.
4. How would you summarize your chances for success?
5. What are some risks that you should guard against?

◆ **Bibliography**

The following list of references will help you solve these cases:

Augustine NR (1995). Managing the crisis you tried to prevent. Harvard Bus Rev Nov/Dec, 147–158

Chinn PL (1992). Where and When Does Change Begin? Nurs Outlook 40(3):102–103

Curtin L (1993). Looking the Snake in the Eye. Nurs Manage 24(7):7–8

Edwards PA and Roemer L (1996). Are nurse managers ready for the current challenges of healthcare? J Nurs Admin 26(9):11–17

Hagerman AJ, and Tiffany CR (1994). Evaluation of Two Planned Change Theories. Nurs Manage 25(4):57–62

Hall FS (1994). Managing the dysfunctional manager in times of change. Aspen's Adv Nurse Exec 10(2):1–3

Hendry J, Johnson G, and Newton J (eds) (1994). Leadership and the Management of Change. New York: Wiley

Issel LM and Anderson RA (1996). Take charge: managing six transformations in health care delivery. Nurs Econ 14(2):78–85

Kirrane DE (1995). Significant system change continues despite the absence of national healthcare reform. Healthcare Exec 10:7–11

Lutjens LR and Tiffany CR (1994). Evaluating planned change theories. Nurs Manage 25(3):54–57

Manion J (1993). Chaos or transformation? Managing Innovation. J Nurs Admin 23(5):41–48

McClellan MA, Henson RH, and Schmele J (1994). Introducing new technology: confusion or order? Nurs Manage 25(7):38–41

McSwain CJ and White OF (1993). A transformational theory of organizations. Am Rev Pub Admin 23(2):81–98

Silber MB (1993). The "Cs" in excellence: choice and change. Nurs Manage 24(9):60–62

Simpson RL (1996). Managing the social and behavioral impact of technology change. Nurs Manag 27(6):26–27

Tiffany CR, Cheatham AB, Doornbos D, Loudermelt L, and Momadi GG (1994). Planned change theory: survey of nursing periodical literature. Nurs Manage 25(7):54–59

Trofino J (1996). Vision—a professional model for nursing practice. Nurs Manage 27(93):43–48

Valanis B (1995). Leadership for the 21st century: transforming the skills and competencies of the future nursing work force. Capsules Comments Nurs Leadership Manage 3(92):101–104

PERSONAL NOTEBOOK

1. Identify a change that you would like to make in your personal life. Examples might include studying more, saving more money, exercising daily, or stopping smoking. List the driving and restraining forces. Devise methods that allow you to increase the driving forces and decrease the restraining forces.

2. Try to remember a time in your life that involved unnecessary change. Why did you feel the change was unwarranted? What types of turmoil did it cause?

3. Have you ever resisted a change that you later came to accept? Describe the stages you went through before acceptance came about.

4. Think back to changes you have undertaken in your personal life. Describe the types of imbalances in the system that provided the catalyst for you to alter your life.

Fiscal Planning

Scarce resources and soaring health care costs have strained all health care delivery systems. There has never been a time when health care organizations needed to operate more efficiently or be more aware of cost containment. *Cost containment* refers to effective and efficient delivery of services while generating needed revenues for continued organizational productivity. Cost containment is the responsibility of every health care provider and the very survival of many health care organizations depends on their ability to do so (Campbell and Dowd, 1993).

◆ Role of the Manager in Fiscal Planning

Of all the forms of planning, fiscal planning is often perceived as the most difficult and thus may be avoided by managers. Although familiar with the basics of fiscal planning, unit managers may encounter difficulty with forecasting costs based on current and projected needs. Sometimes this occurs because the manager has had little formal education or training on budget preparation. Fiscal planning, is a learned skill as is all planning, and improves with practice.

With the current focus on cost containment and fiscal responsibility by all health care providers, it is essential that nurses develop expertise in managing and understanding costs. "Even today, with the increasing emphasis on finance in most nursing graduate programs, well-prepared nurse executives are not as sophisticated in economic matters as this finance-driven health care system requires" (Manthey, 1992; 14).

Historically, nursing management has played a limited role in determining resource allocation in health care institutions. Because nursing is a service and is not usually classified as "income producing" in itself, nursing input has been shortchanged in the budget process. Today, the nursing budget frequently accounts for at least half of the total expenses in health care institutions. "People who have no idea of nursing's culture and belief system, principles, and values make financial decisions about it every day, and nurses continue to let this happen" (Manthey, 1992; 14). Nurses must be involved in fiscal planning to see that appropriate resources are available to provide nursing services. A study by Hodges and Poteet (1991) indicates a continuing problem with authority for chief nurse executives in matters germane to resource allocation. Participating in fiscal planning should be viewed as a fundamental and powerful tool for nursing.

◆ Budgeting

A *budget* is defined as a plan that uses numerical data and predicts the activities of an organization over a set period of time. Although budgets are usually associated with financial statements, such as revenues and expenses, they may also be nonfinancial statements covering output, materials, and equipment (Marriner-Tomey, 1996).

The desired outcome of budgeting is the optimal use of resources. The value of the budget to the institution is directly related to its accuracy. The more accurate the budget forecast, the more closely the organization can plan the most efficient use of its resources. However, as with all planning, fiscal planning requires flexibility. A budget is at best a prediction, a plan and not a rule, thus flexibility must be included, as well as ongoing evaluation and revision.

Marriner-Tomey (1996) identified three conditions necessary for the development and implementation of a budgetary program. First, there is a need for a sound organizational structure with clearly delineated lines of authority and responsibility. Budgetary authority and responsibility can then parallel the corresponding hierarchical pattern of authority and responsibility.

Second, a clearly designated individual must be responsible for collecting and reporting statistical data. Nonmonetary data, such as number of admissions, average length of stay, percentage of occupancy, and number of patient days, is important in the budgetary process.

Third, a condition necessary for the development and implementation of a budgetary program is adequate managerial support. Although budgeting is done at the unit level, it must be valued by top-level administrators. This requires that top-level administrators adequately educate unit-level managers concerning how to budget. Formal budgeting policies and procedures, budgetary objectives, and the requisite responsibility for budgeting must be clearly stated.

Managers should involve as many individuals as is feasible in the budgetary process, because personnel who are asked to participate in fiscal planning are more apt to be cost conscious and will have a better understanding of how their unit must function to meet the overall long- and short-term goals.

DISPLAY 7-1 *(Continued)*
Fiscal Terminology

also available to certain groups of individuals with catastrophic or chronic illness, such as patients with renal failure requiring hemodialysis, regardless of age.

NONCONTROLLABLE COSTS—Indirect expenses that you cannot usually control or vary. Examples might be rent, lighting, and depreciation of equipment.

NOT-FOR-PROFIT ORGANIZATION—This type of organization is financed by funds that come from several sources, but the providers of these funds do not have an ownership interest. Profits generated in the not-for-profit organization are frequently funneled back into the organization for expansion or capital acquisition.

OPERATING EXPENSES—The daily costs required to maintain a hospital or health care institution.

PATIENT CLASSIFICATION SYSTEM—A method of classifying patients. Different criteria are used for different systems. In nursing, patients are usually classified according to severity of illness.

PREFERRED PROVIDER ORGANIZATION—A health care financing and delivery program with a group of providers such as physicians and hospitals who contract to give services on a fee-for-service basis that provides financial incentives to consumers to utilize a select group of preferred providers and pay less for services. Insurance companies usually promise the preferred provider organization a certain volume of patients and prompt payment in exchange for fee discounts (Streff, 1994).

PRODUCTION HOURS—The total amount of regular time, overtime, and temporary time. This may also be referred to as actual hours.

REVENUE—A source of income or the reward for providing a service to a client.

RIM—One minute of nursing resource use. RIMs were developed in New Jersey to allocate nursing resources in such a way as to address the complaints that DRGs inadequately represent variability of nursing care requirements (Marriner-Tomey, 1996).

STAFFING DISTRIBUTION—A determination of number of personnel allocated per shift. Example: 45% days, 35% evenings, and 20% nights. Hospitals vary on how staff is distributed.

STAFFING MIX—The ratio of RNs to other personnel. For example, a shift on one unit might have 40% RNs, 40% LPNs/LVNs, and 20% other. Hospitals vary on their staffing mix policies.

TURNOVER RATIO—The rate at which employees leave their jobs for reasons other than death or retirement. The rate is calculated by dividing the number of employees leaving by the number of workers employed in the unit during the year and then multiplying by 100.

VARIABLE COSTS—Costs that vary with the volume. Payroll costs are variable costs, for example.

WORKLOAD UNITS—In nursing, workloads are usually the same as patient days. For some areas, however, workload units might refer to the number of procedures, tests, patient visits, injections, and so on.

(Continued)

DISPLAY 7-1 *(Continued)*
Fiscal Terminology

ZERO-BASED BUDGETING—A type of budgeting system that begins at zero each year. That means that every dollar that is to be spent needs to be justified. Established costs are not automatically continued from one year to the next. This style of budgeting ensures that the activities aren't continued simply because they were carried out in the past. In zero-based budgeting, objectives are very important and they are listed according to priority. Zero-based budgeting also indicates what will happen if an objective is eliminated as well as which objectives could be accomplished for less money.

expect some fluctuation from the anticipated budget, large deviations must be examined for possible causes and remedial action taken if necessary. Some managers artificially inflate their department budgets as a cushion against budget cuts from a higher level of administration. If this unsound practice is employed by several departments within the same institution, the entire budget may be ineffective. If a major change in the budget is indicated, the entire developmental process must be repeated. Top-level managers must watch for unrealistic budget projections and correct them before they are implemented.

The budget is reviewed periodically and minor modifications are made as necessary throughout the fiscal year. With each successive year of budgeting, managers become better able to accurately forecast the financial needs of their unit. They develop a more historical approach to budgeting as they become better able to predict seasonal variations specific to the population they serve or their particular institution.

◆ Cost Effectiveness

The desired end product of careful fiscal planning is *cost effectiveness.* Cost effective does not imply "cheap." It means getting the most for your money or that the product is worth the price. Buying a very expensive piece of equipment may be considered cost effective if it can be shown that a sufficient need existed and that it was the best purchase to meet the need at that time. Cost effectiveness also takes into account factors such as anticipated length of service, the need for such a service, and the availability of other alternatives.

◆ The Prospective Payment System

Historically, heath care institutions placed little or no emphasis on budgeting. When budgeting was performed the incremental form was used. There was little motivation to save costs and budget effectively, as private insurance carriers reimbursed fully on a virtually limitless basis. Thus, the more the institution spent, the more reimbursement it received.

With the advent of Medicare and Medicaid in the 1960s, health care costs skyrocketed. As a result, the government began establishing regulations requiring organizations to justify the need for services, as well as to monitor the quality of those services. Health care providers were forced for the first time to provide Big Brother-type surveillance, and the introduction of external controls has had a tremendous effect on the industry (Marquis and Huston, 1996).

The advent of Diagnostic Related Groupings (DRGs) in the early 1980s added to the need for monitoring cost containment. DRGs were predetermined payment schedules that reflected historical costs for the treatment of specific patient conditions. The first version of the diagnostic related group system included 383 categories. Four hundred sixty-eight different DRGs or "product lines" had been established by 1989. As a result, DRGs have joined the prospective payment system (PPS), whereby agencies receive a prespecified amount of each patient's admission costs, regardless of the actual cost of care. As a result of the PPS and the need to maintain costs, the length of stay for most hospital admissions has decreased greatly. The PPS has saved billions of health care dollars, even with the adjustments needed to accommodate the shift in geographic site of care to outpatient settings (Swansburg and Sowell, 1992).

However, many experts argue that quality standards have been lowered and that patients are being discharged before they are ready. Other experts feel that some categories lack homogeneity and may be applicable only to the population originally tested; length of stay is not very applicable to actual costs; some physicians have differences in therapeutic philosophies and may vary their treatment of the same disease; different treatments cost different amounts; and some diseases do not have common treatment regimens (Marriner-Tomey, 1996).

Today, a significant number of patients treated by hospitals and other health care agencies are eligible for some type of federal or state health care reimbursement. Accompanying this increase in federal and state funding has come an increase in regulations for health care facilities treating those patients, as well as a system that rewards cost containment. Health care providers are encountering financial crises as they attempt to meet seemingly unlimited health care needs and services with limited fiscal reimbursement. In addition, rapidly changing federal and state reimbursement policies make long-range budgeting and planning very difficult for such facilities.

◆ Capitation, Preferred Provider Organizations, and Managed Care

Although the PPS brought much needed attention to health care costs run amok, and slowed the growth of health care costs, it alone was unable to keep health care expenses from approaching 15% of the gross national product by the mid-1990s. Although general economic recession and inflation played a part in rising health care costs, critics charged that the historical use of fee-for-service reimbursement (cost-based reimbursement) was the culprit, and a movement began toward capitated payment systems (Blancett and Flarey, 1995).

In *capitated* payment systems, predetermined payments are negotiated with health care providers who agree to provide specified services to an individual over a period of time. If the cost of caring for a specific individual is less than the capitated amount, the provider profits. If the cost of caring for a specific individual is greater than the capitated amount, the provider suffers a loss. The goal then for capitated providers is to see that patients receive the essential services needed to stay healthy or to keep from becoming more ill, but to eliminate unnecessary use of health care services. Predictions are that capitation may decrease inpatient utilization by 50% (Cerne, 1994).

Capitation is characteristic of *health maintenance organizations* (HMOs) and other managed care systems. HMOs provide health care in an organized system to subscribing members in a geographical area with an agreed-on set of basic and preventive supplemental health maintenance and treatment services for a fixed, prepaid charge (Streff, 1994). Over 50 million Americans were enrolled in HMOs by the end of 1995 (Stahl, 1995).

Another way that hospitals and physicians have coped with constantly changing reimbursement levels while ensuring an adequate population for services is to contract to become preferred providers. *Preferred provider organizations* (PPOs) render services on a fee-for-service basis, but offer financial incentives to consumers (the consumer pays less) when the preferred provider is used.

To further reduce their individual financial risk, many hospitals, physicians, and even HMOs have formed *strategic partnerships, alliances,* and *networks.* Such alliances allow providers to more adequately integrate a broader range of patient care services and to share the risks and rewards of capitation. The formation of new alliances will continue as providers search for ways to share risks, to reconfigure themselves into price-competitive delivery systems, and to lock in patient revenues and market share (Grimaldi, 1995).

Managed care is a term used to describe a variety of health care plans designed to contain the cost of health care services delivered to members while maintaining the quality of care. In managed care, case managers such as physicians, nurses, and other health care experts oversee the management of a member's care and are usually held accountable to some standard of cost effectiveness and quality (Zander, 1994). Case managers frequently use *critical pathways* to assess both the efficiency and effectiveness of the care provided. Critical pathways are standardized plans of care that identify predictable outcomes that should be achieved within a specific time frame (Catalano, 1996). In other words, they are blueprints for providing and monitoring care. When the patient does not progress as anticipated, the resulting variance must be identified and analyzed to determine its cause.

Managed care programs will continue to proliferate in the coming decade. Not only will the economic motivation persist, but such programs hold the potential for improved coordination of multidisciplinary health care services.

◆ The Shifting Health Care System

With capitation and managed care, provider profits from in-patient hospital care have declined significantly. Thus, hospitals are increasingly being viewed as cost centers, rather than revenue producers. As a result, the hospital is rapidly moving away from the center of the health care system. Fralic (1995) suggests that future profit in health care will come from not using hospitals; instead, care will be provided along a continuum, in multiple sites, and in many modes. Kerfoot (1995) concurs, suggesting that all nurses in the health care system are challenged to make the switch from hospital and illness-based activities to leading and managing in integrated networks.

◆ Summary

It is necessary for all managers to have some understanding of fiscal principles, to be cognizant of their budgetary responsibilities, and to remain accountable to the organization for managing a cost-effective unit. In budgeting, managers must be able to assertively and professionally articulate unit needs to ensure that funds for adequate nursing staff, supplies, and equipment will be sufficient.

The ability to proactively forecast the fiscal needs of the unit with sensitivity to the organization's economic, social, and legislative climate poses a challenge to all managers. It can best be met by, whenever possible, including all individuals in the budgetary process who will be affected by the plan. In addition, the manager must be creative in the identification of budgetary alternatives, flexible in their implementation, and skillful in the monitoring aspects of budget control.

◆ References

Blancett SS and Flarey DL (1995). Reengineering Nursing and Health Care. Gaithersburg, MD: Aspen

Campbell JM and Dowd TT (1993). Success stories- capturing scarce resources: documentation and communication. Nurs Econ 11(2):103–106

Catalano JT (1996). Contemporary Professional Nursing. Philadelphia: FA Davis

Cerne F (1994). Shaping up for capitation. Hosp Health Networks 68(7):28–37

Fralic MF (1995). Abstracted review of "Hospitals become cost centers in managed care scenario." Capsules Comments Nurs Leadership Manag 3(1):30

Grimaldi PL (1995). Variations on the capitation theme. Nurs Manag 26(12):12–13

Hodges LC and Poteet GW (1991). J Nurs Admin 21(10):30–33,45

Kelly LY (1992). The Nursing Experience, 2nd ed. New York: McGraw-Hill

Kerfoot K (1995). Abstracted review of "The leadership challenge of integrated delivery systems." Capsules Comments Nurs Leadership Manag 3(1):41

Manthey M (1992). Budgeting: controlling the ominous art. Nurs Manag 23(3):14

Marquis B and Huston C (1996). Leadership Roles and Management Functions: Theory and Application, 2nd ed. Philadelphia: JB Lippincott

Marriner-Tomey C (1996). Guide to Nursing Management, 5th ed. St. Louis: Mosby

Stahl DA (1995). Merger mania, alliances and subacute care. Nurs Manag 26(11):16–19

Streff MB (1994). "Third-Party Reimbursement Issues for Advanced Practice Nurses in the '90s," in McCloskey J and Grace H (eds): Current Issues in Nursing. 4th ed. St. Louis: Mosby

Swansburg RC and Sowell RL (1992). A model for costing and pricing nursing service. Nurs Manag 23(2):33–36

Zander K (1994). "Nurses and Case Management," in McCloskey J and Grace H (eds): Current Issues in Nursing, 4 ed. St. Louis: Mosby

SAMPLE CASE ANALYSIS

THE CASE ◆

You are a nurse in the coronary care unit and your flexible-nursing-care hours per patient day (NCH/PPD) are budgeted at 16 NCH/PPD. It is your job to determine the NCH/PPD each day at midnight by using the midnight patient census and the standard formula for figuring NCH/PPD. The standard formula is

$$\text{NCH/PPD} = \frac{\text{nursing hours worked in 24 hours}}{\text{patient census}}$$

Today's date is 1/31. At midnight it will be 2/1. You are calculating the NCH/PPD for 1/31. The patient census at midnight is five patients. In checking staffing, you find the following information.

Shift	Staff on duty	Hours worked
11 P.M. to 7 A.M. (last night)	2RNs	8 hours each
	1 LVN/LPN	8 hours
7 A.M. to 3 P.M.	3 RNs	8 hours each
	1 ward clerk*	8 hours
3 P.M. to 11 P.M.	2 RNs	8 hours each
	1 LVN/LPNs	8 hours
11 P.M. to 7 A.M. (on duty tonight)	1 RN	8 hours
	2 LVNs/LPNs	8 hours each

*Ward clerks are generally included in calculating NHC/PPD.

••

Assignment

1. Calculate the NCH/PPD for 1/31.

SAMPLE CASE ANALYSIS (CONTINUED)

••

Analysis

Although ideally you would use 12 midnight to 12 midnight to compute the NCH/PPD for 1/31, most staffing calculations are made beginning with 11:00 P.M. and ending with 11:00 P.M. the following night, to more closely align with work schedules. So in this case, it would be acceptable to figure the NCH/PPD for 1/31 using numerical data from the 11 to 7 shift last night, 7 to 3 shift, and 3 to 11 shift.

The first step in this calculation requires a computation of total nursing-care hours worked in 24 hours. This can be calculated by multiplying the total number of individuals on duty each shift by the hours each worked in their respective shift. Each shift total is then added together to get the total number of nursing hours worked in all three shifts or 24 hours.

In this case:

11 P.M. to 7 P.M. (last night)	3 staff @ 8 hours each = 24 hours
7 A.M. to 3 P.M.	4 staff @ 8 hours each = 32 hours
3 P.M. to 11 P.M.	3 staff @ 8 hours each = 24 hours

The nursing hours worked in 24 hours is 80 hours.

The second step in solving the NCH/PPD problem requires that you divide the nursing hours worked in 24 hours by the patient census. The patient census in this case is five patients. Therefore,

80 divided by 5 = 16; the NCH/PPD for 1/31 is **16.**

••

Assignment

Calculate the NCH/PPD if the midnight census remained the same, but the following were the hours worked.

12 midnight to 12 noon	4RNs	12 hours each
12 noon to 12 midnight	4 RNs	12 hours each

••

Analysis

In this situation, the 24 hour period that we are using for our calculations does extend from 12 midnight to 12 midnight. Again, the same equation is used with the following results:

12 midnight to 12 noon	4 staff @ 12 hours each = 48 hours
12 noon to 12 midnight	4 staff @ 12 hours each = 48 hours
	total = 96 hours

The nursing hours worded in 24 hours is 96. Thus, 96 hours divided by the census of 5 = 19.2. The NCH/PPD in this situation is **19.2.**

SAMPLE CASE ANALYSIS (CONTINUED)

••

Assignment

Calculate the NCH/PPD if the following staff were working.

12 midnight to 12 noon	3 RNs	12 hours each
	1 LVN/LPN	12 hours
12 noon to 12 midnight	2 RNs	12 hours each
	1 LVN/LPN	12 hours
	1 ward clerk	4 hours

••

Analysis

Using the same formula, it is necessary to first compute the number of nursing hours worked in a 24-hour period.

12 midnight to 12 moon	4 staff @ 12 hours each = 48 hours
12 noon to 12 midnight	3 staff @ 12 hours each = 36 hours
	1 staff @ 4 hours = 4 hours
	total = 88 hours

The nursing hours worked in 24 hours is 88 hours. 88 divided by 5 (the census) = 17.6. The NCH/PPD in this situation is **17.6.**

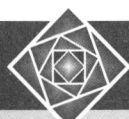 **CASES FOR PROBLEM SOLVING**

CASE 1

One of your goals as the new supervisor of the oncology unit is to prepare all your nurses to be certified in administering chemotherapy. You currently have 10 staff nurses who need this certification.

You find you can hire someone to teach the required course for $600. However, you are responsible for the cost of reproducing all the educational materials that will be needed in addition to providing the secretarial time for preparing these materials. The cost per participant will be less for a group larger than 15 and the total classroom time needed for certification is 15 hours. You will also need to allow for the cost of renting a facility in which the classes can be held. In addition, the staff nurses needing certification have requested that they be reimbursed for attending the classes if they are held after work hours.

CASE 1 (CONTINUED)

. . . .

Assignment

1. Define your goals for this educational program.
2. Determine how you will organize the classes.
3. Decide how much you will charge each participant receiving certification.
4. Will you hold these classes during work hours or at other times?
5. Can this program be cost effective?

CASE 2

An oncologist on your unit (Dr. Jones) has offered to give you his old photocopier since his office is purchasing a new machine. He has requested that all the oncologists and radiologists be allowed to use it free of charge. Should you accept Dr. Jones' gift? What are some of the factors influencing your decision?

. . . .

Assignment

1. Justify acceptance or rejection of the gift. What factors influenced your choice?
2. What are the direct and indirect costs?
3. What are the controllable versus uncontrollable costs?

CASE 3   (From Marquis and Huston, 1996)

You are a unit manager in an acute care hospital. You are aware that staff occasionally go home at the end of their shift with forgotten hospital supplies and small equipment in their pockets. You recall how as a staff nurse, you would often forget and take items home, such as rolls of adhesive tape, syringes, pen lights, and bottles of lotion. Usually you remembered to return them, but other times you did not.

Recently however, your budget has shown a dramatic and unprecedented increase in unaccounted for supplies. These supplies have included ace wraps, blood pressure cuffs and stethoscopes, surgical instruments, and personal hygiene kits. Although this increase represents only a fraction of your total operating budget, you feel it is necessary to identify the users. An audit of patient charts and charges reveals that these items were not used in patient care.

When you ask your charge nurses for an explanation, they state that a few employees have openly expressed their feelings that taking a few small supplies is in effect an expected and minor fringe benefit of employment. Your charge nurses do not feel that the problem is widespread, but cannot objectively document which employees they feel are involved in pilfering the supplies. They suggest that you ask all of your employees to document in writing when they see other employees removing supplies and that they report such incidents to you anonymously for follow-up action.

. . . .

Assignment

Because supplies are such a major part of the operating budget, you feel that some response is required. You must determine just what that action should be.

CASE 3 (CONTINUED)

Analyze your actions in terms of the desirable and undesirable effects on the employees, both involved as well as uninvolved in taking the supplies. Is the amount of the fiscal debit in this situation a critical factor? Is it worth the time and energy that would be required to truly eliminate the problem?

CASE 4

You are the Director of the local Aging Agency that cares for both the ill and well elderly. You are funded by a private corporation grant which requires matching of city and state funds. You have received a letter in the mail today from the state that says that state funding will be cut by $15,000 effective in 2 weeks, when the state's budget year begins. This means that your private funding will also be cut $15,000 for a total revenue loss of $30,000. It is impossible at this time to seek alternative funding sources.

In reviewing your agency budget, you note that as in many health care agencies, your budget is labor intensive. More than 80% of your budget is attributable to personnel costs and you feel that the cuts must come from within the personnel budget. You may reduce the client population that you serve, although you do not really want to do so. You briefly discuss this communication with your staff and no one is willing to voluntarily reduce their hours and no one is planning to terminate their employment at any time in the near future.

Assignment

Given the following brief description of your position as well as each of your five employees, decide how you will meet the new budget restrictions. What is the rationale for your choice? What decision do you believe will result in the least disruption of the agency? Of the employees in the agency? Should group decision-making be involved in fiscal decisions such as this one? Can fiscal decisions such as this be made without value judgments?

Your position is Project Director. As the Project Director, you coordinate all the day-to-day activities in the agency. You are also involved in long term planning and a major portion of your time is allotted to securing future funding for the agency to continue. As the Project Director, you have the authority to hire and fire employees. You are in your early 30s and have a Master's Degree in Nursing and Health Administration. You enjoy your job and feel you have done well in this position, since you started there 4 years ago. Your yearly salary as a full-time employee is $48,000.

Employee #1 is Mrs. Potter. Mrs. Potter has worked at the agency since it started 7 years ago. She is an RN with 30 years experience working with the geriatric population in public health nursing, care facilities, and private duty. She plans to retire in 7 years and travel with her independently wealthy husband. Mrs. Potter has a great deal of expertise she can share with your staff, although at times you feel that she overshadows your authority with her experience and because of your young age. Her salary as a full-time employee is $40,000.

CASE 4 (CONTINUED)

Employee #2 is Mr. Boone. Mr. Boone has BS degrees in both Nursing and Dietetics and Food Management. As both an RN and RD, he brings a unique expertise to your staff that is highly needed in dealing with a chronically ill and improperly nourished elderly population. In the 6 months since he joined your agency, he has proven to be a dependable, well-liked, and highly respected member of your staff. His salary as a full-time employee is $36,000/year.

Employee #3 is Miss Barns. Miss Barns is the receptionist/secretary in the agency. In addition to all the traditional secretarial duties such as typing, filing, transcription of dictation, and so on, she screens incoming telephone calls, and directs individuals who come to the agency for information. Her efficiency is a tremendous attribute to the agency. Her full-time salary is $16,000/year.

Employee #4 is Mrs. Lake. Mrs. Lake is an LPN/LVN with 15 years of work experience in a variety of health care agencies. She is especially empathetic to patient needs. Although her technical nursing skills are also good, her caseload frequently is more focused around those elderly who need companionship and emotional support. She does well at patient teaching because of her outstanding listening and communication skills. Many of your clients request her by name. She is a single mother supporting 6 children and you are aware that she has great difficulty in meeting her personal financial obligations. Her full-time salary is $24,000.

Employee # 5 is Mrs. Long. Mrs. Long is an "elderly help aide." She has completed nurse aid training, although her primary role in the agency is to assist well elderly with bathing, meal preparation, driving, and shopping. The time Mrs. Long spends in performing basic care has decreased the average visit time for each of your staff workers by 30%. She is widowed and feels that she needs this job to meet her social needs as well as esteem needs. Financially, her resources are adequate and the money she earns is not a motivator for working. Mrs. Long works 3 days a week and her salary is $10,000/year.

CASE 5

Today is April 1 and you have received the following budget printout. Your charge nurses are requesting an additional RN on each shift since the acuity has increased dramatically over the last 2 years. Dr. Robb has requested two new continuous limb movement machines for the postoperative orthopedic patients on your unit at a cost of $3,000 each. In addition, you would like to attend a national orthopedics conference in New York in August at a projected cost of $1,000. The registration fee is $350 and is due now.

	Annual budget	Expended in March	Expended year to date *	Amount remaining
Personnel	300,000	25,000	175,000	125,000
Overtime	50,000	0	50,000	0
Supplies	18,000	1500	13,500	4,500
Travel	1000	0	300	700
Equipment	5000	0	5000	0
Staff development	1000	200	600	400

*Fiscal year begins July 1.

CASE 5 (CONTINUED)

....

Assignment

How will you deal with these requests based on the budget printout? What expenses can and should be deferred to the new fiscal year? In what budgeting area were your previous projections most accurate? Most inaccurate? What factors may have contributed to these inaccuracies? Were they controllable or predictable?

◆ **Bibliography**

The following is a list of references to help you solve these cases:

Arford PH and Allred CA (1995). Value = quality + cost. J Nurs Admin 25(9):64–69

Aspling DL and Lagoe R (1996). Benchmarking for clinical pathways in hospitals: a summary of sources. Nurs Econ 14(2):92–97

Curtin L (1996). The bottom line be damned. Nurs Manag 27(9):7–8

Davis K, Collins KS, and Morris C (1994). Managed care: promise and concerns. Health Affairs 13(fall):178–185

Devers KJ, Shortell SM, Gillies RR, Anderson DA, Mitchell JB, and Erickson KLM (1994). Implementing organized delivery systems: an integration scorecard. Health Care Manage Rev 19(3):7–20

Felteau AL (1992). Budget variance analysis and justification. Nurs Manag 23(2):40–41

Foley Pierce S and Luikart C (1996). Managed care—will the healthcare needs of rural citizens be met? J Nurs Admin 26(4):28–32

Grimaldi PL (1996). Is that HMO federally qualified? Nurs Manage 27(1):12–15

Keegan AJ (1994). Hospitals become cost centers in managed care scenario. Healthcare Financ Manag 48(Aug):37–40

Kowal NS and Delaney M (1996). The economics of a nurse-developed critical pathway. 14(3):156–161

Lowe A (1996). Reducing variation in patient care. J Nurs Admin 26(1):14–20

Stahl DA (1995). Capitation: implications for subacute care. Nurs Manage 26(10):18–22

Weilitz P and Potter P (1993). A managed care system: financial and clinical evaluation. J Nurs Admin 23(11):51–57

West DA, Hicks LL, Balas EA, and West TD (1996). Profitable capitation requires accurate costing. Nurs Econ 14(3):162–170

Wilburn D (1992). Budget response to volume variability. Nurs Manag 23(2):42–44

Zachry BR, Gilbert RL, and Gragg, G and M (1995). Director of nursing finance: controlling health care costs. Nurs Manag 26(11):49–53

Zuckerman HS, Kaluzny AD, and Ricketts TC III (1995). Alliances in health care: what we know, what we think we know, and what we should know. Health Care Manage Rev 20:54–65

PERSONAL NOTEBOOK

1. List the ways you spend money in order of importance.

2. Do your priorities for spending money reflect your values system?

3. If you found $5,000 (and it was yours to keep) would you use it to travel, purchase new clothes, buy a car, or would you put it in the bank? How would you spend the money?

4. Would your two best friends decide as you did in question #3?

5. How do you rate your ability to manage your personal finances?

ORGANIZING

One of the most beautiful moments a coxswain has is when all eight oars are clicking at the same time. You don't always get all the divisions of a company clicking together but that's what you strive for.

—*Thornton Bradshaw*

Planning has given the manager a clearly understood purpose, objectives to meet that purpose, and standards to be used for control. Organizing follows planning as the second step in the management process and includes both a formal and an informal structure. The formal structure establishes the method of coordination and effective use of all available resources. In the organizing phase relationships are defined, procedures are outlined, equipment is readied, and tasks are assigned.

in contrast to formal structure, the organization's informal structure is unplanned and covert. Individuals need to be aware that informal authority and lines of communication exist in every group, even when they are never formally acknowledged.

Professional people spend most of their lives in organizations. Understanding how organizations are structured enhances employees' understanding of their role, as well as their responsibilities. Organizations are necessary because they allow work to be completed that could not be accomplished through individual efforts.

In addition to looking at the organization on a system level, it is important to look at how work is organized on the unit level. Nursing care is frequently organized into one of several modes of patient care, and the optimum mode for any given unit depends on such factors as the skill and expertise of the staff, the availability of professional nursing staff, the acuity of the patients, and the complexity of the tasks to be accomplished.

Understanding how the organization has evolved and how it is currently functioning allows an individual to begin to plan strategically how to gain personal power within that structure. Managers need both an understanding of power and skill in the art of politics. They need to develop a political awareness of the organization and its subcultures before they will be able to obtain the power necessary to function effectively within that organization.

Organizational Structure

CHAPTER

8

Organization structure refers to the way a group is formed, its lines of communication, and its means for channeling authority. Formal organizational structure through departmentalization and division of work provides a framework for defining managerial authority, responsibility, and accountability. Hein and Nicholson (1990) maintain that the organizational structure is a lifeline that assists the manager and the organization in meeting its goals. Since most organization structures differ in some manner, it is important for managers to understand the structure where their management takes place.

Max Weber, referred to in Chapter 3, is known as the father of organizational theory and first wrote about organizations in the 1920s. In his study of organizations he used the term *bureaucracy* to identify an organizational design he described as rational, had a clear chain of command, and was impartial. Weber felt a bureaucracy was the ideal tool to be used to cope with the industrial revolution (Marquis and Huston, 1996).

Although an appropriate idea at the time, Weber's work did not take into account the complexity involved in managing contemporary organizations. Worker motivation was taken for granted during the time of Weber's research, and his simplification of the respective roles of the manager and the employee did not allow for the bilateral relationships between employee and manager prevalent in most organizations today. Modern management theorists have learned much about human behavior and most organizations have modified their structure accordingly to render it less rigid and impersonal. However, almost 100 years after Weber's publications, components of bureaucratic structure continue to be found in the design of most large organizations.

Almost everyone acknowledges the difficulties inherent in bureaucracies, that is, faceless decision making, impersonal management, lack of accountability, lack of flexibility, and the establishment of organizational barriers in meeting professional and personal goals (Naisbitt and Aburdene, 1987; Kanter, 1989). However, it has been very difficult for organizations to move away from the Weberian bureaucratic model of organization.

There is no single, widely acceptable alternative model for organizational structure that eliminates the problems of bureaucratic institutions while also promoting an efficient operation (Tappen, 1995). Less rigid organizational designs have not been widely adopted for use in health care organizations. There has been some movement toward a shared governance model of organizational structure, and Maas and Specht (1994) predict that future health care organizations will be more flexible, decentralized, and have authority derived from competence. However, there is little evidence that this will occur soon.

◆ Components of the Organizational Chart

The overall framework for an organization is commonly depicted in the form of an *organizational chart.* A sample organizational chart is show in Figure 8-1. The organizational chart is a visual picture of an organization. By observing such things as which departments report directly to the chief executive officer (CEO), the manager can make some inferences about the organization. For instance, an organization that has the top-level nursing manager reporting to an assistant executive officer rather than to the CEO might be representative of the value that organization places on nursing (Huston and Marquis, 1989).

In addition to formal relationships, the organizational chart identifies lines of formal communication and authority. These formal relationships are diagrammed and depicted by either a horizontal or vertical unbroken line. Horizontal unbroken lines would represent communication between individuals with similar spheres of responsibility and power, but different functions. Vertical unbroken lines between positions denote the official *chain of command.* Those having the greatest decision-making power and authority are located at the top and those with the least are located at the bottom.

Dotted or broken lines on the organizational chart represent *staff* positions. Staff positions are advisory in nature. An individual employed in a staff position provides information and assistance to the manager as needed, but does not have any real authority to make decisions. Staff positions are used to increase a manager's sphere of influence, as well as ability to handle more activities and interactions, while providing specialization that would be impossible for any one manager to achieve alone. Staff positions can make line personnel more effective, but organizations can function without staff authority.

Unity of command is indicated by the vertical solid line between individuals on the organizational chart. The concept of unity of command is best described as "one person–one boss." Each individual has one manager to whom they report and to whom they are responsible. This makes the manager–employee relation-

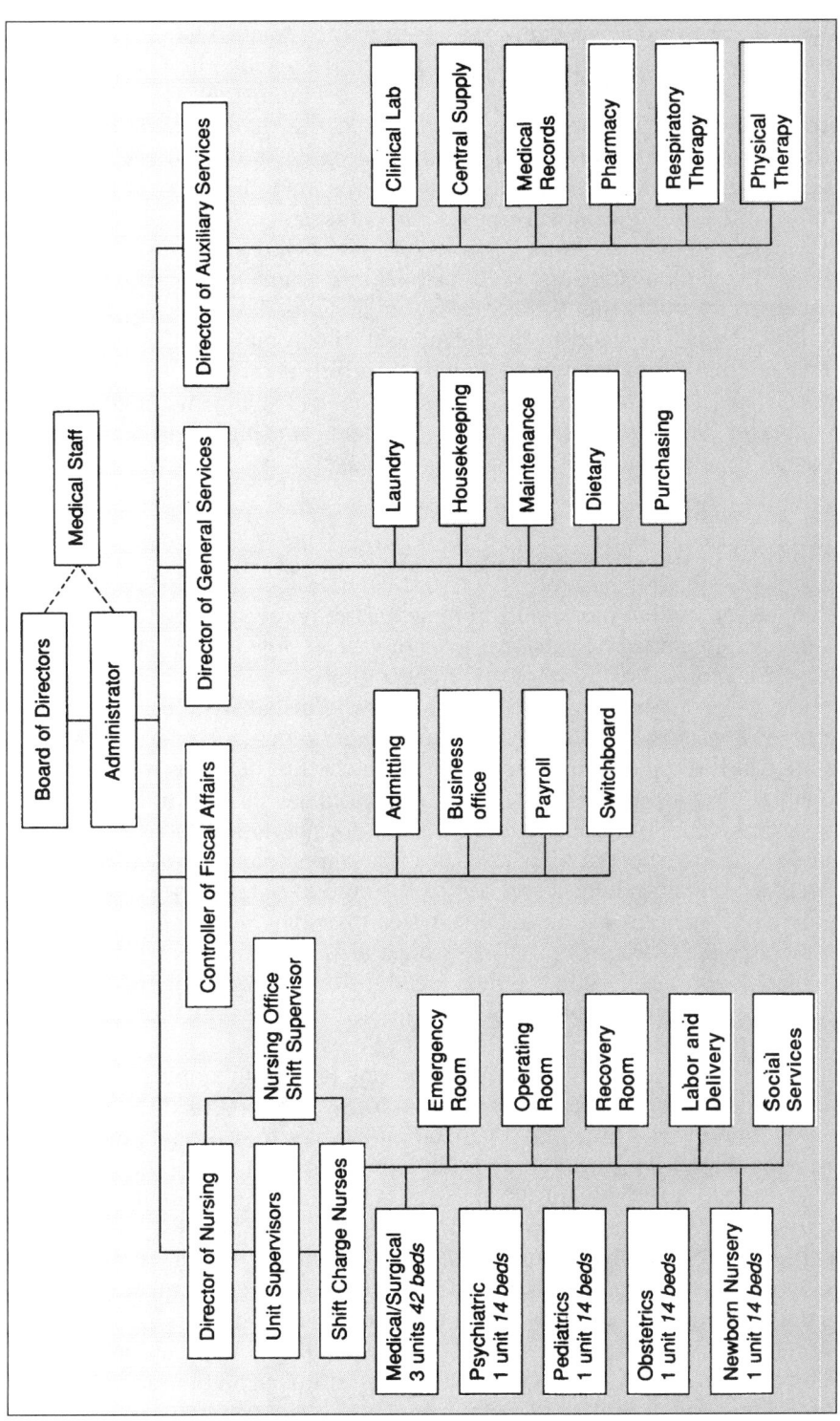

FIGURE 8-1.
Sample organizational chart—Memorial Hospital.

ship as simple as possible, as employees need only maintain a minimum number of relationships and accept the directives of only one person, their boss.

In reviewing the organizational chart, it is also important for the manager to determine where decisions are made within the management hierarchy. Authority must be designated in the management hierarchy. In organizations with *centralized decision making,* all decisions are made by a few at the top of the hierarchy. *Decentralized decision making* diffuses decision making throughout the organization and allows problems to be solved at the level at which they occur. Decision making and responsibility are assigned to the lowest practical managerial level within the organization. In general, the larger the organization, the greater the need to decentralize decision making. Large organizations face complex questions that can best be addressed by a variety of people with specialized areas of expertise. Understandably, leaving such decisions to a few managers in a large organization represents a tremendous burden and could result in devastating decision-making delays.

◆ Limitations of Organizational Charts

There are limits to what an organizational chart may reveal about an organization, since it depicts only formal relationships. The organizational chart does not show the *informal structure* of the organization.

Within every organization there is a dynamic informal structure that can be powerful and motivating. Knowledgeable leaders never underestimate its importance in the organization. The informal structure includes interpersonal relationships of employees, the formation of primary and secondary groups, and the identification of group leaders without formal authority.

The informal structure also has its own communication channel, often referred to as "the grapevine," and has its own group of leaders. These groups serve an important purpose in organizations; providing a feeling of belonging to members of the work group. These groups also wield a great deal of power in an organization, as they can either facilitate or sabotage planned change. Their ability to determine norms and acceptable behavior for a unit has a great deal to do with the socialization of new employees.

Informal leaders are frequently found among long-term employees, or individuals in select gatekeeping positions, such as secretary to the director of nursing. Frequently the informal organization evolves from social activities or from relationships that develop outside the work environment.

Other limitations of organizational charts include their inability to depict the degree of authority held by each line position. Additionally, there is frequent confusion caused by equating *status* with authority. The degree of status is usually determined by the distance from the top of the organizational hierarchy; the closer to the top, the higher the status. Status is also influenced by skill, education, specialization, level of responsibility, autonomy, and salary accorded a position. Individuals frequently have status in an organization, with little accompanying authority.

Last, because organizations are dynamic environments, an organizational chart becomes obsolete very quickly, and is frequently outdated. It is also possible that the organizational chart may depict how things are supposed to be, when in reality the organization is functioning under a different structure, and the people in the organization have not yet accepted the new lines of authority. See Display 8-1 for the advantages and limitations of an organizational chart.

◆ Levels of Management

In an organization with decentralized management, there are often several levels of managers. *Top-level managers* look at the organization as a whole, coordinating both internal and external influences on the organization and generally making decisions with few guidelines or structure. Examples of top-level managers would include the chief executive officer (CEO) and the chief nursing administrator. Current nomenclature for top-level nursing managers varies from one organization to the next. This individual might be called the nurse administrator, the director of nursing, the chief nurse, the assistant administrator of patient care services, or other similar titles. Likewise, the CEO in any organization might be shown on the organization chart with a title of President or Director. It is only necessary to remember that the CEO is the highest ranking individual in the organization and that the top-level nurse manager is the highest ranking nurse in the organization.

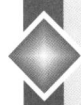

DISPLAY 8-1
Advantages and Limitations of the Organizational Chart

Advantages
1. Maps lines of decision-making authority.
2. Helps people understand their assignments and those of their coworkers.
3. Reveals to managers and new personnel how they fit into the overall organization.
4. Contributes to sound organizational structure.
5. Shows formal lines of communication.

Limitations
1. Shows only formal relationships (not informal or informational).
2. Does not indicate level of authority.
3. May show things as they are supposed to be or used to be rather than as they are (becomes obsolete fairly quickly).
4. Introduces the possibility of confusing authority with status.

Middle-level managers coordinate the efforts of lower levels and act as the channel between employees and top-level managers. Middle-level managers are more involved in day-to-day operations than top-level managers and may have limited input in the development of strategic planning and policy formulation. Examples of middle-level managers include department heads, supervisors, head nurses, and unit managers.

First-level managers are concerned mainly with the work flow through their specific unit of the organization. They deal with immediate problems encountered in the day-to-day operations of the unit and are concerned with meeting both organizational and staff needs. Examples of first-level managers might be a primary care nurse, team leader, or charge nurse.

Managers should also examine the *span of control* when examining the organizational chart. The number of people reporting to any one manager represents that person's span of control. The span of control delineates the number of interactions expected of any one given manager. Management theorists do not agree as to the optimum span of control for any one manager. Attempts have been made to develop quantitative formulas for determining this optimum span of control, with suggested ranges from three to 50 employees. In determining an optimum span of control within an organization, it is necessary to consider the abilities of the manager, the maturity of the employees, the complexity of tasks to be accomplished, the geographic location, and the level in the organization at which the work in question takes place.

The organizational structure has a resounding impact on the effectiveness of the manager. Singleton and Nail (1988) maintain that changing nomenclature in organizational charts, such as modifying a director of nursing service title to administrator of patient care, often carries with it increased responsibilities. They caution that this can lead to a harmful effect on nursing leadership within the organization by increasing the span of control and fostering ineffectiveness (Singleton and Nail, 1988).

◆ Authority, Responsibility, and Accountability

Although the organizational chart may indicate authority, responsibility, and accountability are not defined. All managers must have an understanding of the interrelationship as well as unique differences of these three terms. *Authority* is defined as the official power to act. It is power given by the organization to direct the work of others. A supervisor may have the authority to hire and fire employees.

A *responsibility* is a duty or assignment related to a job. It is comprised of the duties of a position. For example, one responsibility common to many charge nurses is establishing the patient care assignment for a specific unit that day. Managers should always be assigned responsibilities with concomitant authority. If responsibilities are assigned and authority is not given commensurate to the responsibility, role confusion occurs for all the individuals involved. For example, a supervisor may have the responsibility for maintaining high professional standards of care of a unit, but if the supervisor is not given the authority to discipline employees as needed, this responsibility may be difficult or impossible to implement.

Accountability involves morally internalizing responsibility for the job that you have done; you agree to face the consequences of your actions. A nurse who reports a medication error, despite adverse potential personal consequences, is being accountable to patients and for the care provided. A manager cannot force employees to be accountable for their actions. Unfortunately, individuals can and do accept responsibility without accepting the accompanying accountability.

◆ Types of Formal Organization Structures

Most health care organizations use one of the following structural patterns: line organization, line and staff organization (shown in Figure 8-1), functional organization, ad hoc organization, matrix organization, or self-governance (shown in Figure 8-2). The type of organizational structure used affects the individual's self-image, communication style, advancement opportunities, social contacts, assertiveness, and job satisfaction.

Line organization structure and *line and staff structure* are the two most common types of formal structure utilized in large health care organizations. Because

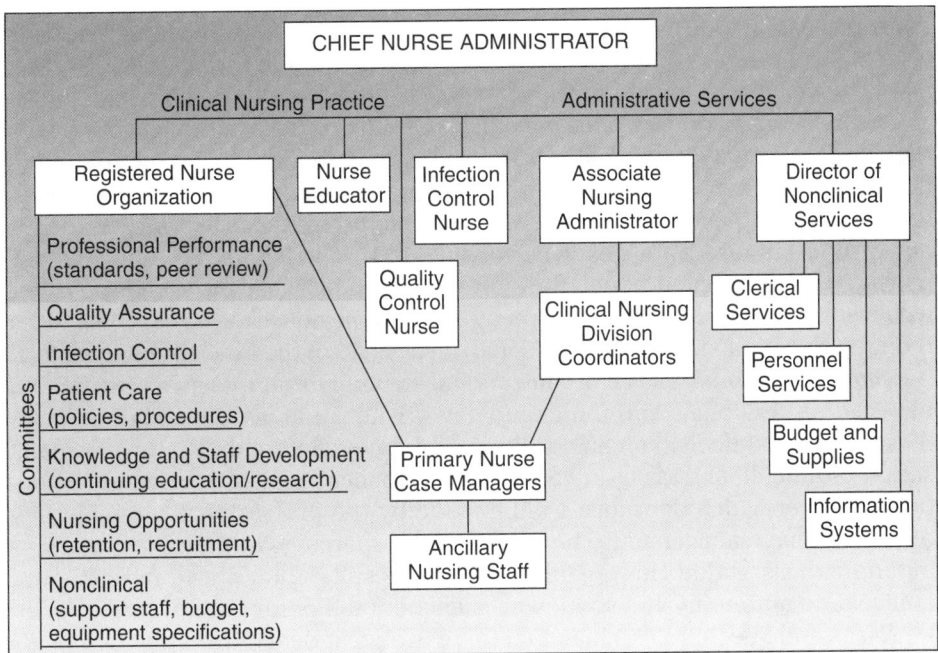

FIGURE 8-2.
Shared governance model.

of the familiarity of most individuals with these types of structures, there is little stress associated with orientation. Accountability and responsibility are clearly defined and there is efficiency and simplicity of relationships.

However, these types of formal structure also have disadvantages. They often produce monotony as well as worker alienation and it is difficult for the organization to adjust rapidly to altered circumstances. Another difficulty with line and line and staff structure is the requirement for chain of command communication, which restricts upward communication. Many top-level managers encourage upward communication in order to compensate for this disadvantage of the line structure. However, when line positions are clearly defined, most employees will not risk going outside the chain of command for upward communication. Therefore, several other types of organizational structure are now being utilized in health care organizations.

The *functional organizational structure* allows advisory (staff) positions to have some control over line employees. This is frequently seen with the director of in-service and nursing education, or the infection control or risk managers in a hospital. By giving these advisory positions some line authority they are able to use that authority to more effectively apply their special expertise. In the functional structure the advisory staff are never given total line authority.

The *ad hoc organizational structure* is a means of overcoming the inflexibility of line structure and facilitates individuals ability to handle the increasingly large amounts of information available to professionals. The ad hoc structure uses a project team or task approach to organizational structure. These teams operate within a more formal organization, but allow for more flexibility and cohesiveness among workers than line structure. The disadvantages to this type of structure are that it decreases the strength of the formal chain of command as well as the loyalty of the employee to the parent organization.

A *matrix organizational structure* utilizes the ad hoc team approach, but builds the team into a fully functional hierarchical organization. In this structure, there is a formal vertical as well as a formal horizontal chain of command. Although there are less formal rules and fewer levels of hierarchy in a matrix structure, it is not without its disadvantages. For example, in this structure, the nurse whose patient has complained about the noise of the housekeeping vacuum cleaner would not be allowed to speak directly to the unit housekeeper, but would be required to communicate with the department head of the housekeeping staff.

Shared Governance is an organizational structure that fosters a partnership between professionals and the employing organization via the use of committees and shared decision making. Sharing of power and authority in an organization is difficult, and Maas and Specht (1994) ascertain that there is much controversy over which decisions will be made by the professional and which by organizational management. The stated aim of shared governance is empowering individuals within the organization. The results should give nurses more control and autonomy. It also increases accountability for employees.

Maas and Specht (1994) maintain there is a great deal of variation in models of shared governance currently in use in health care organizations. Therefore, it is necessary that policies be clearly written concerning accountability and decision making in any shared governance structure in order for it to be implemented successfully. Additionally, management at all levels must understand that if positive outcomes are to occur they must be willing to give up some control and commit the time and financial resources necessary for shared governance to be implemented (DeBaca, Jones, and Torabeni, 1993).

◆ Effects of Organizational Structure

It is helpful for individuals to understand that the structure has a direct bearing on various concepts within an organization. Organizational structure impacts on our self-perception of our role identity and the expectations we and others have of a specific role.

Additionally, status is greatly influenced by placement on an organizational chart. The level of status is closely related to the distance from the top of the organizational hierarchy. Status is also influenced by skill, education, specialization, level or responsibility and autonomy, and salary accorded to a position. Status is closely related to the concept of power. Because power building and political awareness are so essential to functioning effectively in any organizational structure, a separate chapter will discuss those organizational components in depth.

Centrality refers to the location of a position on an organizational chart where frequent and various types of communication occurs. Those employees with a moderate relative organizational distance from either end of the organizational chart will thus be more central and will be able to receive more information in an organization than those individuals who are more peripherally located.

As all communication involves a sender and a receiver, it is easy to understand that messages may not be received clearly because of the hierarchical position of the sender. Often, status and power influence the ability of the receiver of information to be accurately informed.

The difficulties with upward and downward communication are more fully discussed later, in Unit 5, Chapter 17 on organizational communication. Still, it is important to be cognizant of how the formal structure of an organization affects interpersonal and organizational communication. This is especially necessary because organizations change their structure frequently, which results in new communication lines and reporting relationships. Unless an individual comprehends how to interpret a formal organizational chart, much confusion and anxiety can result when organizations are restructured.

◆ Organizational Culture

The organizational chart helps shape the organizational culture, which is a system of symbols and interactions. Each organization has its own unique culture (Thomas, Ward, Chorba, and Kumiega, 1990). It is the sum total of values, language, the past history of *sacred cows*, formal as well as informal communication networks, and the rituals of an organization. *Sacred cows* is a term sometimes used to describe those few things present in each institution that are never to be discussed or changed.

Organizational culture should not be confused with organizational climate. How employees perceive an institution is termed *organizational climate.* The organizational climate and culture may be similar or different.

Successful managers must be knowledgeable about their own organization's culture (Hein and Nicholson, 1990). Managers also need to be sensitive to the culture and norms present in their units. Much of an organization's culture is not accessible to staff in a retrievable source and must often be related by others. For example, beliefs about collective bargaining, nursing education levels, nursing autonomy, and nurse–physician relationships differ from one organization to another. Yet these positions and values are not written down, and rarely appear in a philosophy. Managers should assist subordinates in understanding the culture of the organization. It is possible for organizational culture to evolve over time, but it is unlikely that such change would ever be abrupt.

Managers also have an obligation to accurately assess the perception individuals hold of the organization. When the beliefs of the employee are consistent with the organizational culture the employee will perceive the organizational climate as "good," but when the beliefs are in conflict with those of the institution's culture the employee will perceive the climate as "poor."

◆ Organizational Effectiveness

The effectiveness of the organization will depend to some degree upon how well the organization is structured. Although slow in redesigning the organization to facilitate new technological advances Strasen (1991) and del Bueno (1991) report that some health care organizations are seeking new methods of restructuring in order to promote better communication, increase productivity, and improve quality. It is hoped that health care organizations will eventually move away from the bureaucratic design. The following are the minimal requirements for a sound nursing unit organizational design.

1. The structure should be clearly defined so nurses know where they belong and where to seek assistance.

2. The smallest possible number of managers should be used to keep the unit operating.

3. The unit staff should to be able to recognize where their tasks fit in with the tasks of the organization.

4. The organizational structure should facilitate, not impede, communication.

5. The organizational structure should facilitate decision making at the unit level that results in productivity and efficiency.

6. Staff should be arranged in a manner that facilitates informal groups, so that a sense of community and belonging can develop.

7. Nursing services should be organized in a way that will foster the development of future leaders.

◆ Symptoms of Poorly Structured Organizations

One of the major symptoms of poor unit organizational design is recurring problems. If managers find that their energy continues to be focused on secondary problems, the organizational structure should be reevaluated. Swansburg (1990) maintains that ineffective structure results in malorganization.

Another symptom of malorganization is an excessive number of management levels. The goal of the unit design should be to require the least possible management levels and use the shortest possible chain of command. This eliminates friction, stress, and inertia.

Last, a unit is poorly designed if there is a heavy reliance on committees. Committees are necessary in large organizations, but should result in communication and productivity. Numerous committee assignments exhaust staff and may be poor tools for accomplishing work. An alternative to this approach, that will also meet the goal of participation, is to make individual assignments and meet in committee only to make a report. The appropriate use and structure of committees will be reviewed in Chapter 10.

◆ Summary

Managers need to view organizational structure as the road map that specifies who to communicate with, and who has authority in an organization. This structure enables managers to accomplish the goals of the organization. Without organizational structure individuals would work in a chaotic environment; therefore, structure becomes an important tool in facilitating order and enhancing productivity.

◆ References

DeBaca V, Jones K, and Tornabeni J (1993). A cost–benefit analysis of shared governance. J Nurs Admin 23(7/8):50–57

del Bueno DJ (1991). Managers function and form in the new organization. J Nurs Admin 21(5):7–8,24,46

Hein EC and Nicholson MJ (1990). Contemporary Leadership Behavior, 3rd ed. Glenview, IL: Scott, Foresman/Little Brown Higher Education

Huston CJ and Marquis BL (1989). Retention and Productivity Strategies for Nurse Managers. Philadelphia: JB Lippincott

Kanter RM (1989). When Giants Learn to Dance: Mastering the Challenges-Strategy, Management and Careers in the 1900s. New York: Simon and Schuster

Maas ML and Specht JP (1994). Shared governance in nursing: what is shared, who governs and who benefits? In McCloskey J and Grace HK (eds): Current Issues in Nursing. St. Louis: Mosby

Marquis BL and Huston CJ (1996). Leadership Roles and Management Functions in Nursing, 2nd ed. Philadelphia: JB Lippincott

Naisbitt J and Aburdene P (1987). Reinventing the Corporation. New York: Random-Warner Books

Singleton KE and Nail FC (1988). Nursing leadership—the effects of organizational structure. J Nurs Admin 18(10):10–14

Strasen L (1991). Redesigning hospitals around patients and technology. Nurs Econom 9(4):233–238

Swansburg RC (1990). Management and Leadership for Nurse Managers. Boston: Jones and Bartlett

Tappen RM (1995). Nursing Leadership and Management: Concepts and Practice, 3rd ed. Philadelphia: FA Davis

Thomas C, Ward M, Chorba C, and Kumiega A (1990). Measuring and interpreting organizational culture. J Nurs Admin 20(6):17–24

S A M P L E C A S E   A N A L Y S I S

THE CASE ◆

You have been working at the county health department for 6 months. You are very impressed with the doctor who is the county health administrator. She seems to have a genuine concern for patient welfare. She has a tea for new employees each month and talks with them about the philosophy of the health department and her own management style. She says she has an "open door policy" meaning employees are always welcome to come and visit her.

Since you have been assigned to the evening immunization clinic as charge nurse you have become concerned with a persistent problem: the housekeeping staff often spend part of the evening sleeping on duty or socializing for long periods of time. You have found them sleeping on several occasions, as have other members of your team. You have reported this to your health department supervisor on two separate occasions.

Last evening you discovered the housekeeping staff having another social get-together. The primary reason for concern is that the clinic is chronically in dire need of cleaning. At times the public bathrooms get so untidy that they become an embarrassment to you and your staff. You frequently must remind the housekeepers to empty overflowing waste baskets. You believe this type of environment is demeaning to your clients.

This is also upsetting because you and your staff work hard all evening and rarely have the opportunity to sit down; you feel it is unfair to everyone that the housekeeping staff are not contributing their share.

As you arrive at the health department parking lot this afternoon you see the county health administrator approaching her car. She stops to chat with you, and asks how things are going with your job.

••

Assignment

Should you tell her about the problem with the immunization clinic housekeeping staff? Are you following an appropriate chain of command? What

SAMPLE CASE ANALYSIS (CONTINUED)

should you do? List all available choices and alternatives. Make a decision and explain your rationale.

....

Analysis

The nurse should choose a goal before proceeding. If the aim is to relieve the immediate frustration of the situation, then going outside the chain of command might accomplish this. However, that goal appears to be selfish and meets only the nurse's immediate needs. A more appropriate goal would be to have the clinic clean and tidy.

The first step then is to assess the data and identify possible risks. An assessment of available information and the rationale for decision making in this case is outlined as follows.

....

Assessment of Data

1. A copy of the organizational chart had been given to the nurse on hiring. The formal structure is a line and staff organization. The housekeeping department head is below the health department nursing director and the nursing section supervisor, but is at the same level as the immediate clinic supervisor. The housekeeping department head reports directly to the maintenance and engineering department head.
2. The county administrator has stated she has an "open door policy." The nurse does not know if this means that it is acceptable to bypass department heads with problems, or merely that the administrator is interested in the employees. An important reason for not skipping intermediate supervisors when communicating is that they must be informed about what is going on in their respective departments. Their position, value, and status are strengthened if they serve as vital and essential links in the vertical chain of command.
3. The nurse has made two attempts to discuss the matter with an immediate supervisor; however, there is no indication the nurse returned for feedback regarding the outcome of the complaint.
4. The nurse is new and therefore probably unaware of how the formal or informal structure works. The nurse's newness might render the complaints less credible.
5. Possible risks include (a) creating "trouble" for others in housekeeping and/or their immediate supervisor, (b) being labeled a "troublemaker" by others in the organization, and (c) alienating the nurse's immediate supervisor.
6. Before proceeding the nurse needs to assess personal values and determine what the motivation is to pursue this issue.

....

Alternatives for Action

There are many choices available to this nurse.

1. Do nothing. This is often a wise choice and should always be one of the alternatives for any problem. Some problems solve themselves if left alone, and occasionally it is not the "right" time to solve the problem.
2. Use the opportunity to talk with the county health administrator. Although this involves some elements of risk, there is a possibility the administrator

will be able to do something. At the very least the nurse may feel less burdened having discussed the issue with someone.

3. Speak to the individual housekeepers. Attempt to rectify the situation by going directly to the housekeeping staff and using "I" messages. Perhaps if feelings and frustrations were shared the nurse would gain some additional insight into the problem. Possibly there is a reason for their behavior; maybe their only opportunity to socialize is during their break time. Note, there is some risk involved here as the housekeeping staff may look upon the nurse as a troublemaker.

4. Request that the evening clinic staff circulate a petition and give it to the immediate supervisor. Forming a coalition often produces results. However, the supervisor could view this as an overreaction or somewhat meddlesome, and might feel threatened by such an action.

5. Go to the department head of the housekeeping staff and report the offenders. In this way, the nurse is saving some time and going directly to the person who is responsible for the problem. However, this might be unfair to the housekeepers and certainly will create some enemies for the nurse.

6. Return to the immediate supervisor and inquire as to the status of the problem. The nurse could request permission to personally take action and ask how best to proceed. This would involve the immediate supervisor and keep the nurse informed. However, it shows that the nurse is willing to take some risks and to devote some personal time and energy to solving the problem.

Selecting an Alternative

There is no correct answer here and under certain conditions, various solutions could be used. Under most circumstances it is more equitable to others as well as more efficient for the nurse to select alternative #3. However, because the nurse is new and has little knowledge of the formal and informal organizational structure, her wisest choice would be alternative #6. New employees need to seek guidance from their immediate supervisors. In order for this third session with the supervisor to be successful, the nurse needs to do the following:

1. Talk with the supervisor at an opportune time.
2. Admit to personally "owning" the problem. Do not involve other colleagues.
3. Acknowledge that there may be legitimate reasons for the actions of the housekeepers.
4. Request permission to talk directly with the housekeepers and through role playing with the intermediate supervisor select an appropriate approach.

However, the nurse must accept the consequences of her actions; by trying to correct the problem, her efforts may result in her supervisor pursuing the problem directly with the supervisor of the housekeeping staff. If this is the action the nurse's supervisor decides to take, the nurse first should request an opportunity to speak with the housekeeping staff directly. If, after talking with the housekeeping staff, the nurse decides there is still a problem and elects to address that problem, then she should return to her immediate supervisor before proceeding.

SAMPLE CASE ANALYSIS (CONTINUED)

••

Analysis of the Problem Solving

Would you have solved this problem differently? What are some other alternatives that could have been generated? Have you had experiences where you went outside the chain of command and had a positive experience as a result?

Is it ever appropriate to ignore the chain of command? Of course, there are isolated circumstances when the chain of command must be broken. However, those conditions are rare, and usually involve a question of ethics. In most instances when the chain of command is bypassed, those being skipped should be forewarned. Remember that unity of command provides the organization with a workable system for procedural directives and orders so that productivity is increased and conflict is minimized.

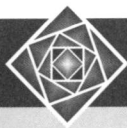 **CASES FOR PROBLEM SOLVING**

The first three cases in this section will refer to some portion of the organizational chart (see Figure 8-1).

CASE 1

Because Memorial Hospital is expanding, the board of directors has made several changes which make modification of the organizational chart necessary. The board has just announced the following changes:

1. The name of the hospital has been changed to General Hospital and Medical Center.
2. State approval has been granted for open heart surgery.
3. One of the existing medical-surgical units will be remodeled, and will become two critical care units (one six-bed coronary and open heart unit, and one six-bed trauma and surgical unit).
4. A part-time medical director will be responsible for medical care on each critical care unit.
5. The hospital administrator's title has been changed to executive director.
6. An associate hospital administrator has been hired.
7. A new hospital-wide educational department has been created.
8. The old pediatric unit will be remodeled into a seven-bed pediatric wing and a seven-bed rehabilitation unit.
9. The nursing director will now have the title of Administrator of Patient Care Services.

CASE 1 (CONTINUED)

Assignment

Depict all these changes except #7 on the old organizational chart, showing chart position, and distinguishing either a staff or line position. Be ready to explain your rationale for your decisions. Discuss where you believe there might be potential conflict.

CASE 2

The newly titled Nursing Administrator of Patient Care Services now finds there is too broad a span of control for effective management; and therefore, decides to decentralize the department, but is unsure which direction to take in restructuring. Although this Administrator will continue to be in a line position with the CEO, both the Board of Directors and CEO have supported the decision to restructure the department. Alternatives under consideration are using a matrix structure where each specialty (i.e., medical-surgical, obstetrics, etc.) becomes a complete independent subsystem with its own nursing director or coordinator or implementing a shared governance model as depicted in Figure 8-2.

Many issues must be considered, including the quality of patient care, the cost to the organization, nurse satisfaction, the willingness of the management team to give up control, the commitment from the professional nurse staff to assume accountability, and which of the alternatives is most likely to be successfully implemented.

Assignment

Examine this issue as if you were a professional staff nurse and as if you were a manager in this organization. Which alternative would you choose in each position? Explain and defend your rationale for your decision.

CASE 3

The executive director has asked the four directors to develop a philosophy for staff development at Memorial Hospital (see Display 8-2). This task has been completed and it is now time to decide where the new department should be located on the organizational chart.

Assignment

Where do you believe it should be located and why? What are other possible alternatives? Should the head of this department have line or staff authority? Over which individuals? What should the relationship be between this department and the medical staff? What problems are unique to staff positions?

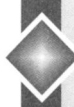

DISPLAY 8-2
Memorial Hospital Education and Staff Development Department Philosophy

1. We believe that all personnel should be offered the opportunity for growth, development, and the advancement of knowledge, understanding, and skills to help them improve their performance.
2. We believe that an active staff development program best serves the interests of the patients, personnel, and the hospital itself.
3. We believe all levels of personnel in all departments benefit from the services of staff development.
4. We believe a patient education program is an essential component of quality patient care.
5. We believe that the success of staff development is influenced by the climate of acceptance and the support engendered by the attitudes and actions of administrative and supervisory personnel at the hospital.
6. We believe the educational process includes the following:

    Assessment: Appraisal of the needs of learners.

    Objectives: Statements of the expected behavior of the learner.

    Evaluation: Method of determining whether objectives have been met and the use of findings in future planning.

CASE 4   (See Huston and Marquis, 1995, in bibliography, for help in solving this case.)

Center City Hospital is a modern, 600-bed nonprofit facility located in an urban area. Sarah Lane is the intensive care unit (ICU) charge nurse on the 3–11 P.M. shift. A new patient, Mr. Johnson, is admitted to the unit at 5 P.M. with a diagnosis of rule out myocardial infarction. Nurse Lane's initial assessment of Mr. Johnson indicates mild hypotension (BP 94/50), cool but dry skin, distant heart sounds, faint bibasilar rales, and general anxiety as verbalized by the patient. Chest pain is denied. The EKG shows early changes indicative of myocardial infarction.

Because Mr. Johnson was admitted directly from the emergency room, he has not yet been seen by his personal physician, Dr. Monroe. After her assessment, Ms. Lane called Dr. Monroe for admitting orders and to report her observations. Dr. Monroe disclosed that he was about to go out for dinner to celebrate his 25th wedding anniversary and therefore would not be in to see Mr. Johnson until later that evening. Dr. Monroe stated that he would write additional orders at that time and to implement ICU standing orders until then (IV morphine prn, bedrest, CPR with all medications, vital signs every hour).

At 6:30 P.M., Mr. Johnson began complaining of some substernal chest pressure. BP was 84/60 and his skin was cool and slightly moist. Heart sounds seemed more distant than during admitting assessments. Mr. Johnson appeared even more anxious, often making references to impending doom and his intense desire to see his physician.

After reassuring Mr. Johnson and relieving his pain with IV morphine, Ms. Lane decided to contact Dr. Monroe concerning what she perceived to be signif-

CASE 4 (CONTINUED)

icant changes in his patient's condition. She called Dr. Monroe's answering service, who said they would have him return his call as soon as possible.

At 6:50 P.M., Mr. Johnson's BP decreased to 80/64; skin was cool and clammy. Lungs–bibasilar rales throughout. He seemed withdrawn and somewhat confused. At 7:10 P.M., Ms. Lane again checked with the answering service and was told that they had been unable to reach Dr. Monroe, but would continue trying.

Nurse Lane felt that Mr. Johnson's condition was rapidly deteriorating and that he was in need of immediate medical attention. She picked up the phone and called the emergency room asking to speak to the physician on duty that night. The ward clerk told Ms. Lane that the ER physician was busy casting the left leg of a young girl involved in a MVA several hours earlier, but that she would ask him to call Ms. Lane as soon as he was free.

At 7:30 P.M., the answering service called back to report that Dr. Monroe apparently had turned off his beeper, but that he should check in within the next 1–2 hours. At the same time, the hospital nursing supervisor for the 3–11 P.M. shift, who was making her regular rounds, walked into Mr. Johnson's room. She cried out, "Ms. Lane, This man is shocky. We are losing him. Why didn't you do something? Why wasn't I notified?"

Assignment

Review the actions of nurse Lane, Dr. Monroe, the answering service, and the shift supervisor. Differentiate the authority, responsibility, and accountability each of them had. Did each of those involved follow an appropriate chain of command?

CASE 5

You are the new head nurse of the long-term care unit at Riverview Long Term Care. You are very pleased to have this position and feel lucky to have been chosen from a field of four candidates. Your best friend Mary Benito, who also works in the unit, applied for the head nurse position as well. She seems sincerely happy for you, but you have some concerns about how your promotion may affect your friendship.

As head nurse, you have direct line authority over all staff on the unit. This authority includes responsibility for hiring, firing, performance appraisal, and discipline.

Shortly after you assume your new position, Mary begins making special requests for days off, extended dinner breaks, and top priority for low census call-offs. In an effort to maintain the friendship, you have responded to these requests with a smile and by lightheartedly saying, "that wouldn't be fair to the other staff now, would it?" She has replied with a smile as she said, "It pays to have friends in high places."

Mary's behavior has become increasingly disruptive. You believe that she is taking advantage of your friendship. In addition, you wonder whether she has been making statements to the other employees implying covert approval of her special privileges. When you attempted to confront her with your concerns, she dismissed them saying, "I wouldn't do anything to hurt you in your new job—you are my best friend." You continue to believe that you are being sabotaged in your new position and your anxiety is beginning to bother you.

> **CASE 5 (CONTINUED)**
>
> ••
> ### Assignment
> What should you do? Discuss how you will resolve this issue. Examine the appropriate place of friendship in a manager's life. This is a very difficult situation and there are no easy answers. In solving this problem be sure to investigate all the issues.

◆ Bibliography

The following is a list of references to help you solve these cases:

Banner DK and Gagne ET (1994). Designing effective organizations: traditional and transformational views. Newbury Park, CA: Sage

del Bueno DJ (1991). Reflections on organizational structure and redesign. J Nurs Admin 21(3):9–10,41

Dirschel KM (1994). Decentralization or centralization: striking a balance. Nurs Manage 25(9):49–51

Dutton JE, Dukerich JM, and Harquail CV (1994). Organizational images and member identification. Admin Sci Quart 39(June):239–263

Grigsby KA (1991). Perceptions of the organization's climate: influenced by the organization's structure? J Nurs Educ 30(2):81–88

Havens DS (1992). Nursing involvement in hospital governance: 1900 and 1995. Nurs Econ 10(5):331–335

Hughes L (1990). Assessing organizational culture: strategies for the external consultant. Nurs For 25(1):15–19

Huston CJ and Marquis BL (1995). Seven steps to successful decision-making. AJN 95(50):65-68

Johnson ELR (1991). Those deadly undiscussables. Heart Lung 20(4):19a–20a

Minnen TG, Berger E, Ames A, Dubree M, Baker W, and Spinella J (1993). Sustaining work redesign innovations through shared governance. J Nurs Admin 23(7/8):35–40

Mularz LA, Maher M, Johnson AP, Rolston-Blenman B, and Anderson MA (1995). Theory M: a restructuring process. Nurs Manage 26(1):49-52

Ott JS and Shafritz JM (1994). Toward a definition of organizational incompetence: a neglected variable in orgainization theory. Public Admin Rev 54(4):370–377

Patz JM, Biordi DL, and Holm K (1991). Middle nurse manager effectiveness. J Nurs Admin 21(1):15–24

Person L (1993). An educational blitz: initiating shared governance. Nurs Manage 24(8):61–62

Peterson SL and Fisher JC (1991). Designing an organizational merger. J Nurs Admin 21(12):42–48

Rizzo JA, Gillman MP, and Messerman CA (1994). Facilitating care delivery redesign using measures of unit culture and work characteristics. J Nurs Admin 24(5):32–37

Schmieding NJ (1992). The complexity of an authority role. Nurs Manage 23(1):57–58

Shah HS, Organek NS, and Lessner MW (1991). Organizational structure: blueprints for action. Nurse Educ 16(3):26–30

PERSONAL NOTEBOOK

1. Have you ever worked in an organization where the lines of authority were unclear, or where your role was undefined? How did it make you feel?

2. If you find your job description or role unclear in an organization, what should you do?

3. Do you feel the "one boss" rule is a good idea? Look at the role of the unit clerk or ward clerk. Do they usually have many bosses?

Organizing Work at the Unit Level

The greatest influence of first- and middle-level managers on the organizational phase of the management process takes place at the unit or departmental level of the organization. It is here that organizing the work to be done and implementing the delivery of patient care occurs. Historically, many variables have influenced the manner in which patient care has been organized. For example, the cost of nursing services, the supply of professional nurses, the requirements of changing demographics, and increased technology have all played a part in changing trends in the design of patient care delivery models. As new models for organizing care appear in the literature, it is important for managers to remain current with the new trends, but it is equally important for managers to discern fads from trends (Curtin, 1994). In the past managers often adopted a new work redesign without fully understanding that particular model of patient care delivery or the necessary resources to implement it, and ended up modifying the model in a manner that rendered it ineffective. Managers must assess their unit environment and financial and personnel resources and have a thorough understanding of the many models of patient care delivery before undertaking work redesign (Fralic, 1992).

A well-designed delivery system helps the manager meet organizational goals in an effective and efficient manner. This involves using resources wisely, coordinating activities with other departments, and appropriately assigning committees. How activities are organized can impede or facilitate communication, flexibility, and job satisfaction.

◆ An Historical Perspective of Modes of Organizing Patient Care

Throughout the history of nursing there have been many methods of organizing nursing care for patients and frequently models were modified from their original design to fit the individual organization. The five most commonly known models are: 1) case method nursing or total patient care, 2) functional nursing, 3) team nursing, 4) primary nursing, and 5) case managed care. Although some of these methods were developed to organize care in hospitals, most can be used in many settings. The "best" organizational mode depends on the skill and expertise of the staff, the availability of registered "professional" nurses, the acuity of the patients being treated, the economic constraints of the organization, and the complexity of the tasks to be completed.

CASE METHOD NURSING

Case method nursing or *total patient* care is the oldest method of organizing patient care. In case method nursing, care providers assume responsibility for meeting all the needs of assigned patients during the time they are on duty. At the turn of the nineteenth century, case method nursing was practiced both at home and in hospitals. A great deal of medical and nursing care for the wealthy and middle class occurred in the home, and hospitals were used primarily by the poor and very acutely ill.

During the Depression of the 1930s people could no longer afford home care and individuals began utilizing hospitals. During that time nurses and student nurses were the caregivers in hospitals and public health agencies. As hospitals grew during the 1930s, case method (total patient care) nursing continued to be the primary means of organizing patient care. A diagram of the case method organizational structure is shown in Figure 9-1.

Case method nursing is still widely used, both in hospital units where there is an all-professional staff such as an intensive care unit, and in home health agencies. It provides high autonomy and responsibility for nurses. The lines of responsibility and accountability are clear and the patient theoretically receives holistic and unfragmented care during the time the nurse is on duty. In terms of assigning patients, it is simple and direct and does not require the coordinating needed in other patient care delivery methods (Tappen, 1995).

Although care is not fragmented while the nurse is on duty, each nurse caring for the patient may modify the care plan. Therefore, if there are three shifts, the patient may receive three different approaches to care. This often results in confusion for the patient. In order to maintain quality care, this method requires more highly skilled and better paid nursing care personnel than some other forms of patient care organization. Many argue effectively that some tasks performed by the primary caregiver could be accomplished by someone with less training and therefore at a lower cost (Dietz, 1994).

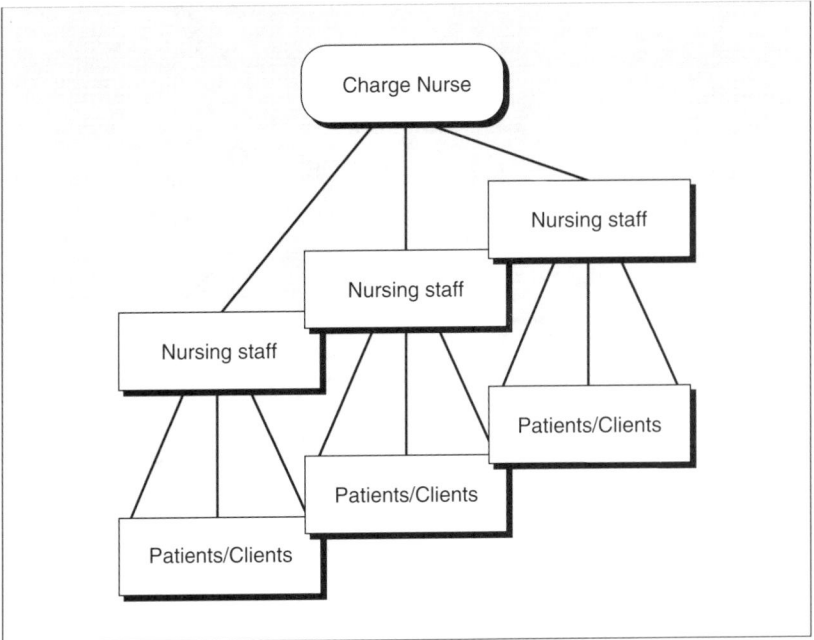

FIGURE 9-1.
Case method or total patient care structure.

Perhaps the greatest disadvantage to this method occurs when the care-giver is inadequately trained/prepared to provide *total* care to the patient. During nursing shortages and economic downturns many hospitals employ health care workers who are not registered nurses as providers of care. A registered nurse is coassigned, but because the RN may also be assigned a heavy patient load, there may be little opportunity for supervision. This has the potential to result in unsafe care.

FUNCTIONAL NURSING

The *functional method* of delivering nursing care evolved as a result of World War II. Nurses were in great demand in both the war effort and at home. Because of the shortage of registered nurses, many ancillary personnel were used to assist in the care of patients. These relatively unskilled workers were trained to perform simple tasks, at which they became quite proficient on repetition (Huston and Marquis, 1989). Personnel were assigned to complete certain tasks rather than care for specific patients. Examples of functional nursing tasks were checking blood pressures, administering medication, changing linen, and bathing patients. Functional nursing structure is shown in Figure 9-2.

This form of organizing patient care was thought to be temporary, as it was anticipated that when the war ended hospitals would not need ancillary work-

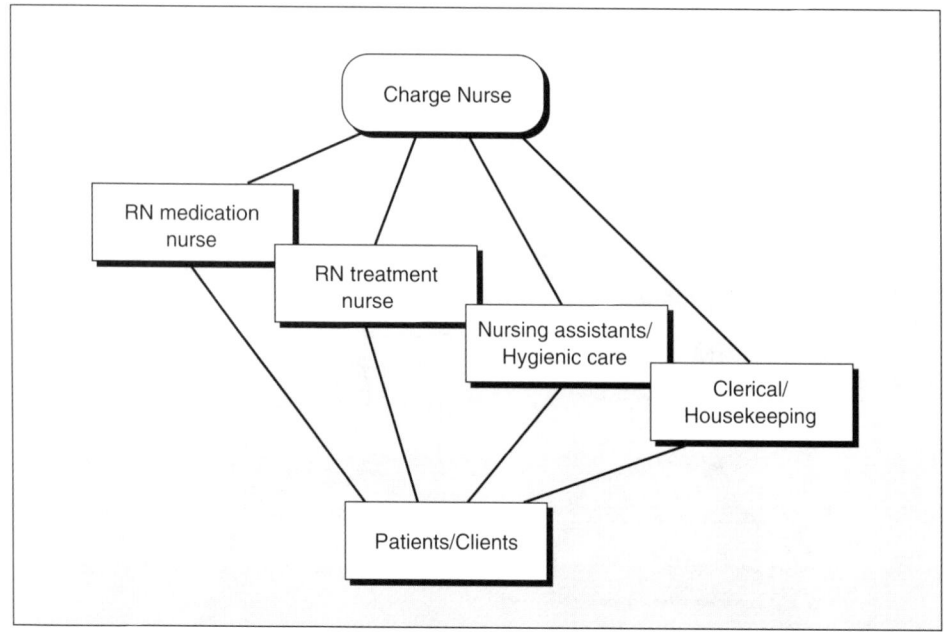

FIGURE 9-2.
Functional nursing organization structure.

ers. However, the baby boom that occurred immediately following World War II continued to leave the country short of nurses. Thus, hospitals continued to use employees with a variety of skill levels and education. Presently, most health care organizations still employ a great many different types of health care workers with varied skills and educational preparation, making it necessary to have different functions or tasks assigned to different skill levels. For instance, one nursing unit might have an unlicensed assistive personnel (UAP) responsible for taking temperatures and a highly trained nurse clinician responsible for maintaining and inserting all intravenous therapy.

Most administrators consider functional nursing to be an economical means of providing care to patients, and increased use of UAP is evident in contemporary hospitals (Huston, 1996). In the past it was felt that quality care and a holistic approach to nursing suffered under functional nursing delivery. However, there are those who argue that by assigning UAP to the nurse, and not the patient, quality of care can be maintained (Joel, 1994). A major advantage to functional nursing is in its efficiency. Tasks are completed quickly and there is little confusion regarding job responsibilities. Functional nursing allows care to be provided for patients with a minimum number of registered nurses. There are many areas within the health care industry where functional structure works well and is still very evident. An example is the operating room.

Functional nursing, however, may lead to fragmented care and the possibility of overlooking priority patient needs. Functional nursing may also result in low job satisfaction, as some workers might feel unchallenged and under-stimulated in their designated functions. Functional organization can also be more costly because of the need for many coordinators, and employees often focus only on their own efforts with less interest in overall results.

TEAM NURSING

Team nursing was introduced in the 1950s in an effort to decrease the problems associated with functional organization of patient care. It was felt that, despite a continued shortage of professional nursing staff, a system for delivering patient care had to be developed that reduced the fragmented care which accompanied functional nursing. Team nursing structure is shown in Figure 9-3.

In team nursing, ancillary personnel work together to provide care to a group of patients under the direction of a professional nurse (the team leader). As the coordinator of the team, the registered nurse is responsible for knowing the condition and needs of all the patients assigned to the team, and for planning the care of each patient. The team leader's duties vary depending on the needs of the patient and the work to be accomplished. These duties may include assisting team members, giving direct personal care to patients, teaching, and coordinating patient activities.

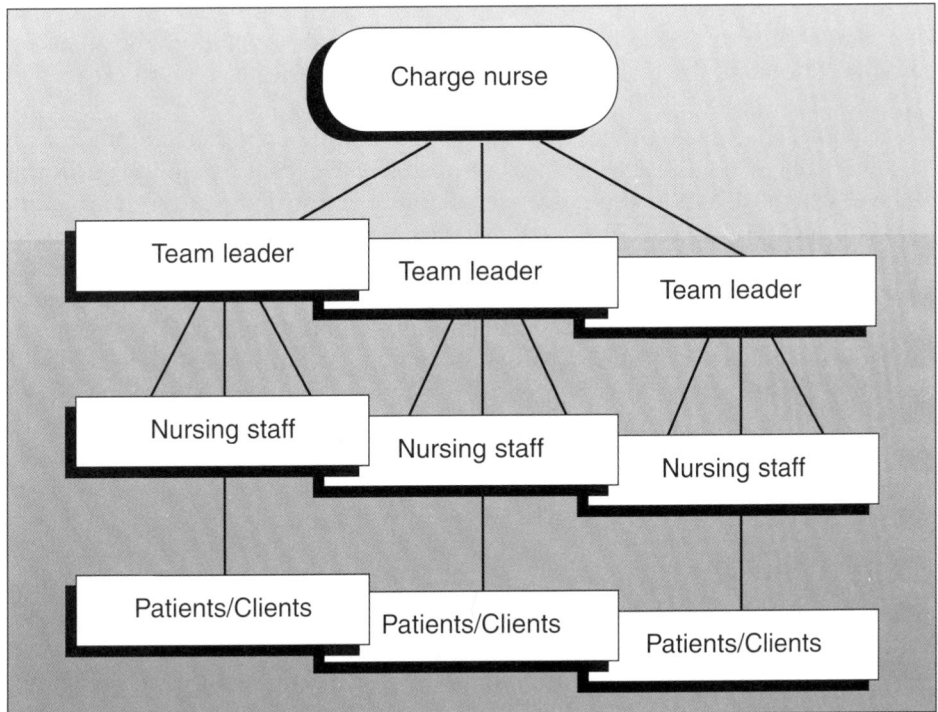

FIGURE 9-3.
Team nursing structure.

Through extensive team communication, comprehensive care can be provided for patients despite a relatively high proportion of ancillary staff. This communication is approached informally by the team leader with individual team members and formally through the regular scheduling of team conferences for patient care planning. A team should be small (four to five members) or it will revert to more function-based organization.

Team nursing is usually associated with a democratic style of leadership. Group members are given as much autonomy as possible while performing assigned tasks, although responsibility and accountability are shared collectively by the team. The necessity for excellent communication and coordination skills makes team nursing organization difficult to implement and requires great self-discipline on the part of team members (Marquis and Huston, 1996).

Team nursing allows team members to contribute their own special expertise or skills in caring for patients, and team leaders should use their knowledge about each specific team member's abilities in making patient assignments. This recognition of the individual worth of all employees as well as the autonomy given to team members results in high job satisfaction.

Disadvantages to team nursing care are associated primarily with improper implementation, rather than with the philosophy itself. Frequently, insufficient time is allowed for team care planning and communication. This can lead to unclear lines of responsibility as well as errors and patient care can become fragmented. For team nursing to succeed, the team leader must be an effective communicator, have good organizational and leadership skills, and be an excellent practitioner. If the team leader does not possess these traits, the team will be ineffective.

The original design of team organization has undergone much modification in the last 25 years. Most team nursing was never practiced in its purest form, but was instead a combination of team and functional structure. Recent attempts to refine and improve team nursing have resulted in the concept of *modular nursing*. This concept uses a smaller group of staff (two or three members) and provides care to a fewer number of patients. It is hoped that by keeping the team very small there will be more involvement of the professional nurse in planning and coordinating care. It is felt that by assigning UAP to the team leader, and not assigning them to the patient to carry out a task, the professional nurse will retain greater control and the care will not be fragmented (Dietz, 1994). Additionally, less communication is required with a small team, which allows team members more efficient use of their time for direct patient care activities.

PRIMARY NURSING

Primary nursing, developed in the early 1970s, utilizes some of the concepts of total patient care, or case method nursing. As originally designed this method required an all-RN staff for implementation. In primary nursing, the registered (primary) nurse assumes 24-hour responsibility for planning the care of one or more patients from the time that patient is admitted or treatment is begun, to the time that patient is discharged or treatment ends. During work hours, the primary nurse provides total direct care for that patient. In the absence of the primary nurse, care is provided by *associate nurses* who follow the care plan established by the primary nurse. Primary nursing structure is shown in Figure 9-4.

Although designed for use in delivering care in hospitals, this structure for care delivery lends itself well to home health nursing, hospice nursing, and other health care delivery enterprises. An integral responsibility of the primary nurse is to establish clear communication between the patient, the physician caring for that patient, the associate nurses, and other members of the health care team. Although the primary nurse establishes the care plan, feedback is sought from other individuals in coordinating the patient's care. The combination of clear interdisciplinary group communication and consistent, direct patient care by a relatively small nursing staff allows for holistic, high-quality patient care.

Job satisfaction is high in primary nursing, although the method is difficult to implement. Implementation difficulties occur because of the degree of responsibility and autonomy required of the primary nurse. However, for these same reasons, once nurses develop skill in primary nursing care delivery they typically feel challenged and rewarded.

The disadvantages of primary nursing, as in team nursing, lie primarily in its improper implementation. An inadequately prepared or insufficiently edu-

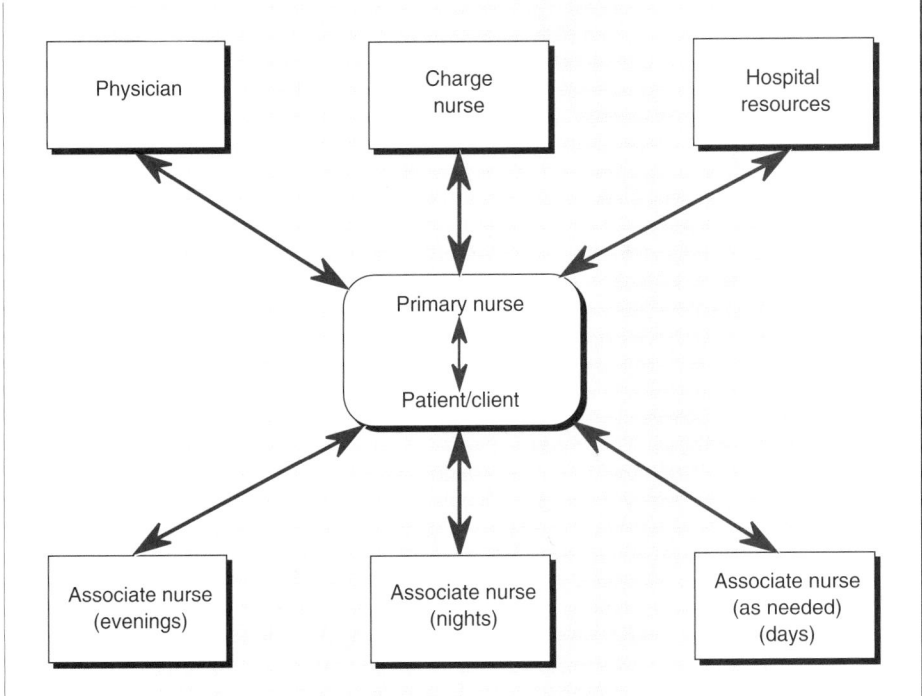

FIGURE 9-4.
Primary nursing structure.

cated primary nurse may be incapable of making the decisions necessary to coordinate a multidisciplinary team or may lack the practitioner skills necessary to identify complex patient needs as well as changes in patient condition.

When originally implemented, an all-RN staff was shown to be no more costly than other modes of delivery, although there has been some difficulty in recruiting and retaining the number of nurses required for this method of care, especially in times of nursing shortages. However, with the increase in registered nursing salaries and studies showing that 23–40% of a nurse's time is spent in work inappropriate to his or her role (Joel, 1994; Huston, 1996) it has become more difficult for managers to justify an all-RN staff. LVNs-LPNs are used as associate nurses in some facilities, and as partners in others (Eriksen et al., 1992), although the function of the primary nurse should be reserved for the registered nurse.

One of the greatest disadvantages in primary nursing has been that many nurses are neither comfortable with nor adequately prepared for the position of primary care nurse. Because the rationale of primary nursing is sound, some organizations are attempting to implement the underlying concepts of primary nursing while differentiating the roles of nurses within their organization. This patient care delivery system is termed *differentiated nursing practice.* Registered nurses are assigned to work within the role structure and responsibilities that correspond to their capabilities. Capabilities are measured by skill, knowledge, and motivation rather than level of education. Differentiated nursing practice is still too new to determine whether it has met the intended goals: to improve nurse retention, quality of care, and fiscal outcomes (Malloch, Milton, and Jobes, 1990).

◆ Case Management

Case management is the latest work design proposed to meet patient needs. There is much confusion regarding the term, as it has had several different meanings since it first came into use. Lyon (1993) makes an effort to clarify and define case management, stating it is not a nursing care delivery model such as team nursing and primary nursing care. Instead, case management is a role that was originally developed in community heath settings and later enlarged as a result of the managed care concept developed by HMOs (Lyon, 1993).

However, hospitals and other health agencies often use the term case management to define a client-centered model of care that uses critical pathways to help plan patient care (Bower, 1992). When used as an organizational model, case management is similar to primary nursing, in that one individual nurse is responsible for coordinating the activities and care of a patient.

Zander (1988) lists four essential components of case management: 1) achievement of clinical outcomes within a prescribed time frame, 2) the caregiver acts as the case manager, 3) episodic nurse–physician group practice that transcends units or departments, and 4) active participation of the patient and family in setting goals and evaluation. However, it differs from primary nursing in two ways. First, although the case manager uses the nursing process, the primary focus is on planning, coordinating, and evaluating care. There is less control of the patient care and more collaboration (Zander, 1994). The case associates assigned to the care deal more directly with assessment and intervention. Second, unlike primary nursing, in case management it is recognized that not every patient needs a case manager (Kramer, 1990).

The limited studies on patient care management have shown positive outcomes for both clients and staff (Lamb and Stempel, 1994). However, the literature continues to show much confusion about both the role of the case manager and the definition of case management, and it remains to be seen how the term will ultimately be defined. Although, Lyon (1993) is probably correct when she says that case management is more a monitoring of client resource utilization and should not be called a delivery system, the reality is that many organizations are using the term to define a system of patient care delivery.

◆ Selecting the Optimum Mode for Organizing Patient Care

In a recent study of health care delivery systems, eight models were identified, but the most common models still in use in hospitals were total patient care, team nursing, and primary nursing care (McLaughlin, Thomas, and Barter, 1995). Unfortunately, many nursing service departments have a history of selecting modes for organizing patient care based on the latest fad rather than by objectively deciding what is the best mode for a particular unit or department. Because change always introduces an element of stress, it is important to evaluate the effectiveness of the current mode of patient care delivery to determine whether there is a need for work redesign prior to instituting change in the organizational structure. The amount of resources necessary for work redesign is tremendous and should not be undertaken lightly (Ritter and Tonges, 1991; Fralic, 1992; Porter-O'Grady, 1996).

In determining the effectiveness of the present system, the following questions should be asked.

1. Is the organization of patient care delivery providing the level of care stated in the health organization's philosophy? Does it facilitate or hinder meeting other goals of the organization?
2. Is the delivery of nursing care organized in a manner that is cost effective?
3. Does the patient care delivery system provide patient, as well as family, satisfaction? (Satisfaction and quality care differ; either may be provided without the other being present.)
4. Does the organization of patient care delivery provide some degree of fulfillment and role satisfaction to nursing personnel?
5. Does the patient care delivery system allow implementation of the nursing process?
6. Does the structuring of care delivery facilitate adequate communication between all members of the health care team?

If the present system of organizing patient care reveals deficiencies, the manager needs to examine the available resources and compare those with the means necessary for the change. Nursing managers often choose a delivery system that requires a high percentage of professional nurses, only to discover adequate resources are unavailable, resulting in a failed plan change. There must be a commitment on the part of top-level administration and a majority of the nursing staff for a change in patient care delivery to be successful.

Because health care is multidiscipinary, the patient care delivery system used will impact heavily on many other individuals outside the nursing unit itself; therefore, those affected by a change in organizing patient care must be involved. This includes other departments, the medical staff, as well as the health care consumer.

Last, the human elements that have great bearing on the success or failure of a change in the work place should be examined before there is a modification in work organization. There are many pitfalls inherent in restructuring job design. Remember that all people are different and not every nurse desires a challenging job with the autonomy of personal decision making. There are a great many simultaneous interacting forces in an employee–job design relationship (Fralic, 1992). Satisfaction in the work place does not only occur because of role fulfillment; it also takes place as a result of social and interpersonal relations. The change agent redesigning the organization of the work needs to consider how the following elements will be changed as a result of the reorganization.

1. How will autonomy as well as individual and group decision making be altered by the reorganization? Who will be affected? Will there be a decrease or increase in autonomy?
2. How will social interactions and interpersonal relationships change?
3. Will there be a modification in what the employee views as their unit of work? Will there be a change from a partial unit of work to a whole unit? (For example, total patient care is a whole unit of work, team nursing is a partial unit of work.)
4. Will the change require a wider or more restrictive range of skills and abilities?
5. Will the redesign produce a change in how employees receive feedback on their performance, either for self-evaluation or by others?
6. Will there be changes in communication patterns?

Whenever the patient care delivery system is altered some or all of the listed elements will be affected. That is not to say that change should not occur, but only that managers must first evaluate all the variables that interact with the job before proceeding with the reorganization of the patient care delivery system.

◆ Committee Structure Within an Organization

An additional responsibility of managers in unit organization is the designation and implementation of appropriate committees. What are the benefits of committees and when are they justified? In order to compensate for some of the difficulty in organizational communication created by line, as well as line and staff structure, committees are widely employed in all institutions as a means of facilitating upward communication. As organizations seek new ways to revamp old bureaucratic structures, many look to the use of committees as a method of sharing organizational governance and increasing staff participation (Maas and Sprecht, 1994).

Committees may be advisory or may have a coordinating or informal function. In the previous chapter a sample of the committee structure found in self governance is shown in Figure 8-2. Committees are an essential part of shared governance organization structure and have a major function in professional practice issues

Committees in any organizational structure are beneficial, as they communicate information in two directions and encourage participation of interested or affected employees. They often generate new ideas and promote creative thinking to solve operational problems or improve services, and upgrade the quality and quantity of work accomplished. They can also be used to pool the talents of people with specific skills and expertise and to help reduce resistance to change.

However, all the positive benefits of committees can only be achieved if they are appropriately organized and led. If not properly managed, the committee becomes a liability to the organizing process, wasting energy, time, and money and possibly deferring decision making and action taking. Committees should not be used to avoid or delay decisions, but to facilitate organizational goals. Since group communication is such an important part of committee effectiveness, it is covered extensively in Chapter 17.

In organizing committees and making appointments there are several factors to be considered.

1. The committee should be composed of individuals who want to contribute to the committee in terms of commitment, energy, and time.
2. The members should have a variety of work experience and educational backgrounds, but composition should have sufficient expertise to ensure that the task of the committee is accomplished.
3. There should be an adequate number of members to accomplish assigned tasks but not so many that discussion cannot occur. Six to eight members is usually ideal.
4. The tasks and responsibilities should be clearly outlined, including reporting mechanisms.
5. Assignments should be given ahead of time, with clear expectations that assigned work will be reported on at the next meeting.
6. All committees should have prepared agendas and effective committee chairs who are comfortable using the group process and have a working knowledge of group dynamics.

It is important for the manager to be aware of the possibility for *groupthink* to occur in any work group or committee structure. In this context, groupthink is the inappropriate conformity to group norms (Swansburg, 1990). It occurs when members fail to take adequate risks by disagreeing, being challenged, or by assessing discussion carefully. If the manager is actively involved in the work group or on the committee, groupthink is less likely to occur. Teaching group members to avoid groupthink by demonstrating critical thinking and by encouraging questioning of all ideas is vital.

◆ Summary

Organizing is an important management function. The work must be ordered in such a manner that the goals of the organization are sustained. Activities must be grouped so that there is full use of resources, people, material, and the time demands of each shift.

The type of patient care delivery selected should bring satisfaction to the nursing staff, provide adequate patient care, and be economically sound. A change in the mode of delivery should not be attempted without adequate resources and an appropriate justification for doing so.

The effective manager has a sufficient knowledge of how to use committees appropriately. Committees are used to increase productivity, not to delay decisions. Groupthink among work groups or in committees should be discouraged.

◆ References

Bower KA (1992). Case Management by Nurses. Kansas City, MO: American Nurses Publishing

Curtin L (1994). Learning from the future. Nurs Manage 25(1):7–9

Dietz EO (1994). Should nurses use assistants? In McCloskey J and Grace HK (eds). Current Issues in Nursing, 4th ed. St. Louis: Mosby

Eriksen LR, Quandt B, Teinert D, Look DS, Loosle R, Mackey G, and Strout B (1992). A registered nurse-licensed vocational nurse partnership model for critical care nursing. JONA 22(12):28–38

Fralic MF (1992). Creating new practice models and designing new roles. J Nurs Admin 22(6):7–8

Huston CJ (1996). Unlicensed assistive personnel: a solution to the dwindling health care resources or the precursor to the apocalypse of registered nursing? Nurs Outlook 44(2):67–73

Huston CJ and Marquis B (1989). Retention and Productivity Strategies for Nurse Managers. Philadelphia: JB Lippincott

Joel JL (1994). Changes in the hospital as a place of practice. In McCloskey J and Grace HK (eds). Current Issues in Nursing, 4th ed. St. Louis: Mosby

Kramer M (1990). The magnet hospitals: excellence revisited. J Nurs Admin (9):2

Lamb GS and Stempel B (1994). Nurse case management from the client's view: growing as insider-expert. Nurs Outlook 42(1):7–13

Lyon JC (1993). Models of nursing care delivery and case management: clarification of terms. Nurs Econ 11(3):163–169

Maas ML and Sprecht (1994). Shared governance in nursing. In McCloskey J and Grace HK (eds). Current Issues in Nursing, 4th ed. St. Louis: Mosby

Malloch KM, Milton DA, and Jobes MO (1990). A model for differentiated nursing practice. J Nurs Admin 20(2):20–26

Marquis B and Huston CJ (1996). Leadership Roles and Management Functions, 2nd ed. Philadelphia: JB Lippincott

McLaughlin FE, Thomas SE, and Barter M (1995). Changes related to care delivery patterns. JONA 25(5):35–46

Porter-O'Grady T (1996). The seven basic rules for succesful redesign. JONA 26(1):46–53

Ritter J and Tonges MC (1991). Work redesign in high intensity environments. JONA 21(12):26–35

Swansburg RC (1990). Management and Leadership for Nurse Managers. Boston: Jones and Bartlett

Tappen RM (1995). Nursing Leadership and Management: Concepts and Practice, 3rd ed. Philadelphia: FA Davis

Zander K (1988). Nursing care management: strategic management of cost and quality outcomes. J Nurs Admin 18(5):23–30

Zander K (1994). Nurses and case management. In McCloskey J and Grace HK (eds). Current Issues in Nursing, 4th ed. St. Louis: Mosby

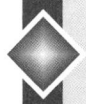

DISPLAY 9-1 (For Sample Case Analysis)
Sample Break and Lunch Schedule Oncology Unit–Memorial Hospital

RN Staff

Break time	Lunch time	Name
8:00 A.M.	11:00 A.M.	_____
8:20 A.M.	11:30 A.M.	_____
9:20 A.M.	12:30 P.M.	_____

LVN Staff

Break time	Lunch time	Name
8:20 A.M.	11:00 A.M.	_____
8:40 A.M.	12:00 Noon	_____
9:40 A.M.	1:00 P.M.	_____

The ward clerk may go to lunch at 12:30 P.M. or 1:00 P.M. Ward clerk morning breaks are always at 9:40 A.M. The float aide takes a morning break at 8:00 A.M. and lunch at 11:30 A.M. The head nurse goes to lunch/break at various times depending on the needs of the unit.

SAMPLE CASE ANALYSIS

THE CASE ◆

In order to accommodate increasing personnel, Memorial Hospital has expanded its cafeteria hours. The cafeteria will now start serving lunch at 11:00 A.M. instead of 11:30 A.M. and will continue serving until 1:15 P.M. instead of 12:45 P.M.

As day charge nurse, you welcome this news, as it will enable the unit to have fewer staff off the floor at any given time, leaving more staff available at lunch time to assist with the passing of trays and the feeding of patients. However, you know that some employees probably will not like taking lunch at 11:00 A.M. and some will dislike waiting until after 1:00 P.M. Note that the cafeteria is open from 8:00 A.M. to 10:00 A.M. for breakfast.

Employees at Memorial Hospital are entitled to one 20-minute break in the morning, one 30-minute break for lunch, and one 10-minute break in the afternoon. During the short afternoon break, the unit is fairly quiet and the staff use the conference room for their brief respite, but the morning and lunch breaks are times when the employees leave the unit.

Each day you have one ward clerk for clerical duties and one floating aide to pass water, run errands, answer lights, and make beds. You do not take a patient assignment. Three RNs, and three LVNs-LPNs are assigned to total patient care for an average of four patients each. Breakfast trays arrive on your floor at 7:45 A.M. and lunch trays arrive at 12:15 P.M.

Assignment

Organize morning and lunch breaks for all personnel in a manner that is efficient and equitable. Support your decision with an appropriate rationale.

Analysis

The plan or goal for solving this case has already been stated. There are many possible alternatives for decision making in this case and most of them would meet the stated objective. Because this case has numerous "right" answers, the users of this text may want to solve this case in other ways. Only one alternative will be presented. The following action and rationale explain the sample schedule provided in Display 9-1.

Action and Rationale

Design a sign-up sheet for lunch and coffee breaks and allow the RNs and LVNs/LPNs to sign up each day. All staff may trade with each other but someone must go at the designated times. This allows the staff to have some control over their environment. By allocating numbers of slots for each time frame, you have made certain that sufficient staff is always present to accomplish unit work. You have also built in flexibility for unforeseen changes in the work environment by allowing staff to trade times.

Use of a sign-up sheet assures adequate staff coverage while providing sufficient personnel for passing breakfast and lunch trays and assisting with meals.

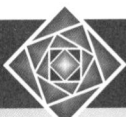

CASES FOR PROBLEM SOLVING

CASE 1

You are the head nurse of an oncology unit. At present, the designated patient care delivery system on the unit is total patient care. You have a staff consisting of 60% registered nurses, 35% practical nurses, and 5% clerical staff.

Your bed capacity is 28, but your average daily census is 24. An example of day shift staffing is the following:

1. One charge nurse who records orders, speaks with doctors, organizes care, makes assignments, and is a resource person and problem solver.
2. Three registered nurses who provide total patient care, including all treatments and medications to their assigned patients, give IV medications to the practical nurses' assigned patients, and act as a clinical resource person for the practical nurses.
3. Two practical nurses assigned to provide total patient care except for IV medications.

Your supervisor called a meeting of all head nurses. She told you the hospital is downsizing registered nurse positions and has decided to hire more nursing assistants. As a result, the registered nurses on your unit will have to assume greater supervisory responsibilities and fewer direct care duties.

She has asked you to reorganize the patient care management on your unit in a way that will best utilize the following day-shift staffing: three RNs including the present charge nurse position, two practical nurses, and two nursing assistants. You may eliminate the previous charge nurse position and divide charge responsibility evenly among all three nurses or delegate the work in any manner you choose.

• •

Assignment

Draw a new patient care organization diagram. Who would be most affected by the reorganization? Present your choice. Explain your rationale, both for your selection as well as those you rejected. How would you go about implementing this planned change?

CASE 2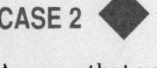

Assume that you are a director in a home health agency. You primarily employ RNs, although there are some LVNs-LPNs on your staff. Most of the nursing care that your agency provides is done on a contractual basis with clients in their home. Although your nurses provide care for a wide variety of patient needs, there seems to be a high incidence of patients who have cancer, irreversible spinal cord injuries, or who are recovering from a CVA.

Because many of these patients require nursing care on an extended basis, you believe there is great potential for your nurses to form therapeutic relationships with these patients and to implement a holistic nursing care plan. Currently, patient assignments are rotated among the staff.

CASE 2 (CONTINUED)

· ·

Assignment

Decide whether an alternative method of patient care management or a modification of the current method would be appropriate. Be sure you consider the makeup of your staff in terms of the motivation nurses need to care for the same patients on a long-term basis. How would you guard against having an inadequately prepared or undereducated nurse assigned to a patient on a long-term basis? What evaluative checkpoints can be constructed to guard against this happening?

CASE 3

You are the supervisor of an intensive care unit. Your staff members are independent and capable. Recently your staff expressed that they would like to be more self-managed. Some of your staff recently attended a conference on shared goverance. You have told them they may begin to work on the structure and bylaws of such a proposed committee, all of which will be subject to your approval.

· ·

Assignment

Refer to the previous chapter and Figure 8-2 for assistance in solving this case. Develop a design for the structure of the committee. Institute a general policy and a few procedures that would help guide the committee. What decisions should the staff be allowed to make and what areas should be reserved for the supervisor? List some of the dangers as well as the benefits of such a committee.

◆ **Bibliography**

The following list of references will help you to solve these cases:

ANA to blue-ribbon panel: RN restructuring puts patient care and safety at risk (1994). Revolution: J Nurse Empowerment 4(4):17–18.

Barter M and Furmidge ML (1994). Unlicensed assistive personnel: issues related to delegation and supervision. J Nurs Admin 24(4):36–40

Bowman G and Carter E (1990). Making sense of primary nursing. Nurs Times 86(27):39–4

Fralic MF (1995). Into the future: new models, new methods. Capsule Commentary. Nurse Lead Manage 3(1):9

Gardner K (1991). A summary of findings of a five-year comparison study of primary and team nursing. Nurs Res 40(2):113–117

Jannotta M and Mandonado T (1992). Self-management for nurses. J Nurs Admin 22(6):59–63

Jung FD, Pearcey LG, and Phillips JL (1994). Evaluation of a program to improve nursing assistant use. J Nurs Admin 24(3):42–47

Le Clair CL (1991). Introducing and accounting for RN case management. Nurs Manage 22(3):44–49

Lulavaagae A (1991). RN–LPN teams: toward unit nursing case management. Nurs Manage 22(3):58–62

Mark BA (1992). Characteristics of nursing practice models. JONA 22(11):57–63

Sheafor M (1991). Productive work groups in complex hospital units. J Nurs Admin 21(5):12–15

Sherman M (1990). Team nursing revisited. J Nurs Admin 20(11):43–46

Waterworth S (1991). A change worth the making: implementing primary nursing. Prof Nurse 6(8):442–445

Wong R, Gordon DL, Cassard SD, Weisman CS, and Bergner M (1993). A cost analysis of a professional practice model for nursing. Nurs Econ 11(5):292–297, 323

PERSONAL NOTEBOOK

1. What has contributed to the committees you have served on that made them productive? Nonproductive? Have you ever served on a committee that made recommendations to a higher authority that were never acted on? How did it affect the work?

2. Many nurses learn organizing "tricks" that assist them in accomplishing patient care tasks. Discuss organizing techniques with veteran nurses and with other students. List 10 ways that a nurse can help organize work and get more accomplished.

3. List the types of patient care delivery systems you have observed and include what you believe are their strengths and weaknesses.

Power and Politics in Organizations

CHAPTER
10

In the first chapter of this unit the reader was introduced to status, authority, and responsibility at different levels of the organizational hierarchy. Authority, or the right to command that accompanies any management position, is a source of legitimate power. The knowledgeable manager exercises the wise use of authority, power, and political strategy and will, in turn, be more successful.

◆ Authority Versus Power

If authority is the right to command, then one must ask, "Why do workers sometimes not follow orders?" The right to command does not ensure that employees will always follow orders. There is sometimes a gap between a position of authority and the response of subordinates to that authority. This is called the *authority–power gap*. The term "manager power" may be used to explain the subordinate response to the manager's authority. The more power subordinates *perceive* a manager to have, the smaller the gap between the right to certain expectations and the resulting fulfillment of those expectations by others (Huston and Marquis, 1988).

Many children are conditioned to *accept* the directives of their parents, teachers, and community leaders. Because of this early socialization, the gap between the manager's authority and the worker's response is relatively small in this country. In other countries it may be larger or smaller, depending on how individuals are socialized to respond to authority.

The authority dependence that begins with our parents is later transferred to our employers and is an important resource for managers. Although the authority–power gap continues to be small, it has grown over the last 20 years.

Both the women's rights movement and the student unrest of the 1960s contributed to the widening of the authority–power gap. An example of this expansion is evidenced by an exchange between a college student of the 1970s and her mother. When asked why she did not protest as a college student, the mother replied, "I didn't know we could."

There are times when authority should be questioned. An example in the health care industry is the questioning of physicians (many who feel they have the authority to command) by nurses, patients, and other health care workers. Figure 10-1 shows the dynamics of relationships in the organizational authority–power response.

The negative effect of a wide authority–power gap is that chaos may develop in the organization. There would be little productivity if every order were to be questioned. The organization rightfully should expect that the goals of the organization will be accomplished. One of the core elements of the dynamics of civilization is that there will always be a small number of authority figures pushing the many for a certain standard of performance.

◆ Bridging the Authority–Power Gap

Sometimes subordinates can begin to feel badgered by conspicuous demonstrations of authority. As each individual has a limited capacity for tolerating authority, its use as a tool of power should be limited to a last resort. It is best not to use arbitrary commands as they can stifle cooperation.

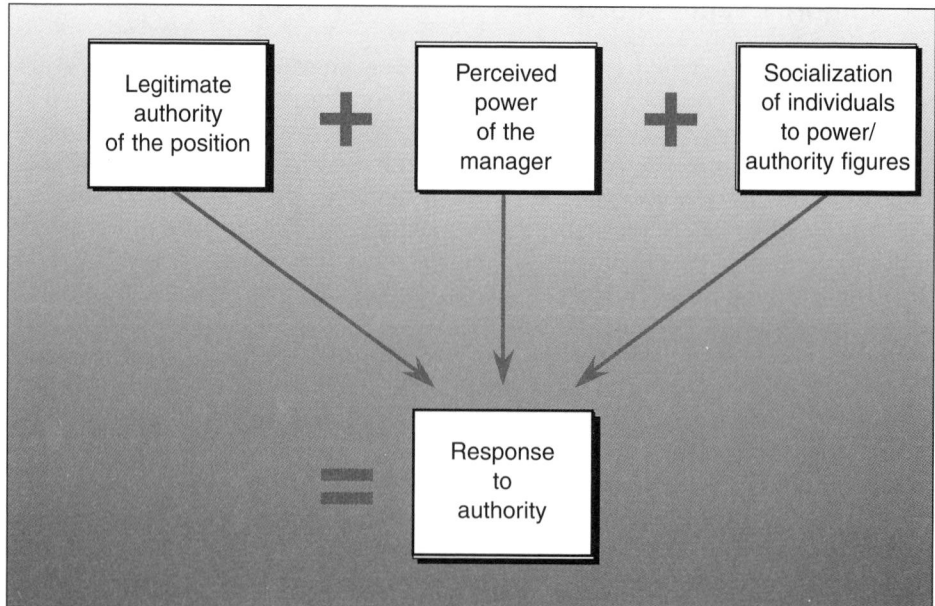

FIGURE 10-1.
Interdependency of response to authority.

Managers can use various techniques to enable the subordinates to distinguish authority from the person who holds it. This can be achieved through the use of ceremony so that respect is given to the office, rather than to the person who holds it.

Another method to bridge this gap is for the manager to instill trust and make the subordinates believe that the organization cares about them. The manager whose followers 1) believe that the manager is doing a good job, 2) trust that the organization has their best interests in mind, and 3) do not feel controlled by authority, will have bridged the authority–power gap.

The manager must also be seen as credible for the authority–power gap not to grow wider. Every manager begins his or her appointment with subordinates ready to believe them. This is because of the socialization process that makes individuals believe that what those in power say is true. However, the deference to authority will erode if the manager handles employees in a careless manner, is dishonest, or seems incapable of carrying out the duties of the job. When a manager begins to lose credibility, the power inherent in his or her authority begins to decrease.

Another dimension of the authority–power relationship is the impact of employee expectations. It is best to be conservative when promises must be made. Managers should *never* guarantee future rewards. If managers inaccurately predict the future, they lose credibility in the eyes of their subordinates. However, managers *should* grant current rewards to buy patronage. This makes the manager more believable and builds greater power into their already existing legitimate authority. The following is an example of the difference in dispensing current and future awards.

> An RN requests an extra day off to attend a wedding. As you are able to replace her, you use the power of your position to reward her and give her the day off. She is grateful to you and this increases your power.
>
> Another RN requests 3 months in advance to have every Thursday off in the summer to take a class. You grant permission, but on June 1, three of your nurses resign and you are unable to keep your promise. This nurse is very upset and you have lost much credibility, and therefore power. It would have been wiser for you to have said you could not guarantee that you could grant her request (underpromising). If the situation had remained the same and the nurses had not resigned, then you could have granted the request.

The key then is for the manager to be able to accomplish three separate tasks. Authority must be used in such a manner that subordinates view what happens in the organization as obvious and necessary. The manager must be viewed as powerful, and astute political strategy must be employed so that power and authority are maintained.

◆ Understanding Power

Power may be defined as the generalized capacity or potential an individual has that enables him or her to get others to do something they would not ordinarily do. Power may also be viewed as the potential of an individual or group to affect or influence the behavior of another (Kippenbrock, 1992). The word power is derived from the Latin verb *potere* (to be able); thus, power may be appropriately defined as that which enables one to accomplish goals.

Power may be feared, worshipped, or mistrusted; it is frequently misunderstood. McCurdy (1988) maintains that our first experience with power occurs in the family unit. Because children's roles are likened to later subordinate roles, and the parental power position is similar to management, the adult views of power in the management–subordinate relationship will be influenced by how power was used in the family unit. Whether the familial power experience was positive or negative will greatly affect an individual's ability to deal with power in adulthood.

◆ Types of Power

All management positions are supported by some measure of power. French and Raven (1959) have postulated that there are several bases, or sources, for the exercise of power: reward power, punishment or coercive power, legitimate power, expert power, and referent power.

Reward power is power obtained by the ability to grant favors, or to reward others with whatever they value. The arsenal of rewards that a manager can dispense to get employees to work toward meeting organizational goals is very broad. The use of rewards tends to foster a great deal of loyalty and devotion on the part of subordinates.

Punishment or *coercive power* is the opposite of reward power and is based on fear of punishment if the manager's expectations are not met. The manager may obtain compliance through (often implied) threats of transfer, layoff, demotion, or dismissal. The manager who shuns or ignores an employee is also exercising power through punishment, as does the manager who berates or belittles an employee.

Legitimate power is position power. Authority is also referred to as legitimate power. It is the power gained by a title or official position within an organization. As previously discussed, the socialization and culture of subordinate employees will influence to some degree how much power a manager has owing to position.

Expert power is power gained through knowledge, expertise, or experience. Possessing required knowledge allows a manager to gain power over others who need that knowledge. This type of power is limited to a specialized area. For example, someone with a vast knowledge of oncology would only be powerful in the area of oncology, not in another area of specialization.

Referent power is power an individual has because others develop an identification with him or her or what he or she symbolizes. Referent power is given to others through association with the powerful. An individual may also develop referent power because others perceive them as powerful. This perception could be based on personal charisma, the way the individual speaks or acts, the related organizations they belong to, or the people with whom they associate. Referent power is enjoyed by those who are accepted by others as role models or ideals. Physicians use referent power very effectively.

Some theorists make a distinction between charismatic power and referent power. Willey (1990) maintains that charisma is a type of personal power, whereas referent power is gained only through association with powerful others.

Heineken and McClosky (1985) added informational power to the French and Raven power sources. This power is obtained when individuals have information that others must have in order to accomplish their goals.

Morrison (1988) refers to the types of power already cited as patriarchal types of power and asserts that they imply power over others. She identifies another category of power as feminist power, which is defined as power over one's own life. This power is the power that resides in a person that comes from maturity, ego integration, security in the individual's relationships with others, and confidence in one's impulsive responses. The various sources of power are summarized in Table 10-1.

◆ Building a Power Base

Managers must build a power base in the organization where they work. This is necessary to further organizational goals, carry out management functions, and meet personal goals. As power implies interdependency, managers must not only understand the organizational structure they work in, but also be able to function effectively within that structure, including dealing appropriately with the inherent organizational politics present. Only when managers understand the power and politics of their organization will they be capable of recognizing both limitations and potential for change.

In addition to understanding power within the organizational structure, the individual manager must be knowledgeable about the essence of power. Successful managers develop a personal awareness of their view of power, its

◆ TABLE 10-1
Sources of Power

Type	Source
Referent	Association with others
Legitimate	Position
Coercive	Fear
Reward	Ability to grant favors
Expert	Knowledge and skill
Charismatic	Personal
Informational	The need for information
Self	Maturity, ego strength

use, and its abuse. Many individuals, particularly women, hold negative connotations of power and never learn to use power constructively.

McCurdy (1988) maintains that women have been socialized to view power differently than men. For women, power is seen as dominance versus submission; it is associated with personal qualities as opposed to accomplishments and is dependent upon personal or physical attributes, not skill. Additionally, women seldom feel they inherently possess power, but instead rely on others for its acquisition. Edwards (1994) states that most women have traditionally demonstrated ambivalence toward the concept of power and usually have had little experience wielding legitimate power.

Although many women believe that power manages them and feel they are incapable of acquiring and managing power, some recent researchers have found that more nurses and women in general are becoming more positive about the concept of power (Porter, 1991; Reimer et al, 1994).

In order to look at power in a different light it is necessary to examine the opposite of power, which is powerlessness. Most individuals agree that they dislike being powerless and everyone needs some control in their lives. It becomes apparent then, that power has a negative as well as a positive face.

The negative face of power is that aspect of dominance versus submission, "I win and you lose." Someone gains while someone loses power. The positive face of power occurs when someone exerts influence on behalf of someone or something rather than over others. Therefore, it is not power itself that is evil, but how it is used and for what purpose that determines if it is good or evil.

Individuals know when they are followers of powerful managers because their own status is enhanced as they become part of the growth and excitement of the organization. Followers of powerful individuals tend to have high morale because their managers delegate more authority and build with a team effort. Most workers find it exciting to be working as a subordinate for someone who has clout in an organization.

On the other hand, powerlessness tends to breed bossiness and the manager who feels powerless often creates an ineffective, petty, dictatorial, and rules-oriented management style. The old adage that power corrupts might be true for some individuals, but it may be more correct to stay that it is not organizational *power* that corrupts but rather organizational *powerlessness.*

Nurses need power to assure adequate resources. The ability to manipulate resources is one of the arts of management and requires political astuteness. Power and politics exist in each organization and if novice nurse managers are going to be able to function effectively, they must develop skill in the three arenas of power: 1) power building, 2) political strategy, and 3) maintaining a small authority–power gap.

◆ Techniques for Building an Organizational Power Base

There are many ways an individual new to an organization can build a base of power. The following are suggestions for enhancing power (Marquis and Huston, 1996).

1. *Expand personal resources.* Self-awareness, vitality, resilience, mental and emotional strength, and the ability to take risks are all characteristics of the powerful person. Therefore, accumulating resources in any of these areas will increase personal power. Likewise, maintaining a healthy mind and body through exercise and good nutrition are simple but often overlooked ways of increasing personal power.

2. *Present a powerful picture to others.* How individuals look, act, and speak influence whether others view them as powerful or powerless. The nurse who stands tall, is poised, assertive, articulate, and well-groomed presents a picture to others of personal control and power.

3. *Pay the entry fee.* Newcomers in organizations who stand out and appear powerful are those who do more, work harder, and contribute to the organization. Neither "clock watchers" nor "nine-to-fivers," they attend meetings, do committee work, attend in-services, and accept their share of night shifts, weekend, and holiday assignments without complaining. A power base is not achieved by slick, easy, or quick maneuvers. It is acquired through hard work.

4. *Identify the powerful in the organization.* It is necessary to understand and work within both the formal as well as the informal power structure. It is important for individuals to be cognizant of their limitations and to appropriately seek counsel. One should know the names and faces of the people with both formal and informal power. The powerful individuals in the informal structure are often more difficult to identify than those in the formal structure. When working with powerful people in organizations, individuals should attempt to identify the similarities and shared values, rather than focusing on the differences.

5. *Learn the language and symbols of the organization.* Each organization has its own culture, as well as its own values. It is necessary for new members to understand this culture and to be socialized into the organization if they are to build a power base. There are certain "taboos" that exist in each organization, and being unaware of what they are often results in embarrassment for the newcomer. The novice employee or new manager must develop a sensitivity to the organization's culture if they expect to become powerful.

6. *Learn how to use the organization's priorities.* Every group has a priority list of goals it wishes to achieve. Individuals seeking to construct a power base must be cognizant of institutional goals and priorities and use this knowledge to meet unit needs. For example, a need for a new manager at a community health service facility might be to develop educational programs on chemotherapy, as some of the patient case load includes this nursing function. If fiscal management is a high priority of the organization, the manager needs to show how the cost of these programs will be offset by additional revenues. If public relations with physicians and clients is a priority in the organization, the manager could justify the same request in terms of additional services to clients and physicians.

7. *Increase professional skills and knowledge.* Because it is expected that employees will perform their job well, one's job performance must be

extraordinary to enhance power. One method of achieving this is by increasing professional skills and knowledge until an advanced level of expertise is reached. Having knowledge and skill others lack greatly enhances an individual's power base. Excellence that reflects knowledge and demonstrates skill enhances the credibility of the nurse and determines how he or she is viewed by others.

8. *Maintain a broad vision.* Because individuals are assigned to a unit or department, they often begin to develop a narrow view of the total organization. Power builders always look upward and outward. The successful manager not only recognizes how the single unit fits in with the larger organization, but also how the organization as a whole fits into the scheme of the entire community. People without vision rarely become powerful.

9. *Use experts and seek counsel.* Newcomers should seek out role models to emulate. By soliciting the advice and counsel of others, new employees demonstrate their willingness to be team players, that they are cautious and welcome advice from experts prior to proceeding, and that they are not rash newcomers who thinks they have all the answers.

10. *Be flexible.* An individual wishing to acquire power should develop a reputation as someone who can compromise. The rigid, uncompromising newcomer is viewed as insensitive to the needs of the organization.

11. *Increase visibility and develop a voice in the organization.* It is important that newcomers become active in powerful committees, or other groups that are recognized by the organization as having clout. When working in groups it is crucial that the newcomer not monopolize committee time. Novice managers must develop observational and listening skills as well as articulate verbal skills.

12. *Learn to toot your own horn.* There is an art to accepting compliments. One should be gracious, but certainly not passive, when attention is forthcoming for extraordinary effort. Additionally, individuals should let others know when some special professional recognition has been achieved. This acknowledgment should be made in such a manner that is not bragging, but reflective of the self-respect of one who is talented and unique.

13. *Maintain a sense of humor.* Appropriate humor is a very powerful tool and the ability to laugh at oneself and not take oneself too seriously is one of the most important power builders.

14. *Empower others.* Empowerment is one of the characteristics of a transformational leader and occurs when power is shared (Strader and Decker, 1995). Just as leaders need to empower others, followers must empower their leaders. When nurses empower each other they gain referent power. If women are frequently bitter and envious of other women, they may withhold support or openly attack. Both individual nurses and the profession as a whole are deprived of their share of power because they allow others to create divisiveness and weaken their power base (Huston and Marquis, 1988). Nurses can empower other nurses by shar-

ing knowledge, maintaining cohesiveness, valuing nursing, and supporting each other (Sohier, 1992).

In contrast to the manager who empowers others is the one who will not teach others and does not want to see others succeed. This individual has been termed the *Queen Bee,* and the activities and behaviors used to keep others from power has been called the *Queen Bee Syndrome* (Staines, Travis, and Jayaratne, 1974). The behavior exhibited by Queen Bees includes identification with others outside of nursing, usually males who hold higher positions in the organization, and a disinterest in improving or changing the profession. The Queen Bee wants to be the main attraction and desires that subordinates remain powerless.

On the other hand, empowerment occurs when those in power communicate their vision; when employees are given the opportunity to make the most of their talents; and when learning, creativity, and exploration are encouraged. Managers empower others when they delegate assignments to provide learning opportunities and allow employees to share in the satisfaction derived from their achievements (Hawks, 1992).

Power is likely to multiply in an ascending cycle, whereas powerlessness will only generate more powerlessness. Having power gives individuals a greater capacity toward accomplishment and therefore enhances their power in the organization. As managers gain power in an organization they are less coercive and less bound to rules, thus their peers and subordinates are more cooperative.

◆ Selecting Appropriate Political Strategies

It is necessary to develop savvy in political strategies so that hard-earned power is not lost through political mistakes. Even seasoned managers occasionally blunder in the political arena, causing power to be lost instead of gained.

Those in power may be attacked from many fronts. When these attacks occur, individuals who hold powerful positions often undermine themselves by regressing rather than progressing, and by being reactive rather than proactive.

It is useless to dispute the ethics or value of politics in an organization. Because politics exist in every organization, one wastes energy and remains powerless by refusing to learn the art and skill of political maneuvering. Instead, Menke and Ogborn (1993) suggest that time be spent learning the intricacies of political behavior. The following list of political strategies will assist the novice manager in developing political effectiveness:

1. *Information and Communication Strategies.* Be aware that facts can be presented seductively and out of context. The manager must be cautious in accepting facts as presented because information is often changed to fit the needs of others. Managers must become adept at the art of information acquisition.

   Decisions should be delayed until adequate and accurate information has been received. Managers must do their homework and should not allow themselves to be trapped into discussing something about which they know little. It is politically astute to say "I don't know" when inadequate information is available.

Grave political consequences can occur from sharing the wrong information with the wrong people at the wrong time. There is a discipline in nurturing the skill of determining who should know, how much they should know, and when they should know it.

Perhaps the most politically damaging communication error is lying to others. Withholding information or refusing to divulge information are good political strategies, but lying is not.

2. *Proactive Strategies.* Nurses have had a long history of being reactive, that is, reacting to what is being done to them. To be reactive is better than being passive, but the goal is to be proactive: to get the job done better, faster, and more efficiently. Proactive individuals see approaching changes in the health care system, and *prepare* to meet those changes.

One way to become proactive is by assuming authority. The proactive manager stops asking, "May I?" and instead assumes he or she may. In this way a powerful image is built. When individuals ask permission they are really asking someone to take responsibility for them. If something is not expressly *prohibited* in the organization or in a job description, the politically astute *assume* that it may be done. However, individuals do need to be aware that when they assume authority and something goes wrong, they will be held accountable, so this strategy is not without risk.

Another method of becoming proactive is by compiling personal resources so that one is prepared to meet the unpredictable future. Such resources include economic stability, higher education, and a broadening of one's skill base. This is often called the political strategy of having maneuverability. That is, the individual who avoids having limited options, who has "money in the bank and gas in the tank," has a political freedom of maneuverability that others do not.

Individuals lose power if others know they cannot afford to make a job change, or do not have the necessary skills to do so. Those who become economically dependent on a position lose political clout.

3. *Alliance and Coalition Strategies.* Nurses can often increase their power by forming alliances with other groups, thereby increasing their influence. Individuals can form associations with peers, sponsors, or subordinates from both within and outside their own group.

One of the most effective methods of forming alliances is through networking. Managers sharpen their political skills by becoming involved with peers outside the immediate organization. In this manner, the manager is able to keep abreast of current happenings and to solicit others for advice and counsel. For the nurse manager, there are probably no groups as valuable as the local and state nursing associations.

Networking and forming coalitions and alliances can also be effective within the organization. This strategy is especially desirable for some types of planned change. More power and political clout results when there are groups of people involved rather than individuals acting alone. When under political attack by others in the organization, group power is very useful.

4. *Conflict Resolution and Negotiation Strategies.* Because inappropriate conflict management can have grave political consequences, Chapter 18 in Unit 5 will examine these skills in depth.

5. *Timing and Sensitivity Strategies.* The successful manager develops a sensitivity to both the timing of certain actions as well as the appropriate actions to take. Occasionally, actions should be delayed, rules should be bent, or factors should be ignored. The individual who submits a request to attend a costly nursing conference on the same afternoon that his or her supervisor just had extensive dental work is insensitive to timing.

   The effective manager must also know when it is the appropriate time to do nothing. The passage of time itself often solves problems.

   The sensitive manager also knows when it is time to stop pressing an issue, before a superior has given a firm "no." Once a firm "no" decision has been reached, it is almost irreversible.

6. *Promoting Subordinate Identification as a Political Strategy.* There are many ways in which a manager can promote the identification of subordinates. Appreciation of a job well done works especially well when expressed in front of others. Writing subordinates sincere thank you notes, placing letters of commendation in employee's personnel files and rewarding employees for excellent work in other ways are also effective political strategies.

7. *Political Strategies for Meeting Organizational Needs.* Even extraordinary and highly visible activities will not result in the desired power unless those activities are used to meet organizational goals. Hard work rooted in purely personal gain will become a political liability.

   Frequently, novice managers think only in terms of their needs and their problems, rather than seeing the big picture. Additionally, individuals often look upward to find solutions to problems rather than attempting to find solutions themselves. When problems are identified it is more politically astute to take the controversy *and* a proposed solution upward rather than simply presenting the problem to the superior. Although the superior may not accept the solution, the fact that an attempt was made will probably be appreciated.

8. *Wellness Political Strategies.* Because political strength comes from the image others have of the individual, it is important to retain that image. Taking sufficient time for oneself to unwind, reflect, rest, and have fun, preserves that powerful image. Managers who do not take care of themselves are likely to begin to make mistakes in judgment. It is important to make time for significant interpersonal relationships and to develop outside interests so that other resources are available to rejuvenate the individual when political forces in the organization drain their energy. The manager who begins to look like a victim will undoubtedly become

one. The politically astute manager will always appear rested, full of energy, and will be articulate, poised, and courteous to both supervisors and subordinates. Power building and political strategies are summarized in Table 10-2.

◆ Summary

A manager's ability to gain and wisely use power is critical to success. To acquire this ability, managers must gain expertise in power building, political strategies, and in bridging the authority–power gap.

The successful manager uses legitimate authority and develops a powerful persona. Managers who recognize the dual pyramid of power will be less apt to abuse power and will use power and authority to increase respect for the position and for nursing as a whole. Those comfortable with power ensure that cooperation will be the goal of political maneuvers, and not personal gain. The successful manager will not seek to have power over others, but instead will empower them.

◇ TABLE 10-2
Power Building and Political Strategies

Power Building Strategies	Political Strategies
Expand personal resources.	Use information acquisition.
Present a powerful persona.	Communicate in an astute manner.
Pay the entry fee.	Become proactive.
Identify the powerful.	Assume authority.
Learn the organizational culture.	Network.
Use organizational priorities.	Expand personal resources.
Increase skills and knowledge.	Maintain maneuverability.
Have a broad vision.	Develop conflict management and negotiation skills.
Use experts and seek council.	Remain sensitive to people, timing, and situations.
Be flexible.	Promote subordinate identification.
Increase visibility and have a voice.	Meet organizational needs.
Toot your own horn.	Expand personal wellness.
Maintain a sense of humor.	
Empower others.	

◆ References

Edwards R (1994). Image practice and empowerment: a call to leadership for the invisible profession. Rev-J of Nurse Empowerment 4(1):18–20, 87

French J and Raven B (1959). The Bases of Social Power. In Cartwright D (ed): Studies in Social Power. Ann Arbor, MI: University of Michigan

Hawks J (1992). Empowerment in nursing education: concept analysis and application to philosophy, learning and instruction. J Adv Nurs, 17:608–618

Heineken J and McCloskey J (1985). Teaching power concepts. J Nurs Educat 24(1)

Huston CJ and Marquis BL (1988). Ten attitudes and behaviors necessary to overcome powerlessness. Nurs Connect 1(2)

Kippenbrock TA (1992). Power at meetings: strategies to move people. Nurs Econ 10(4):282–286

Marquis BL and Huston CJ (1996). Leadership Roles and Management Functions in Nursing, 2nd ed. Philadelphia: JB Lippincott

McCurdy JF (1988). Power is a nursing issue. In Muff J (ed): Socialization, Sexism, and Stereotyping. Prospect Heights, IL: Waveland Press

Menke K and Ogborn SE (1993). Politics and the nurse manager. Nursing Management, 24(12):35–37

Morrison EG (1988). Power and nonverbal behavior. In Muff J (ed): Socialization, Sexism, and Stereotyping. Prospect Heights, IL: Waveland Press

Porter S (1991). A participant observation study of power relations between nurses and doctors in a general hospital. J Adv Nurs 16:728–735

Reimer JM, Morrissey N, Mulcahy KA, and Bernat AL (1994). Power orientation: a study of female nurse and non-nurse managers. Nurs Manage 25(5):55–58

Sohier R (1992). Feminism and nursing knowledge: the power of the weak. Nurs Outlook 40(2):62–66

Staines G, Tavris A, and Jayaratne TE (1974). The queen bee syndrome. Psychol Today 7(8)

Strader MK and Decker PJ (1995). Role transition to patient care management. Norwalk, CT: Appleton and Lange

Willey EL (1990). Acquiring and using power effectively. In Hein EC and Nicholson MJ (eds): Contemporary Leadership Behavior, 3rd ed. Glenview, IL: Scott, Foresman/Little, Brown Higher Education

S A M P L E   C A S E   A N A L Y S I S

THE CASE OF LEMONS ◆

Sally Jones has been nursing director at Memorial Hospital for 2 years. She has made many improvements in the nursing department and is generally respected by the hospital administrator, the nursing staff, and the physicians.

The present situation involves the newly hired Assistant Administrator, Bob Wilson. Previously, the hospital had been too small to require an assistant administrator, but with growth this position was created. Since Mr. Wilson has been hired, he has shown obvious signs that he would like to increase his power and authority. One of the departments Mr. Wilson has been charged with is the personnel and payroll department. Until the present, nursing, which comprises 45% of all the personnel, has done its own recruitment, interviewing, and selection.

Mr. Wilson has now proposed that he hire an additional personnel clerk to do much of the personnel work for the nursing department, although nursing administration will be able to make the final selections in hiring. Mr. Wilson proposes that his department do the initial screening of applicants, check references, and so on.

It has become more and more frustrating for Ms. Jones to deal with what she perceives as the encroachment of Mr. Wilson. She has just received his latest proposal and has requested to meet with the hospital administrator and Mr. Wilson to discuss his plan.

Assignment

1. What danger, if any, is there for the nursing director in Mr. Wilson's proposal?
2. Be able to explain two political strategies you feel she could employ in the upcoming meeting.
3. Is it possible to facilitate a win–win solution to this conflict? If so, how? If there is not a win–win solution, how much *can* Mr. Wilson win?
4. Attempt to solve this case before reading further.

Analysis

In analyzing this case, it is necessary to forgo feelings of resentment regarding Mr. Wilson's obvious play for control and power. In reality, what actual danger does the director of nursing incur from Mr. Wilson's empire building attempts? Is she not simply eliminating clerical duties and interruptions in her time as well as that of her assistants?

There is a certain amount of power that is inherent in the hiring of individuals. It is true that employees develop a loyalty for the person who actually hires them. However, Ms. Jones, or her designee, will still be the individual who makes the final selection. Thus there should be little loss of loyalty or power as a result of Mr. Wilson's request to centralize the personnel and payroll department.

Let us examine what the real nursing director, Sally Jones, did to solve this conflict. She was capable of employing some very proactive strategies once she realized that Mr. Wilson was not depriving her of any power. Here was an opportunity for her to appear compromising, thereby increasing her esteem in the eyes of Jane Smith, the CEO, and at the same time gain political clout in the organization.

SAMPLE CASE ANALYSIS (CONTINUED)

When the nursing director met with the CEO and Mr. Wilson, she began by complimenting him on his ideas. She then suggested that since nurses were in the habit of coming to the nursing department to apply for positions and as personnel offices were rather cold and formal places, it would be more convenient and inviting if Mr. Wilson's new personnel clerk were stationed in the nursing office. She was aware that the new personnel department had inadequate space and that she had some extra room in the office for Mr. Wilson's clerk. She elaborated that some of her unit clerks were very knowledgeable about the hospital organization and he might want to interview several of them for the new clerk position. Although an experienced unit clerk would be difficult to replace, Ms. Jones said she was willing to make this sacrifice in order for Mr. Wilson's plan to succeed.

The CEO was very impressed with the nursing director's generous offer. She turned to Mr. Wilson and said, "I think Sally has an excellent idea. Why don't you hire one of her clerks and put her in the nursing office?" The CEO then said to Ms. Jones, "Now it is understood that the clerk will be Mr. Wilson's employee and will work under him?" The nursing director was in agreement with this, since she felt she had just pulled off a coup. Let's examine what she managed to win in this political maneuver.

1. The nursing director gained by not competing with Mr. Wilson, therefore not making him an enemy.
2. She gained by impressing the CEO with her flexibility and initiative.
3. She gained a new employee. Although the new employee will be working for Mr. Wilson, with the salary charged to his cost center, the clerk would be a former employee of nurse Jones. Since the clerk would be working in the nursing office there would be some allegiance to her. In addition, the clerk would be doing all the work that nurse Jones and her assistants had been doing and at no cost to the nursing department.

When the nursing director first received Mr. Wilson's memo, she was angry and her initial reaction was to talk with the CEO privately and complain about Mr. Wilson. Fortunately, she did not do this. It is most often a political mistake for one manager to talk about another manager behind their back and without their knowledge. This generally reflects unfavorably on the employee, with a loss of respect from the supervisor.

Another option the nursing director had was to compete with Mr. Wilson and be uncooperative. This might have delayed centralization of the personnel department, but in the end Mr. Wilson undoubtedly would have accomplished his goal, and Ms. Jones, at a later date, would not have been able to reap such a great political victory.

The later effects of this political maneuver were even more rewarding. The personnel clerk remained loyal to Ms. Jones and constantly "leaked information" to her regarding the personnel department and Mr. Wilson. He became less of an adversary and began to cooperate more with the director on other issues, and the CEO gave her a sly grin later in the month and said, "Great move with Bob Wilson." This case might be concluded by saying that this is an example of "someone being given a lemon and then making lemonade."

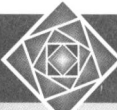 **CASES FOR PROBLEM SOLVING**

CASE 1

You have been a registered nurse for 3 years. Six months ago you left your position as a day charge nurse at one of the local hospitals and took a position at the public health agency. You really miss your friends at the hospital and find most of the public health nurses older and aloof.

However, you love working with your caseload of clients and have decided this is where you want to build a lifelong career. You feel you have some good ideas, but you are aware that since you are so new to the agency you will probably not be able to be a change agent at this time. In the future, you would like to be promoted to the position of agency supervisor and be capable of being a powerful force for stimulating positive growth within the agency. You decide that there are some things you can do to build a power base and you spend a weekend plotting your political design.

Assignment

Make a power building plan. Give specific examples of six to 10 things you would do to build a power base in the new organization. Give your rationale for each selection. (Do *not* merely select from the general lists in the text, but outline *specific* actions *you* would take.) *Note:* It might be helpful to the reader to consider his or her own community and personal strengths when solving this case.

CASE 2

After 5 years as a public health nurse, you have just been appointed supervisor of the western region of the county health department; there is one supervisor for each region, plus a nursing director and an assistant director. You were selected over a field of four other applicants to fill the position. You have eight public health nurses who report directly to you.

The area where you feel there needs to be change involves some of the nurses on various health committees in the area. In the past both the physician–medical director and the nursing director have viewed this community responsibility as part of their job and part of the job of each supervisor. Staff nurses have not been expected to serve on such advisory boards or committees, such as the local hospice advisory board, the cardiac rehabilitation board, the heart association education committee, and many others.

You would like the nurses under your supervision to become more involved on such committees for several reasons. You want them to be more visible and have a greater voice in the organization. Also, you believe that being a nursing professional includes the responsibility to contribute to the community.

You have decided your first planned change will be to increase the number of nurses on these committees. You thought that you would begin by asking one of the regular nursing staff to accompany you when you attended the four committee meetings to which you have been assigned. At present, you are the only public health agency nurse who meets with each group, but other nurses from

CASE 2 (CONTINUED)

the university and local hospitals do attend. Not all the nurses who attend these meetings are classified as administrative.

....

Assignment

1. Devise a political strategy for successfully involving the public health nurses on your committees.
2. Where is the danger of your plan being sabotaged? What change tactics can you use to ensure success?
3. What are the political advantages and disadvantages of making a change fairly soon after being appointed a nurse manager?

CASE 3

You are the charge nurse of the day shift for the small intensive care unit. One of your nurses, Jane Smith, has just requested a week off to attend a conference. She is willing to use her accrued vacation time for this and to pay the expenses herself. The conference is in 1 month and you are a little irritated that she had not made her request sooner. Ms. Smith's request conflicts with the vacation already granted to another nurse. The other nurse requested her vacation 3 months ago.

Therefore, you deny Ms. Smith's request, explaining that you will need her to work that week and you cannot spare her to go to the conference. She protests, stating that the educational conference will benefit the ICU repeating that she will bear the cost of the conference. You are firm but polite in your refusal.

Later, Ms. Smith goes to the supervisor of the unit to request the time. The supervisor upholds your decision, but you are furious that Ms. Smith has not pursued the chain of command.

....

Assignment

1. What, if any, further action will you take with Ms. Smith or her request?
2. Decide what your approach should be and support your decisions with political rationale.

CASE 4 (from Marquis and Huston, 1996)

You are a 3–11 P.M. team leader on a medical unit of a small community hospital. On leaving the report room, John, the day shift team leader, tells you that Mrs. Jackson, a terminally ill patient with cancer, has decided to check herself out of the hospital "against medical advice." John states that he has already contacted Mrs. Jackson's doctor, who expressed his concern that the patient would have inadequate pain control at home as well as undependable family support. He feels that she will die within a few days if she leaves the hospital. However, he did leave orders for home prescriptions and a follow-up appointment.

You immediately go in to Mrs. Jackson's room to assess the situation. She tells you that the doctor has told her that she will probably die within 6 weeks,

CASE 4 (CONTINUED)

and that she wants to spend what time she has left at home with her little dog, who has been her constant companion for many years. In addition, she has many things to put in order. She states that she is fully aware of her doctor's concerns and that she was already informed by the day shift nurse that leaving "against medical advice" may result in the insurance company refusing to pay for her current hospitalization. She states that she will be leaving in 15 minutes when her ride home arrives.

When you go to the nurse's desk to get a copy of the home prescriptions and follow-up doctor's appointment for the patient, the ward clerk states, "The hospital policy says that patients who leave against medical advice have to contact the physician directly for prescriptions and an appointment, because they are not legally discharged. The hospital has no obligation to provide this service. She made the choice—now let her live with it." She refuses to give a copy of the orders to you and places the patient's chart in her lap. Short of physically removing the chart from the ward clerk's lap, it is clear that you have no immediate access to the orders.

You confront the charge nurse, who states that the hospital policy does give that responsibility to the patient. She is unsure what to do, and has paged the unit director, who appears to be out of the hospital temporarily.

You are outraged. You feel the patient has the "right" to her prescriptions because the doctor ordered them, assuming she would receive them before she left. You also know that if the medications are not dispensed by the hospital, there is little likelihood that Mrs. Jackson will have the resources to have the prescriptions filled.

Five minutes later, Mrs. Jackson appears at the nurse's station, accompanied by her friend. She states she is leaving and would like her discharge prescriptions.

• •

Assignment

The power struggle in this scenario involves you, the ward clerk, the charge nurse, and organization politics. Does the ward clerk in this scenario have informal or formal power? What alternatives for action do you have? What are the costs and/or consequences of each possible alternative? What action would you take?

CASE 5

You are the director of a small Native American Health Clinic. Other than yourself and a part-time physician, your only professional staff are two RNs. The remainder of your staff are from the local population and have been trained by you. The following is a description of the two RNs.

Nurse Bennett is a 26-year-old BSN with several years of experience working at a large southwestern community health agency. She is familiar with many of the problems of the local clientele. She is hardworking and extremely knowledgeable, although occasionally her assertiveness is mistaken for bossiness among the Native American workers. However, everyone respects her judgment.

Nurse Mikiou is a 34-year-old male Native American. He began his career as a medic in the Vietnam war and attended several career-ladder external degree programs until he was able to take the registered nursing exam. He does not

CASE 5 (CONTINUED)

have a baccalaureate degree. His nursing knowledge is occasionally limited and he tends to be very casual about performing his duties. However, he is competent and has never displayed unsafe judgment. His humor and good nature often reduce tension in the clinic. The Native American population is very proud of him and this results in a special relationship with them. However, he is not a particularly good role model as his health habits leave much to be desired. In addition, he is frequently absent from work.

Ms. Bennett has come to find Mr. Mikiou intolerable. She feels she has tried working with him but this is difficult because she does not respect him.

As the director of the clinic, you have tried many ways to resolve this problem and to alleviate the many conflicts in this case. You feel especially fortunate in having Ms. Bennett on your staff. It is difficult to find many nurses of her quality willing to come and live on a desolate Native American reservation. On the other hand, you feel that the local work force must be utilized and promoted if the Native American health concept is really going to work. You feel that local Native Americans must be educated and placed in the agencies so that one day they can run their own clinics. However, it is very difficult to find educated Native Americans who wish to return to this reservation.

You are now faced with a management dilemma. A dilemma is often described as a choice between two wrongs. Ms. Bennett has said either Mr. Mikiou must go or she will. She has asked you to decide.

Assignment

What are the power issues involved in this case? Decide which wrong choice will be least damaging. Justify your decision.

◆ **Bibliography**

The following references will assist you in solving these cases:

Alm TG (1991). Power in nursing. J Adv Nurs 16(5):503

Bocchino CA and Sharp NJ (1995). Health care policy issues: Nursing politics and power. In Vestal KW (ed), Nursing Management: Concepts and Issues, 2nd ed. Philadelphia: JB Lippincott

Brown CL and Schultz PR (1991). Outcomes of power development in work relationships. J Nurs Admin 21(2):35–39

Carlson-Catalano J (1992). Empowering nurses for professional practice. Nurs Outlook 40(3):139–142

Chisholm M (1991). Use and abuse of power. Clin Nurse Specialist 5(1):57

Dobos CL (1990). Big fish in a big pool: empowerment, assertiveness and risk taking among nurses. Todays OR Nurse 12(8):12–16

Erlen JA and Frest B (1991). Nurses perceptions of powerlessness in influencing ethical decisions. Western J Nurs Res 13(3):397–407

Hawks JH and Hromek C (1992). Nursing practicum: empowering strategies. Nurs Outlook 40(5):231–234

Kanter RM (1994). Collaborative advantage: the art of alliances. Harvard Bus Rev July/August, 96–108

Kerfoot KM (1990). To manage by power or influence: the nurse manager's choice. Nurs Econom 8(2):117–118

Mason DJ, Backer BA, and Georges A (1991). Toward a feminist model for the political empowerment of nurses. Image: J Nurs Schol 23(2):72–77

Murphy SZ (1994). Don't be a doormat: personal empowerment in nursing. Revolution 4(2):66–68

Sabiston JA and Lascbinger HKS (1995). Staff nurse work empowerment and perceived autonomy: testing Kanter's theory of structural power in organizations. JONA 25(9):42–50

Tebbitt BV (1993). Demystifying organizational empowerment. JONA 23(1):18–23

PERSONAL NOTEBOOK

1. Think back to your childhood. Who did you feel was the most powerful figure in your family? Why did you think that person was powerful?

2. Did you grow up with a very small authority–power gap? Did that change as you grew older? Have your views regarding authority and/or power changed since you were a child, or are your views still very similar to earlier ones?

3. Do you feel that young children today have as narrow an authority–power gap as you did when you were growing up? Support your answer with examples.

4. When have you felt powerful and when have you felt powerless? Which produced the strongest feelings?

STAFFING

Every administrator will be judged by the quality of persons with whom he surrounds himself.

—*Albert Lepanesky*

The health care industry is labor intensive, with a work force composed of a highly skilled professional staff; therefore, managing staff so that the work of the organization is accomplished is an important function for all levels of managers.

The staffing function begins at the planning level of management because the philosophy and fiscal resources of the organization help influence the mix and size of the staff. Likewise, staffing is also affected by the type of patient care delivery system used to manage patient care, since some types of patient care management require a higher percentage of registered nurses to other nursing personnel.

Other factors impacting on the staffing function of management are:

1. The type and number of nursing personnel available.
2. The competitiveness of salaries and benefits offered.
3. The attrition rate of the organization.
4. The ability of managers to select and match personnel to job requirements.
5. The resources available for staff development.
6. The utilization of centralized or decentralized staffing and management.
7. The ability of the manager to create a motivating climate.

Fiscal planning, philosophy, and types of patient care management, all of which impact on the management function of staffing, have been reviewed in previous chapters. The first staffing function is to determine the specific positions and numbers of personnel necessary in order to fulfill the philosophy and goals, while keeping within the budgetary constraints of the organization. The following are the sequential steps of the staffing functions, but each step has some interdependence with all staffing activities.

1. Determine the number and types of personnel needed to fulfill philosophy, meet fiscal planning responsibilities, and carry out the selected method of patient care delivery.
2. Recruit, interview, select, and assign personnel based on established job description performance standards.
3. Use staff development resources to orient, train, socialize, and develop selected personnel.
4. Effect creative and flexible scheduling based on patient care needs to increase productivity and at the same time meet employee needs.

Recruitment, Interviewing, and Selection

In complex organizations, managers cannot function alone, as their time and energies are limited. Work must be accomplished by groups of people, and wise managers attempt to surround themselves with people with ability, motivation, and promise. Managers should seek the most talented individuals available to fill positions and not settle for mediocrity. The ability of the organization to meet its goals and objectives is directly related to the quality of the individuals it employs. Managers who recruit, identify, and hire gifted individuals prevent stagnation, increase productivity, and increase their own value to the organization.

◆ The Role of the Manager in Recruitment, Interviewing, and Selection

Managers may be closely involved with recruitment, interviewing, and selection or their involvement may be minimal, depending on: 1) the size of the institution, 2) the existence of a separate personnel department within the organization, 3) the presence of a nurse recruiter, and 4) the use of centralized or decentralized nursing management.

When management is decentralized and the personnel department is not complex, involvement of lower level managers in recruitment, selection, and interviewing of personnel for their units is greater (Huston and Marquis, 1989).

◆ Recruitment

Recruitment is the process of actively seeking out qualified applicants for existing positions in organizations in a cost-effective manner. Recruitment requires long-term planning and continuous efforts if the organization is to be proactive in recruiting and retaining a highly qualified staff. Unfortunately, many institutions fail to assess their staffing needs adequately and do not plan well for the future. In the last 25 years there have been acute nursing shortages, often followed by a nursing surplus, with a later reoccurrence of a nursing shortage. During shortages and surpluses organizations often use reactive strategies to bring about a quick resolution of the immediate problem. These reactive strategies have included major layoffs of nurses during organization downsizing and offering excessive hiring bonus during periods of nursing shortages.

Although at any given time an organization may have an adequate supply of registered nurses to meet demand, historical data supports the idea that recruitment should generally constitute an ongoing process (Stratton et al., 1991). Recruitment is critical when organizations restructure because skills needed for a job may be complex and it becomes even more important that there be a good fit between the individual and the job. A successful match between individual and job begins with recruitment efforts (Wells and Mueller, 1996).

◆ Recruitment Variables

Successful recruitment of an adequate workforce is dependent on many variables, including:

1. Resources available for advertisement, recruitment literature, and visits to career day programs.
2. Number of new and experienced nurses available.
3. Competitiveness of the organization's salaries and benefits.
4. Attractiveness of the setting to the potential workforce.
5. The reputation of the organization regarding past employment practices and quality of patient care.
6. The status of the national and local economy.

It is easier to recruit adequate numbers of nurses when there are several local schools of nursing, a progressive community with a mild climate, and an organization that has a good reputation for quality patient care and fair employment practices. It is much more difficult to recruit nurses to rural areas that historically have experienced less appropriation of health care professionals per capita than urban areas (Stratton et al., 1991). Factors contributing to the maldistribution of nurses include substandard salaries, fewer opportunities for professional development and continuing education, and a shortage of ancillary health care professionals (ANA, 1989).

The manager should understand the impact of the national and local economy on the ability of the institution to maintain an adequate work force (Buerhaus, 1993). When the national economy is on an upswing there is usually a nursing shortage nationwide. However, when the economy worsens nursing jobs become more scarce, often making it difficult for new graduate nurses to obtain positions (Marquis, 1988).

◆ Steps in the Recruitment Process

Lyles and Joiner (1986) identified the following five steps in the recruitment process.

1. Organizational policies regarding recruitment should be reviewed prior to the advertisement of job positions.
2. All possible sources of potential applicants must be identified.
3. The optimum mode of publicizing job vacancies must be determined.
4. The recruitment need and qualifications required must be stated.
5. The response to the recruitment effort should be evaluated and adjusted as needed.

◆ Recruitment Challenges: 1990–2000

Because nursing shortages are cyclical, some experts predict a shortage again by the end of this decade. Styles and Holzemer (1986) predict that by the year 2000, there will be about one-half as many nurses as needed. Aiken (1990) predicts that future nursing employee pools will be inadequate. This is especially true for the baccalaureate degree nurses.

Prior shortages consisted of inadequate numbers of working nurses in specialized areas and in specific parts of the country. The nursing pool itself was adequate to meet the need, thus the solution centered on recruiting inactive nurses and drawing from the new graduate nurse pool (Neubs, 1991).

These predictions are very different from other reports that many hospitals will continue to downsize and use more unlicensed assistive personnel, creating a large surplus of registered nurses (Pew, 1991). Buerhaus (1993) sees the registered nurse market as unpredictable, extremely difficult to accurately forecast, varying by region, complex, and influenced by intertwined forces.

Presently, it appears that entry-level positions for the most part are being adequately filled. However, critical care and home health positions continue to require recruitment to meet demand. Additionally, because of the increased competitiveness of health care facilities there is an even greater need to be able to recruit and replace key people in an organization in a timely manner (Wells and Mueller, 1996). Perhaps the greatest challenge for recruitment is in obtaining an adequate diversified candidate pool to meet the needs of a culturally diverse patient population. The need for nurses with multiple language skills and in-depth understanding of other cultures will become increasingly important by the year 2000.

◆ The Relationship Between Recruitment and Retention

Although retention is not the primary focus of this chapter, it is important to remember that retention and recruitment are very closely linked. Longo and

Uranker (1987) stated that hospitals should adopt the premise, "A nurse retained is a nurse recruited," and that the retention of a nurse exemplifies the hospital's protection of its investment. Many organizations could vastly decrease the need for external recruitment if retention–recruitment programs were more closely aligned and given equal priority.

Retention is more than reducing the rate of turnover to some preordained level (Young and Hayne, 1988). Some turnover is normal, and in fact desirable. Turnover rids the organization of undesirable employees and infuses the organization with fresh ideas. It also reduces the probability of groupthink, where all individuals in the organization share similar thought processes, values, and goals. However, excessive or unnecessary turnover is not only expensive, but reduces the ability of the organization to produce its end product.

Competent, proficient, and expert-level nurses promote needed revolutionary and evolutionary changes. Their value must be recognized with financial differentiation for experience and longevity. Furthermore, they deserve the added prestige of having their value recognized by their membership and leadership in participative management and shared governance (Sovie, 1988). These strategies will increase retention in the organization.

◆ Interviewing

Interviews are still the most common method used for the selection of new employees. Interviews usually involve an exchange of information between the person applying for the job and an individual representing that organization. Organizations differ regarding who interviews candidates for positions. However, it is becoming quite common for first- and middle-level managers to have some input into the interview process since this is an appropriate time to create a bond between the employee and their immediate supervisor. Regardless of who does the interviewing, there are some guiding principles that will aid the interviewer in conducting successful interviews.

◆ Prior to the Interview

1. Review the application and note any points that may require further investigation.
2. Develop standardized interview questions to be asked of each applicant. These should be nondirective, open-ended questions. Avoid superficial questions. Devise questions that give you an insight into the applicant's understanding of the organization's values, his or her philosophy of nursing, and interpersonal and communication skills. Examples of such questions are:
   a. Why did you apply to this facility?
   b. What key issues do you see this organization and the health care industry on the whole facing in the next few years?

c. What do you find most challenging about working with other people?

d. What do you think separates nursing from all the other health care professions? What makes nursing unique?

e. What have you learned about yourself since you became a nurse that keeps you motivated in this profession?

f. What is your greatest strength?

In addition to determining in advance what should be asked of the applicant, the interviewer needs to understand recent civil rights legislation that limits what can be asked in the interview. By law, the interviewer cannot ask questions about age, marital status, children, race, sexual preference, financial or credit status, national origin, or religion (Swansburg, 1990). Often this information will be volunteered by the applicant in response to questions from the interviewer, but this information should not be used as a basis for making a hiring decision. Table 11-1 summarizes legal and illegal interview inquiries.

3. Have enough time allotted to conduct the interview without interruptions (allow at least 20–30 minutes for each applicant).

◆ At the Time of the Interview

1. Maintain uninterrupted privacy and a comfortable environment.

2. Use a standardized interview outline.

3. Listen actively and be aware of the applicant's nonverbal communication.

4. Do not fully describe the available position until after you have explored the candidate's background and future plans. It is important to note that in the suggested interview format, all information from the applicant is collected prior to giving much detail about the position requirements and the organization. This is done to avoid leading the applicant into giving answers based on what he or she thinks the interviewer wants to hear.

5. Give written material as well as verbal information regarding the position, as applicants frequently forget important details.

6. Identify both the positive and the negative aspects of the position.

7. Be gracious throughout the interview. The applicant might not be right for the position or the applicant could decide the position is not right for himself or herself, but this is an important public relations connection and you are representing your organization to an individual, often for the first time.

8. In concluding the interview, be certain that the candidate knows what the subsequent steps are in the selection process.

◆ Following the Interview

1. Follow up with each applicant as soon as possible, thanking him or her for the application and informing the applicant if he or she is being offered the position.

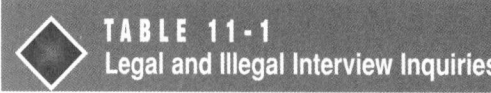

TABLE 11-1
Legal and Illegal Interview Inquiries

Subject	Acceptable Inquiries	Unacceptable Inquiries
Name	If applicant has worked for the company under a different name. If school records are under another name. If applicant was convicted of a crime under another name.	Inquiries about name that would indicate lineage, national origin, or marital status.
Marital and family status	Whether applicant can meet specified work schedules or has commitments that may hinder attendance requirements. Inquiries as to anticipated stay in the position.	Any question about applicant's marital status, or number or age of children. Information about child care arrangements. Any questions concerning pregnancy.
Address or residence	Place of residence and length resided in city or state.	Former addresses, names or relationships of persons with whom applicant resides, or if owns or rents home.
Age	If over 18 or statement that hire is subject to age requirement. Can ask if applicant is between 18 and 70.	Inquiry into specific age or date of birth.
Birthplace	Can ask for proof of U.S. citizenship.	Birthplace of applicant or spouse or any relative.
Religion	No inquiries allowed.	
Race or color	Can be requested for affirmative action, but not as employment criteria.	All questions about race are prohibited.
Character	Inquiry into actual convictions that relate to fitness to perform job.	Questions relating to arrests.
Relatives	Relatives employed in company. Names and addresses of parents if applicant is a minor.	Questions about relatives not employed in company. Number of dependents.
Notice in case of emergency	Name and address of a *person* to be notified.	Name and address of a *relative* to be notified.
Organizations	Professional organizations.	Requesting a list of all memberships.
References	Professional and/or character reference.	Religious references.
Physical condition	All applicants can be asked if they are able to carry out the physical demands of the job.	Employers must be prepared to justify any mental or physical requirements. Specific questions regarding handicaps are forbidden.
Photographs	Statement that a photograph may be required *after* employment.	Requirement that a photograph be taken *prior to* interview or hiring.
National origin	If necessary to perform job, languages in which applicant is fluent.	Inquiries about birthplace, native language, ancestry, date of arrival in United States, or native language.
Education	Academic, vocational, or professional education, schools attended. Ability to read, speak, and write foreign languages.	Inquiries into racial or religious affiliation of a school. Inquiry into dates of schooling.

(continued)

TABLE 11-1 (CONTINUED) Legal and Illegal Interview Inquiries		
Subject	Acceptable Inquiries	Unacceptable Inquiries
Sex	Inquiry or restriction of employment is only for bona fide occupational qualification, which is interpreted very narrowly by the courts.	Cannot ask sex on application. Sex cannot be used as a factor for hiring decisions.
Credit rating	No inquiries.	Questions about car or home ownership are also prohibited.
Other	Notice may be given that misstatements or omissions of facts may be cause for dismissal.	

(Adapted from Huston and Marquis, 1989.)

2. A candidate not offered a position should receive some explanation regarding the reasons for his or her elimination.
3. Inform applicants who receive job offers what the preemployment procedure is (i.e., physical exam, chest X-ray) and dates to report to work.
4. Request that applicants being offered positions confirm in writing their intention to accept the position.

◆ Weakness of Interviews

Although interviews remain the most common selection process (Dorio, 1994), research has shown that there is little correlation between how an applicant is rated in interviews and later job performance. In fact, some studies have indicated that managers often make up their minds about a potential applicant within the first 60 seconds of the interview (Marquis and Huston, 1996). Interviews contain many hazards. Among those hazards are the biases, prejudices, and subjective emotions of the interviewer. Another hazard involves "the halo effect" or being overly impressed with one aspect of the applicant. Or there may be a "horns effect" of being overly critical based on one aspect of the applicant. However, perhaps the greatest weakness in interviews lies in the failure of the interviewer to listen.

◆ Methods to Overcome Weaknesses of Interviews

In addition to the principles listed previously for conducting successful interviews, the following will assist the interviewer in overcoming some of the weaknesses of the interview process.

1. Have the applicant interviewed on two separate occasions.
2. Have the applicant interviewed and rated by more than one person.
3. Use a planned, structured, nondirective interview format.
4. Use other data to make the final selection in addition to the interview, such as:
   a. school records
   b. prior employment records
   c. letters of reference

◆ Selection

Selection is the process of choosing from among applicants the best qualified individual(s) for a particular position or job. Jernigan (1988) maintains that the selection process is difficult because you must find the best qualified individual who is willing to accept the position using only an application form and often slanted references.

Selection as the last step in the employment process can only be successful if recruitment and interviewing have been done appropriately. Successful recruitment yields an adequate pool of qualified applicants. A carefully implemented interview process provides invaluable feedback to both the employer and the applicant regarding the expectations of the position and the unique strengths, weaknesses, needs, and desires of each applicant.

Figure 11-1 illustrates a typical selection process. The applicant pool is generated in response to recruitment and should yield an adequate number of qualified and motivated applicants. The applicant pool then undergoes preemployment screening. This screening is usually done on a one-on-one basis (although it may be done in small groups) and involves the employer sharing information about minimum qualifications required of potential applicants, as well as a brief outline of employer expectations for a given position. If both the potential employee and employer feel that there is a match between expectations, the candidate should continue through to the completion of the application. Information given in the application is then used in following up on references and in the interview process. Preemployment testing and physical examinations may be required by the employer. The last step of the selection process is employer decision and notification of applicants.

There should be a good match between the qualifications of the applicant and the position requirements. Often more than one individual is well qualified, so a greater weight may be placed on which of the final candidates would best fit into the present work group. Mills and Oie (1992) suggest that selection teams made up of staff nurses provide a better selection for fit than does a nursing manager.

Placement of the employee in an appropriate position in the organization is the end result of a carefully implemented selection process. Faulty placement can result in sacrifices to organizational efficiency, threats to institutional integrity, frustration of personal and professional ambitions, and feelings of failure. Conversely, proper placement promotes personal and organizational growth, satisfaction, stability, and prosperity. Ideal placement represents an integration of

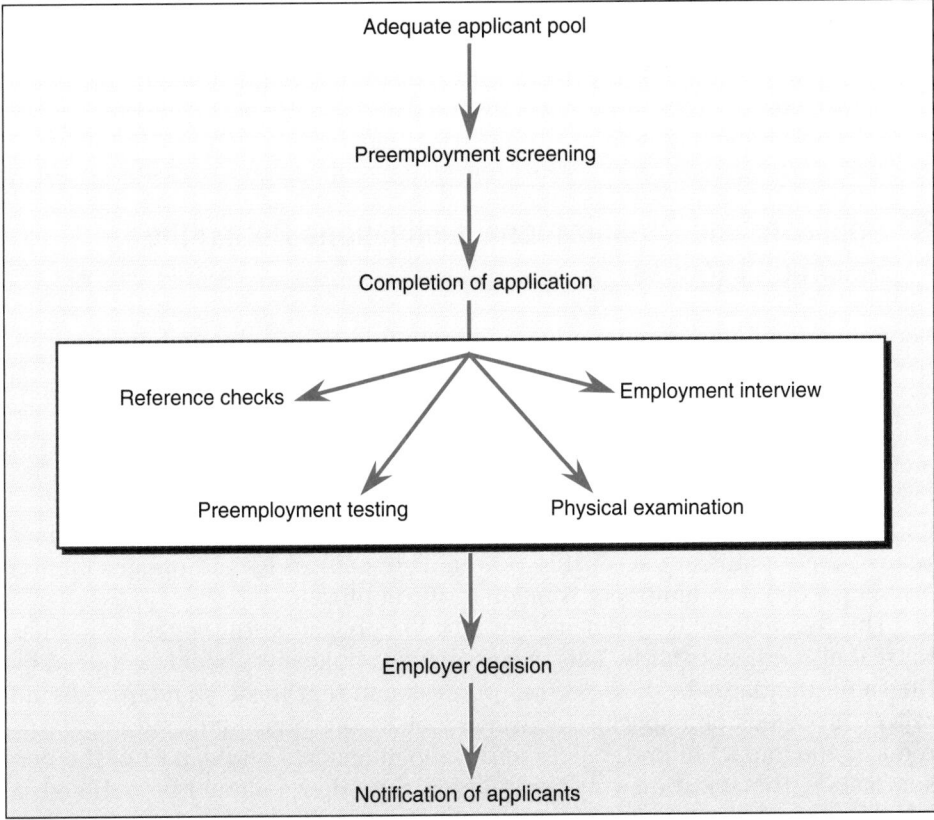

FIGURE 11-1.
The selection process.

organizational and individual goals and is obvious by the subsequent productivity and success of the employee and the meeting of organizational goals.

◆ Processing the Application

All applications should be examined to see if they are complete and to ascertain that the applicant is qualified for the position. This is also the time when references and verification of former employment are requested. Usually, the personnel department carries out some of these functions. Once this data has been received, all qualified candidates should be scheduled for interviews and/or testing to complete the selection process.

◆ The Paper Trail of the Selection Process

Four primary sources of information are available to use in the selection process. These include the application form and/or resume, interview impressions, test results, and references from past employers. Dorio (1994) warns that academic and professional credentials are the least checked applicant items. No single source of information should be weighed disproportionately in the selection decision. Of these four sources, two are composed mostly of a paper trail. These are the application form and/or resume, and references from past employers.

◆ Applicant and Organizational Obligations During the Selection Process

Because selection involves a process of reduction, that is, diminishing the number of candidates for a particular position, the individual making the final choice for the organization has two vital concerns: control and responsibility. The "control" element refers to the control the organization has in selecting the employees that it wants. The individual(s) making the selection decision has control over decisions that have a tremendous impact on individual lives. It is imperative that selectors recognize how much power they have and guard against any unethical use of this power. This control by the organization is given up when a commitment is made to the applicant.

The "responsibility" element refers to the obligation the organization has to treat all applicants fairly. This means that all applicants should be judged by the same standards in the selection process and that these standards should reflect the needs of a specific job. Having clear-cut, preestablished standards reduces the impact of preferences and value judgments on the part of the person making the selection. Any flexibility in the criteria should be outlined in advance for all individuals.

It is important to remember that the final selection decision involves human beings and thus is never a totally objective process. There are always circumstances that modify selection as a scientific process, such as urgency of need, ratio of applicants to the number of openings, rigidity of the selection criteria, and the appeal, promises, and needs of the applicants.

The organization is also compelled to bring a complete and timely closure to the selection process. All applicants should be notified in writing of the selection decision in as timely a manner as possible. Individuals being offered positions should receive formal notification at the same time as those who are not. The applicant also has the responsibility to be honest and forthright regarding his or her qualifications, needs, and wants.

◆ Selecting an Assistant

Because managers must delegate so many aspects of work it is especially important for the manager to carefully select individuals for positions close to them in the chain of command. This might be a supervisor appointing charge nurses for each shift, or selecting an assistant manager. It could be a manager appointing a supervisor or a director of nursing choosing an assistant, or even hiring a ward clerk or secretary.

Regardless of the level of appointment, the effective manager will examine all available candidates for any assistant position carefully. Del Bueno and Freund (1986) maintain that such selection has far-reaching implications, including a possible struggle for power at some future date. The manner of the selection of individuals for these positions is often watched closely by members of the staff and therefore every effort must be made to ensure fairness. The following suggestions are helpful in selecting an assistant:

1. Select an individual with a compatible philosophy. It is very difficult to work closely with someone who has a completely different view of nursing and life than you have. The manager ends up wasting time convincing the assistant of the value of every decision. However, the candidate should not be a clone of the existing manager.
2. Choose individuals with different strengths and weaknesses than your own. Selecting someone different from the existing manager makes it possible both to compensate for each other's weaknesses and to complement each other's strengths. It is especially helpful when accomplishing the total work necessary in any organization for there to be differences in leadership styles and abilities among those in management positions.
3. Select an individual who can be a good follower. This does not mean a blind follower. A good follower is loyal, but will tell leaders when they are in error, demonstrating the ego strength and wisdom to question inappropriate decisions of leaders.

◆ Summary

The productivity and potential of any organization is directly related to the quality of the personnel it employs. Ongoing recruitment allows institutions to bring the most qualified personnel to an institution. After applicants have been recruited, the nursing manager, using prespecified criteria, has the critical responsibility of seeing to it that the best applicant is hired for the position. This requires skill in interviewing and other selection processes to ensure that all applicants are evaluated against the same standards and that personal bias is minimized.

Selection is the final step in the employment process and epitomizes the goals of human resource planning. When an employee is selected and placed appropriately within the organization, goals become shared and worker satisfaction is high. Employee and organizational productivity rises and retention increases.

◆ References

Aiken LK (1990). Charting the future of hospital nursing. Image 22(2):72–78

American Nurses Association (1989). Statement on Rural Nursing. Kansas City, MO

Buerhaus P (1993). Effects of RN wages and non-wage income on the performance of the hospital RN labor market. Nurs Econ 11(3):129–135 del Bueno DJ and Freund CM (1986). Power and Politics in Nursing Administration: A Casebook. Owing Mills, MD: National Health Publishing, Rynd Communications

Dorio M (1994). Staffing: Problem Solver for Human Resource Professionals and Managers. New York: Wiley

Huston C and Marquis B (1989). Retention and Productivity Strategies for Nurse Managers. Philadelphia: JB Lippincott

Jernigan DK (1988). Human Resource Management in Nursing. Norwalk, CT: Appleton and Lange

Longo RA and Uranker MM (1987). Why nurses stay: a positive approach to the nursing shortage. Nurs Manage 18(7):78–79

Lyles RI and Joiner C (1986). Supervision in Health Care Organizations. New York: Wiley

Manio EB (1995). Cross-cultural issues in the hiring and selection of Asian staff. Semin Nurse Manag 3(1):40–42

Marquis BL and Huston CJ (1996). Leadership Roles and Management Functions, 2nd ed. Philadelphia: JB Lippincott

Marquis B (1988). Attrition: the cost effectiveness of retention activities. J Nurs Admin 18(3):25–29

Mills J and Oie M (1992). Autonomous staff selection teams. JONA 22(12):57–63

Neubs HP (1991). The nursing shortage: Crisis as opportunity. JONA 21(3):5,36

Pew Health Professions Commission (1991). Healthy America: Practitioners for 2005. Durham, NC

Sovie MD (1988). Clinical nursing practices and patient outcomes: evaluation, evolution, and revolution. Nurs Econom 7(2)

Stratton TD, Dunkin JW, Juhl N, Ludtke RL, and Geller JM (1991). Recruiting and retaining registered nurses in rural community hospitals. J Nurs Admin 21(11):30–34

Styles MM and Holzemer WL (1986). Educational remapping for a responsible future. J Profess Nurs 2(1):30–34

Swansburg R (1990). Management and Leadership for Nurse Managers. Boston: Jones and Bartlett

Wells RW and Mueller JF (1996). Revisioning the recruitment of talented professionals. JONA 26(1):21–30

Young LC and Hayne AN (1988). Nursing Administration: From Concepts to Practice. Philadelphia: WB Saunders

SAMPLE CASE ANALYSIS

THE CASE ◆

As a new manager of the oncology unit at Hillside Hospital you must *plan* your staffing needs. You begin by drawing up a list of five minimum criteria that RNs must have before they will be considered for hire.

••

Assignment

Would new graduates meet the criteria? If you were that head nurse, what would be your five minimum criteria? Include any special requirements, years of experience, education, and so on. Justify your selection for each criteria. Remember there are both pros and cons to very selective criteria.

••

Analysis

In order to set minimum criteria, it is essential that the manager have an understanding of the job at hand. The position should be analyzed and the qualifications necessary to complete each task should be identified.

A job description should be developed if this has not already been done. In this situation, the following might be identified as the duties of the job.

1. Administration of oral, intravenous, and intramuscular medications, including chemotherapeutic drugs.
2. Assisting patients with activities of daily living (eating, bathing, hygiene, comfort measures).
3. Planning, supervision, and evaluation of the care of all patients. This includes supervision of unlicensed personnel and vocational or practical nurses.
4. Conducting patient education as specified by hospital policy and in the individual patient care plan.
5. Working collaboratively with physicians in the planning and implementing of patient care.
6. Communicating clearly using both verbal and written documentation of nursing assessments, interventions, and needs.
7. Assisting patients and significant others in coping psychologically with the oncological disease process. Actively participating in hospice counseling.

Once the job requirements have been identified, it becomes easier to recognize the qualifications needed to perform those duties. Usually, hiring criteria fall within three distinct categories—skills, knowledge, and personal attributes. Skills indicate a person's ability to do something, whereas knowledge refers to learning obtained through education or experience. Personal attributes refer to personal characteristics that promote a cooperative and productive work environment. Based on the cited job requirements, the manager might choose the following minimum criteria for hiring.

The applicant must:

1. Be a graduate of an accredited school of nursing.
   Rationale: Assumes that applicant has achieved at least an acceptable minimum nursing knowledge and experience level.

SAMPLE CASE ANALYSIS (CONTINUED)

2. Possess a valid and current license to practice nursing in the state of practice.
   Rationale: Meets legal and licensing requirements for the institution.
3. Have the ability to direct and supervise the work of subordinate personnel.
   Rationale: The oncology unit utilizes RNs, LVNs/LPNs, and nonlicensed personnel in the administration of patient care. A registered nurse is responsible for overseeing the care of subordinate personnel.
4. Have 2 years experience in medical-surgical nursing. Oncology nursing experience is highly preferred.
   Rationale: Oncology patients are frequently acutely ill, requiring the assessment and intervention expertise gained only through nursing experience.
5. Have completed a Chemotherapy Certification Course approved by the Hillside Hospital Education Department.
   Rationale: The administration of chemotherapeutic drugs on an oncology floor is a frequent practice. Such drugs have specific indications for use, as well as special precautions in their preparation and use. A requirement of staff to complete such a course prior to their being considered for hire could also be an indication of the staff's interest in the subject area and motivation to become a part of the oncology unit.

The five listed criteria suggest that the philosophy of the head nurse and the institution is that oncology nursing is a complex type of nursing that requires nursing expertise and some prerequisite knowledge in the subject area. Therefore, it would not be appropriate to hire new graduate nurses. These criteria, however, are not so restrictive as to discourage the motivated new graduate with an interest in oncology from pursuing the educational and work experience required for oncology nursing in the future. Having selective criteria will limit the number of potential applicants, but results in a greater probability that the abilities of the applicant and the requirements of the job will be more closely matched.

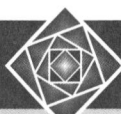

CASES FOR PROBLEM SOLVING

CASE 1 (From Marquis and Huston, 1996)

You are the ICU/CCU supervisor and are interviewing Sam Haught, a prospective charge nurse for your evening shift. Mr. Haught is currently the critical care director at Daleview Hospital, the other local facility and your organization's primary competitor. He is leaving Daleview Hospital because of personal reasons.

Mr. Haught, well qualified for the position, has strong management and clinical skills. Your evening shift requires an assertive manager with excellent clinical skills. You feel very fortunate that he is applying for the position.

Just before the close of the interview, however, Mr. Haught shuts the door, lowers his voice secretively, and tells you he has vital information regarding

CASE 1 (CONTINUED)

Daleview Hospital's plans to expand and reorganize its critical care unit. He states he will share this information with you if you hire him.

Assignment

How would you respond to Mr. Haught? Will you hire him? Identify the major issues in this situation. Support your decision with your rationale. Do you see any possible conflicts between your personal values and those of the organization in such a situation?

CASE 2

You are the administrator of nursing at Valley Home Health. The manager of one of the major client districts (district 2) has just given 8 weeks notice of her intent to resign and the CEO has called an executive cabinet meeting to discuss her replacement. You have been given full authority to execute the selection process.

You are aware that the current manager of the Home Aides and Equipment Rental Division of Valley Home Health would like to have the job. She is well qualified and energetic, and you have had a close and supportive working relationship with her over the last 7 years. You have every reason to believe that this relationship will continue if she is promoted to client manager. The staff is highly supportive of hiring from within the organization.

However, you are also aware that hiring from within can lead to internal stagnation and that the organization can only be as strong as the managers who represent it. There is adequate time to do a thorough search. A job search outside the organization could yield additional applicants who are highly qualified for the job, but also brings the risk of "the unknown."

Assignment

Determine an appropriate course of action. What are the greatest risks of hiring within? The greatest benefits? If an outside applicant had the same qualifications as the current director at Valley Hospital, which employee would you hire? How did your personal values impact your decision making?

CASE 3

As the director of nursing, you are frequently asked to write letters of reference for those who have terminated their employment. The information you use in composing these letters comes from performance evaluations, personal interviews with staff and patients, evidence of continuing education, and your personal observations. You have collected the following information on Mary Dorland, an RN who worked at your facility for 3 months before abruptly resigning with a 48 hour notice.

CASE 3 (CONTINUED)

Performance Evaluation

Three month evaluation scant. The following criteria were marked competent: 1) amount of work accomplished, 2) relationships with patients and coworkers, 3) work habits, and 4) basic skills.

The following criteria were identified as needing improvement: 1) quality of work, 2) communication skills, and 3) leadership skills. No criteria were marked either unsatisfactory or outstanding. Narrative comments were limited to the following:

Has a bit of a chip on her shoulder.

Works independently a lot.

Assessment skills improving.

Interviews with Staff

1. *Coworker RN Cortland:* "She was OK. She was a little strange—she belonged to some kind of traveling religious cult. In fact, I think that's why she left her job."
2. *Coworker LVN/LPN Mesa:* "Mary was great. She got all her work done. I never had to help her with her medications or A.M. care. She took her turn at floating, which is more than I can say for some of the other RNs."
3. *Coworker RN Hill:* "When I was the charge nurse, I found I needed to seek her out to find out what was going on with her patients. It made me real uncomfortable."
4. *Coworker LVN/LPN Schooster:* "Mary hated it here—she never felt like she belonged. The charge nurse was always hassling her about little things and it really seemed unfair."

Patient Comments

1. "She helped me with my bath and got all my pills on time. She was a good nurse."
2. "I don't remember her."
3. "She was so busy—I appreciated how efficient she was at how she did her job."
4. "I remember Mary—she told me she really liked older people. I wish she had had more time to sit down and talk to me."

Notes from Personnel File

Twenty-four years old. Graduated from 3 year diploma school 2 years ago. Has worked in three jobs since that time. Divorced, the mother of two small children.

Continuing Education

Current CPR card. No other continuing education completed at this facility.

Assignment

Nurse Dorland's prospective employer has requested a letter of reference to accompany her application to become a hospice nurse-counselor. No form has been provided. Decide which information you should include in your letter and which should be omitted. Will you weight some information more heavily than

CASE 3 (CONTINUED)

other? Would you make any recommendations about Ms. Dorland's suitability for the hospice job? Be prepared to read your letter aloud to the class and justify the rationale for its content.

CASE 4 ◆

You are the supervisor of a critical care surgical unit. For several years you have been experimenting with placing four newly graduated nurses directly into the critical care unit; two from each spring and fall graduating classes. These nurses are from local BSN programs and you consult their former nursing faculty and employer closely prior to making a selection.

Overall, this experiment has worked well. You have thus far had only two new graduates who were unable to develop into critical care nurses initially. However, both of them transferred back after 2 years on a medical-surgical unit.

Because of their motivation and enthusiasm, the new graduates have been a nice compliment to your experienced critical care staff. You feel your success with this program has been owing to your: 1) well-planned and structured 2 month orientation and education program, 2) careful selection, and 3) appropriate shift placement.

This spring, you have narrowed the selection down to four acceptable and well-qualified candidates. You plan to place one on the 3–11 P.M. shift and one on the 11 P.M.–7 A.M. shift. You sit in your office and review the "culture" of each shift, as well as your notes on the four candidates. You have the following information:

3–11 P.M. shift: Very assertive all female staff: 85% RNs and 15% LVNs/LPNs. This is your most clinically competent group. They are highly respected by everyone and although the physicians often have confrontations with them, they also frequently tell you how good they are. These nurses are known as a group that lacks humor and who are not openly welcoming of newcomers. However, once the new employee earns their trust, they are very supportive. They are very intolerant of anyone not living up to their exceptionally high standards. Your two unsuccessful new graduate placements occurred on this shift.

11 P.M.–7 A.M. shift: Very cohesive and supportive group: 65% RNs and 35% LVNs/LPNs. Although competent overall, this shift has some of your more clinically weak staff. However, it is also the shift that rates the highest with families and patients. They are caring and compassionate and every new graduate you have placed on this shift has been successful. There is a large number of male nurses (30%) on this shift. The group tends to be very close and has a high number of outside social activities together.

Your four applicants consist of the following:

John Davis—30-year-old male. Has had a great deal of experience as an emergency room medical technician. Appears somewhat aloof. Has definite career goals (i.e., 2 years in critical care, 3 years in the emergency room, and then flight nursing). Instructors praised his independent judgment, but felt he needed to be more of a "team player" in school. Former employers have called him an independent thinker and very capable.

Jennie Cho—22-year-old female. At the top of her class, both clinically and academically. Has not had much work experience until the last 2 years as a summer nursing intern at a major medical center, where her performance appraisals were very good. Instructors felt she lacked some maturity and interpersonal skills, but praised her clinical decision making ability. Does not want to work in a regular medical-surgical unit and feels "she can adapt to critical care."

CASE 4 (CONTINUED)

Joan Feld—38-year-old female. Has had a great deal of health-related experience in counseling, but limited clinical nursing experience (only nursing school). Former employers praised her attention to detail and her general competence. Instructors praised her interpersonal skills, maturity, and intelligence. She is willing to work elsewhere if not selected for the critical care position. Has a long-term commitment to nursing.

Susan Young—28-year-old female. Was previously an LVN/LPN and returned to school to get her bachelor's degree. Did less well academically owing to working and family commitments. Former employers and instructors spoke of her energy, organization, and interpersonal skills. Appears to have fewer independent decision-making skills than the others. Has previously worked in a critical care unit.

Assignment

Select the two new graduates you will hire. Place them on the appropriate shift. Support the decisions with your rationale.

CASE 5

Gina Long is the supervisor of a 16-bed ICU/CCU in the 200-bed Metro Hospital. She has been the supervisor for 8 years and is respected and well liked by her staff. Her staff retention level and productivity are higher than any other unit in the hospital.

Supervisor Long relies heavily on Mark Rudd, her permanent charge nurse on the day shift for the last 6 years. He is bright, motivated, and has excellent clinical and management skills. It is fair to say that Mr. Rudd's work has greatly increased her scope of power and enhanced the reputation of the unit. He seems satisfied and challenged in his current position, although she has not had any formal career planning meetings with him to discuss his long-term career goals.

Recently, one of the physicians approached supervisor Long regarding wanting to open an outpatient cardiac rehabilitation program. The program will require a strong leader and manager who is self-motivated. It will be a great deal of work, but also provides many opportunities for advancement. He suggests that Mr. Rudd would be an excellent choice for the job, although he has given supervisor Long full authority to make the final decision.

Supervisor Long is aware that Lynn Ingram, a bright and dynamic staff nurse from the open heart surgery unit, would also be very interested in the job. Nurse Ingram has only been employed at Metro Hospital for 1 year, but has a proven track record and would probably be very successful in this position. In addition, there is a staffing surplus right now on the open heart surgery unit, as the census has declined. It would be time-consuming and difficult to replace Mr. Rudd as charge nurse in the ICU/CCU.

Assignment

What process should supervisor Long use to determine who should be selected for the position? Should the position be posted? When does the benefit of using transfers/promotions as a means of reward outweigh the cost of reduced productivity? Is an autocratic decision justified? State why or why not.

CASE 6 ◆

You are the manager of an inner-city drop in medical clinic that is partially subsidized by the city. The majority of your clients are Blacks, Asians, and Hispanics. The majority of your RN nursing staff are Caucasians.

Recently you have felt that some of the problems with lack of compliance with prescribed medical regimen and frequent no-shows at appointments is owing to cultural and language issues. You would like to increase the cultural and ethnic diversity of your staff but do not know what is an appropriate and fair method to meet this goal. The city has given you a $5,000 budget to be used in any way in order to assist with meeting your goal.

Assignment

Make a list of at least five methods that would assist you in meeting your goals. Determine if they are fair and nondiscriminatory to all concerned. Will the use of these methods result in your ability to select the best qualified applicants for the positions available?

◆ Bibliography

The following is a list of references to help you solve these cases:

Birkenstock M (1991). Recruitment and retention: strategies for keeping good nurses. Assoc Operat Room Nurses J 53(1):110–114, 116–118

Cassidy J (1991). Desperately seeking nurses: recruitment and retention strategies. Health Progr 72(4) May:14–16

Curtain LL (1995). Job security: is nothing sacred anymore? Nurs Manage 26(7):7–9

Jackson BS (ed) (1996). The job that didn't fit. JONA 26(1):9–11, 30

Labig CE Jr. (1990). Effectiveness of recruiting sources for staff nurses. J Nurs Admin 20(7/8):12–17

McCluskey RL and Erickson B (1990). Selection of talented employees is no accident. Provider 16(4):26–27

Muller-Smith P (1995). Management. Tomorrow's workplace: no jobs . . . just work to be done. J Post Anesthesia Nurs 10(3):172–174

Nash J (1990). Turn it around: make the interview work for you. Todays OR Nurse 12(11):12–16

Ott MJ, Esker S, and Caserza C (1990). Peer interviews: sharing the hiring process. Nurs Manage 21(11):32–33

Pattan JE (1991). Nurse recruitment: from selling to marketing. J Nurs Admin 21(9):16–20

Perspectives on the changing job market (1995). Nurs Econ 13(1):23

Sanniti JK, McAliley LG, and Urbancic CJ (1990). Selection, promotion and development of employees. Nurs Manage 21(1):30–1, 34

Schaffner M (1990). Interviewing orientation and evaluation. Gastroenterol Nurs 12(3):172–178

Smeltzer CH, Tseng S, and Harty LM (1991). Implementing a strategic recruitment and retention plan. J Nurs Admin 21(6):20–28

Zimmerman PG (1994). Nursing layoffs are not the answer. J Emerg Nurs 20(6):468–474

PERSONAL NOTEBOOK

It is the policy at North Creek Hospital to limit the hiring of new graduate nurses to 10 per year. The remaining open positions are held for experienced nurses. In addition, North Creek Hospital believes that the new graduates they do hire should represent a variety of schools so that inbreeding will not occur. Therefore, competition is extremely high among your classmates.

You have been called for an interview. You want a job at North Creek Hospital very much. Outline what your approach will be during the job interview. What can you say and do that will convince the nursing director to hire you? Outline your plan and your rationale for selecting that particular approach. Be sure to list your strengths and weaknesses for the position.

Staff Development

CHAPTER
12

The knowledge levels and capabilities of employees have a direct correlation to the number of staff required to carry out the goals of the unit. Therefore, the development and education of staff is an important function of management. The better trained the work force, the fewer numbers are required. Thus, staff development is a cost-effective measure for increasing productivity.

Early staff development emphasis was on orientation and in-service training. In the last 20 years, however, other forms of education have become commonplace in health care organizations. Management development, certification classes, and continuing education courses to meet relicensure requirements are now a part of many staff development programs.

In most organizations, staff development consists of three separate but interrelated activities: 1) induction, orientation, and socialization, 2) in-service training, and 3) continuing education. The manager has varying degrees of responsibility regarding each of these areas, depending on the size and type of organization, the resources available, and the manager's job description. The responsibilities for these activities are usually shared with the personnel department and the staff development or in-service department.

◆ Induction, Orientation, and Socialization

Those activities that help a new employee to "fit in" or become socialized to the organization are induction, orientation, and socialization. They also provide employees with enough information and training to be able to perform the responsibilities of the position for which they were hired. Induction, orientation, and socialization are as necessary for individuals acquiring a new position within their present organization as it is for new employees. Therefore, it is important that employees who are transferred or promoted also receive staff development.

INDUCTION

The first phase of staff development is induction and takes place after the employee has been selected, but prior to performing the job role. The induction process includes all activities that educate the new employee about the organization as well as employment and personnel policies and procedures.

Induction activities are often performed during the placement and preemployment functions of staffing or may be included as part of orientation. The information and activities that should be included during the entire induction, orientation, and socialization process are shown in Display 12-1.

The employee handbook is an important instrument of induction. Handbooks are usually written by the personnel department, but managers should be aware of what they contain and have some input into their composition. Most employee handbooks contain a form that must be signed by the employee, verifying that they have received and read it, and this signed form is then placed in the employee's personnel file.

To ensure understanding, the information presented in the handbook must be followed by a discussion with various knowledgeable individuals during the orientation process. The most important link in promoting comprehension of personnel policies is the first-level manager.

ORIENTATION

There is a wide variety of orientation programs to choose from, and many larger organizations offer more than one type. For example, a hospital may have a first-day orientation conducted by the personnel department. This includes a tour of the hospital, in addition to all of the items listed in Display 12-2. The next phase of the orientation program could take place in the staff development department, where aspects of concern to all employees such as fire safety, accident prevention, and health promotion would be presented. Orientation to each unit or department is the third phase. Specific departments, such as dietary, pharmacy, and nursing would each be responsible for their own programs of orientation.

Because induction and orientation involve many different individuals from a variety of departments, they must be carefully coordinated and planned to achieve preset goals. The overall goals of induction and orientation include providing employees with information that will smooth their transition into the new work setting. New employees who take part in a formal orientation program reach independent and adequate functioning sooner and remain in the organization longer than employees who receive none (Alspach, 1990). Orientation programs also increase retention and productivity as well as prevent burnout by promoting the situational support that has been shown to reduce work stress (Brooks, Wilkinson, and Popkess-Vawter, 1994).

DISPLAY 12-1
Employee Orientation Content

1. Organization history, mission, and philosophy.
2. Organization service and service area.
3. Organizational structure, including department heads, with an explanation of the functions of the various departments.
4. Employee responsibilities to the organization.
5. Organizational responsibilities to the employee.
6. Payroll information, including how increases in pay are earned and when they are given. (Progressive and/or unionized companies publish pay scales for all employees.)
7. Rules of conduct.
8. Tour of the organization and of the assigned department.
9. Work schedules, staffing, and scheduling policies.
10. When applicable, a discussion of the collective bargaining agreement.
11. Benefit plans, including life insurance, health insurance, pension, and unemployment.
12. Safety and fire programs.
13. Staff development programs, including in-service, and continuing education for relicensure.
14. Promotion and transfer policies.
15. Employee appraisal system.
16. Work load assignments.
17. Introduction to charting.
18. Review of selection policies and procedures.
19. Specific legal requirements, such as maintaining a current license, reporting of accidents, and so on.
20. Introduction to fellow employees.
21. Establishment of a feeling of belonging and acceptance, showing genuine interest in the new employee.

Note: Much of this content could be provided in an employee handbook, and the fire and safety regulations could be handled via a media presentation. *Appropriate* use of video tapes or film strips can be very useful in the design of a good orientation program. All indoctrination programs should be monitored to see if they are achieving their goals. Most programs need to be revised at least annually.

It is important to examine productivity and retention as the orientation program is planned, structured, and evaluated. Organizations should periodically review their induction and orientation program to determine if it is continuing to meet ultimate goals. Programs that are not satisfying organizational concerns should be restructured. For example, if employees consistently lack information regarding the institution's benefits program, this part of the induction process should be evaluated to determine the cause. Too often, various

DISPLAY 12-2
Responsibilities for Orientation

1. *Personnel Department:*
   Perform salary and payroll functions, insurance forms, physical exams, income withholding forms, tour of the organization, employee responsibilities to the organization and vice versa, additional labor–management relationships, and benefit plan.
2. *Staff Development Department:*
   Hand out and review employee handbook, discuss organizational philosophy and mission, review history of the organization, show media presentation of various departments and how they function (if a media presentation is not available, introduce various department heads and share how departments function), organizational structure, fire and safety programs, CPR certification and verifications, discussion of available educational and training programs, review selected policies and procedures, and general charting of medication and treatment policies.
3. *The Individual Unit:*
   Tour of the department, introductions, review of specific unit policies that differ in any way from general policies, review of unit scheduling and staffing policies and procedures, work assignments, promotion and transfer policies, review appraisal system, and establishing a feeling of belonging, acceptance, and socialization.

individuals having partial responsibility for induction and orientation "pass the buck" regarding the failure of, or the weaknesses in, their given program. It is the joint responsibility of the personnel department, the staff development department, and each nursing service unit to work together to provide an orientation mechanism that meets employee and organizational needs.

An adequate orientation program minimizes the likelihood of rules violations, grievances, and misunderstandings, fosters a feeling of belonging and acceptance, and promotes enthusiasm and morale. A sample 2 week orientation schedule is shown in Display 12-3.

SOCIALIZATION

Orientation is usually inadequate in itself to ensure that employees are properly socialized into the organization. Socialization differs from orientation in that it involves little structured information. Rather, it is a sharing of the values and attitudes of the organization by the use of role models, myths, and legends. It is during socialization that the leader introduces employees to the special values and culture of the organization.

Much has been written about the importance of socializing new members into their professional role, and research has documented the importance of this process in the prevention of burnout and the promotion of retention and a

DISPLAY 12-3
Sample Two-Week Orientation Schedule
for Experienced Nurses

Week One
Day one, Monday:

8:00 A.M.–10:00 A.M.	Welcome by Personnel Department; employee handbooks distributed and discussed.
10:00 A.M.–10:30 A.M.	Coffee and fruit served; welcome by staff development department.
10:30 A.M.–12:00 M.	General orientation by staff development.
12:00 M.–12:30 P.M.	Tour of the organization.
12:30 P.M.–1:30 P.M.	Lunch.
1:30 A.M.–3:00 P.M.	Fire and safety films; body mechanics demonstration.
3:00 P.M.–4:00 P.M.	Afternoon tea and introduction to each unit supervisor.

Day two, Tuesday:

8:00 A.M.–10:00 A.M.	Report to individual units. Time with unit supervisor; introduction to assigned preceptor.
10:00 A.M.–10:30 A.M.	Coffee with preceptor.
10:30 A.M.–12:00 M.	General orientation of policies and procedures.
12:00 M.–12:30 P.M.	Lunch
12:30 P.M.–4:30 P.M.	CPR recertification.
Day three, Wednesday:	Assigned all day to unit with preceptor.
Day four, Thursday:	Assigned all day to unit with preceptor.
Day five, Friday:	Morning with preceptor, afternoon with supervisor and staff development for wrap-up.

Week Two

Monday to Wednesday:	Work with preceptor on shift and unit assigned, gradually assuming greater responsibilities.
Thursday:	Assign 80% of normal assignment with assistance and supervision from preceptor.
Friday:	Carry normal workload. Have at least a 30 minute meeting with immediate supervisor to discuss progress.

professional identity (Kramer, 1974; Lynn, McCain, and Boss, 1989; Strader and Decker, 1995).

It is not only for the novice professional that organizational socialization is critical. Adequate socialization of *all* employees has been shown to reduce attrition. It is during the socialization phase that employees should be instilled with high morale and enthusiasm. Employees must be socialized and molded so there is a good fit between the employee and the organization (Johnson, 1994).

The impressions an employee forms during the first weeks in a new job are significant because sensitivity is heightened by the normal anxiety experienced in a new environment. Therefore, it is essential that the manager be supportive during this time.

Kramer and Schmalenberg (1988) state that one of the major roles of leaders in magnet hospitals is to generate enthusiasm down to the very last worker. The ability to instill and clarify the values system of the organization to new employees is a part of the socialization process that creates the team approach found in excellent organizations.

◆ The Socialization Process

Among sociologists, the phenomenon of socialization has generally revolved around role theory. That is, we learn the behaviors that accompany each role via two simultaneously occurring processes. One is referred to as an *interactional process* and involves both groups and significant others in a social context. The other is referred to as a *learning process* and includes such mechanisms as role playing, identification, modeling, operant learning, instruction, observation, imitation, trial and error, and role negotiation (Hardy and Conway, 1988).

Brim (1966), an early pioneer in resocialization, believed that efforts toward this end would be more effective if it could be determined why the individual was having difficulty. He maintains that there are usually three areas where problems occur, which include:

1. *ignorance of the particular role prescriptions and expectations,*
2. *inability to meet role demands,* and
3. *deficiencies in motivation.*

Some employees have little difficulty with the process of resocialization, but most experience some stress when there is role change. Organizations can plan in advance to ease the stress of resocialization by the conscious use of appropriate interventions.

Effective interventions for role clarification include well-written job descriptions and the use of role models, preceptors, and mentors. Mentors are discussed in Chapter 14.

1. *Role Models.* Individuals who are role models serve as examples of experienced employees who are competent in performing their role. The relationship between the new employee and the role model is passive. That is, employees see that role models are skilled and attempt to emulate them, but the role model does not actively seek this emulation. One of the exciting aspects of role models is their cumulative effect. The greater the number of excellent role models available for new employees to emulate, the greater the possibilities for them to perform well (Kramer and Schmalenberg, 1988).

2. *Preceptors.* Although the educational process in role modeling is passive, preceptoring is active and purposeful. A preceptor is an experienced nurse who both provides emotional support and is a strong clinical role model for the new nurse. A preceptorship provides both role socialization for the new nurse and recognition of the preceptor's excellence in nursing practice (Coudret et al., 1994). The preceptor should serve as both role model and teacher in the clarification of role expectations. Preceptors need an adequate knowledge of adult learning theory if they are to fulfill their role in the socialization process. Careful selection of preceptors will assist the organization in role definition.

If difficulties in resocialization occur as a result of motivational deficiencies, then a planned program of reorientation to the defined goals should occur through the use of rewards and punishment. These and other forms of motivational strategies and interventions will be discussed in Chapter 14.

◆ Employees with Special Needs

Positive socialization is directly related to retention and productivity of employees. Although Kramer's (1974) research has been used as a foundation for new graduate intern programs, little attention has been paid to the resocialization needs of other employees. Resocialization occurs when:

1. New graduates leave nursing school and enter the work world.
2. The experienced nurse undertakes a new role and undergoes role status change.
3. The experienced nurse changes work settings, either within the same organization or by moving to a new organization.

◆ The New Nurse

Kramer (1974) described special fears and difficulties in adapting to the work setting common to new graduate nurses. Kramer called this phenomenon "reality shock" and stated it occurred as a result of a conflict between the new graduate's expectations of the nursing role and its reality in the actual work setting.

The four phases of role transition from student nurse to staff nurse are: the honeymoon phase, followed by the shock, recovery, and resolution phases. They maintain that cultural conflict occurs because the values in the school and work subcultures differ.

There are few difficulties in the honeymoon phase, as long as the novice nurse is sincerely welcomed into the work place. However, during the second phase of reality shock, there is often great personal conflict, as the nurse discovers that many nursing school values are not appreciated in the work place. Usually the new graduate will be correctly resocialized if the manager and the organization takes appropriate action during the recovery and resolution phases.

There are several mechanisms managers employ to ease the role transition of new graduates. Anticipatory socialization carried out in educational settings should prepare the new nurse for the inevitable reality shock. Managers should also build into their orientation program opportunities for sharing and clarifying values and attitudes about the nursing role overall. Use of the group process is an excellent means of promoting the type of sharing that provides support for new graduates and assists them in recovering from reality shock (Schumacher and Meleis, 1994).

Additionally, managers should be alert for the signs and symptoms of the shock phase of role transition and intervene by listening to new graduates and assisting them in coping with the real world. Some of the values of the new nurse should be supported and encouraged, so that there is a blending of work and academic values. New professionals need to understand the universal nature of the process they are experiencing and realize it is not limited to nurses. Providing a class on role transition may also be helpful in assisting new graduates in resocialization.

Kramer's work has been substantiated by other researchers who have studied professionals in their first year of employment. No one is immune to a loss of idealism and commitment in response to stress in the work place, but it is during the first year of employment that the greatest change in attitude and behavior takes place (Johnson, 1994; Schumacher and Meleis, 1994).

Following the publication of Kramer's work, many hospitals began to look at methods that could be used in their orientation programs to alleviate some of the shock experienced on entering nursing. Some hospitals developed prolonged orientation periods for new graduates that lasted from 6 weeks to 6 months. This extended orientation, called an *internship,* contrasts sharply from the routine 1–2 week orientation normal for other employees. During this period the graduate nurse is usually assigned to work with a preceptor and gradually takes on a patient assignment equal to that of the preceptor. Presently, many hospitals have discontinued internship programs owing to their expense, but have continued with the preceptor concept of teaming a new graduate with another nurse.

◆ Employees with a Role Status Change

Although the orientation of new managers is often neglected, there is growing recognition that good managers do not emerge from the work force without a great deal of conscious planning on the part of the organization. A management development program should be ongoing and every individual should receive some instruction prior to an appointment to a management position (Verbey, Valentine, and Harrison, 1992).

The orientation by the outgoing manager should be relatively short, especially when the newcomer is familiar with the organization. If the new manager has been recruited from outside the organization, the period may need to be extended. A short orientation by the outgoing manager allows the newly appointed manager to quickly gain control of the unit and establish their own management style.

Frequently, a new manager will be appointed to a position that is vacant, or one that is newly established. In either case, there will be no one readily available to orient the new manager. In such cases it is necessary that the immediate superior appoint someone to orient the new manager.

The orientation does not cease following the short period spent introducing them to the various tasks of their job. Every new manager needs guidance, direction, and continued orientation and development during their first year in this new role. This kind of direction comes from several sources in the organization, specifically:

1. *The new manager's immediate superior*
2. *A group of the new manager's peers*
3. *A mentor*

Nurses undergoing a change in status often experience guilt as they leave the bedside for other nursing duties. When employees and physicians see a nurse manager assuming the role of caregiver, they often make disparaging remarks such as, "Oh, you're working as a *real* nurse today." This tends to reinforce values conflict of the nurse in the new role.

Nurses moving into positions of increased responsibility also experience stress created by ambiguity and overload. *Role ambiguity* describes the stress that occurs when job expectations are unclear. *Role overload* occurs when the demands of the role are excessive. Scalzi (1988) demonstrated that role overload is a major stress factor for nurse managers. All of these elements of stress make the transition of nurses moving into higher status positions difficult.

The second most valuable mechanism that organizations use to assist in this type of resocialization is a clear understanding of role expectations. As nurses move into increased status positions their job descriptions tend to become increasingly vague. Therefore, clarifying job definitions becomes an important tool in the resocialization process.

◆ The Experienced Nurse in a New Position

Another transition occurs when an experienced nurse decides to make a lateral transfer within the same organization, takes another position that is considerably different from the previous role, or takes a similar position in another organization. These nurses have specific orientation needs that arise from: 1) transition from expert to novice, and 2) transition from the familiar to the unfamiliar.

The managers of departments receiving frequent transfers should prepare a special orientation program for experienced nurses transferring to that department. In addition to providing necessary staff development content, these orientation programs should focus on efforts to promote the self-esteem of these nurses as they learn the skills necessary for success in their new roles.

For example, when a nurse moves from a medical floor to labor and delivery, the nurse does not know the group norms, is unsure of expected values and behaviors, and goes from being an expert to being a novice. All of these create a great deal of role strain. This same type of role stress occurs when experienced nurses move from one organization to another. Nurses often sense a feeling of powerlessness during these role transitions, which may culminate in anger and frustration, as they seek to become socialized to a different role.

Managers should not assume that the experienced nurse is aware of the expected role attitudes necessary for a new role. Excellent hospitals have leaders who take responsibility for shaping the values of all employees. By instilling and clarifying organizational mores to new employees, managers are able to create a homogeneous staff who work as a team (Kramer and Schmalenberg, 1988).

◆ Education and Training

The pendulum tends to swing back and forth regarding who is responsible for the education and training within a department. At one time this was a shared responsibility between managers and in-service education, but in the 1970s, education departments enlarged and managers willingly relinquished their responsibilities for the education and training of their personnel.

Managers assumed that between the personnel and staff development (or in-service) department, orientation of the new employee would be complete. This often resulted in much frustration on the part of the employee, because although they received an overview of the organization, they received little orientation to the specific unit. Since each unit has many idiosyncrasies, the new employee was left feeling inadequate and incompetent. The latest trend in orientation is for the nursing unit to take a greater responsibility for individualizing the orientation to their unit (Tucker, 1987; Asselin and Barber, 1991).

This has occurred as a result of fiscal concerns, the awareness of the need to socialize new employees at the unit level, and the recognition of the positive effect well-skilled workers have on the productivity of employees. It is now generally accepted that the ultimate responsibility for staff training and education rests with the manager, although the manager does not personally provide all aspects of staff development.

There are some difficulties associated with decentralized staff development (Gillies, 1994). One of these difficulties is the conflict caused by role ambiguity created whenever two people share responsibility. Role ambiguity is sometimes lessened when staff development personnel and managers distinguish the difference between training and education.

Early staff development emphasis was on orientation and in-service training. However, in the last 20 years, other forms of education have become commonplace in health care organizations. Management development, certification classes, and continuing education courses to meet relicensure requirements are now a part of many staff development programs.

Education and training are cost-effective measures for increasing productivity. Only since World War II has a systematic program of education and training become a part of business and industrial management functions.

EDUCATION

Education is more formal and broader in scope than training. Although training has an immediate use, education is designed to develop the individual over time. Recognizing educational needs and encouraging educational pursuits is the responsibility of the manager. However, unless managers have expertise in a particular area, they would not normally be responsible for the formal education of an employee. Managers may appropriately be requested to give a formal class, if qualified to do so, but this would be not be considered a regular management function.

TRAINING

Training may be defined as an organized method of ensuring that people have knowledge and skills to satisfy a specific purpose. This means acquiring the necessary knowledge to perform the duties of the job. The knowledge may require an increase in affective, motor, or cognitive skills. It is expected that newly learned skills will be used to increase productivity and/or create a better product. Every manager at every level must assume some responsibility for the training of the employees they supervise.

◆ Theories of Learning

Since all managers teach employees as a normal part of their role, it is necessary that they be familiar with adult learning theories. Use of the following teaching–learning principles enable the trainer to alter employee behavior, which is the end goal of all employee training.

◆ Adult Learning Theory

Many managers attempt to teach adults as they themselves were taught in school, using pedagogy or child learning strategies. This type of teaching is usually ineffective for adult learners, who have special needs. Knowles (1970) distinguished the concept of androgogy or adult learning, separating the adult from the child learner. Table 12-1 summarizes the basic differences between the two learners. Adult learners are mature, self-directed individuals who have acquired a great deal of knowledge from life experiences and are focused on solving problems that exist in their immediate environment.

By understanding the assets the adult learner brings to the classroom and the obstacles that might interfere with their learning, trainers and educators

TABLE 12-1
Pedagogy and Androgogy Characteristics

Pedagogy	Androgogy
Learner is dependent.	Learner is independent.
Learner needs external rewards and punishment.	Learner is internally motivated.
Learner's experience is unimportant or limited.	Learner's experiences are valued and varied.
Subject-centered.	Task- or problem-centered.
Teacher-directed.	Self-directed.

are able to create a learning environment that is effective. Table 12-2 depicts the obstacles to and assets for adult learning and Table 12-3 shows how the child and adult learning environment should differ.

Sullivan and Decker (1988) suggest that Knowles' studies have the following implications for trainers and educators.

1. A climate of openness and respect will assist in the identification of what the adult learner wants and needs to learn.
2. Adults enjoy taking part in and planning their learning experiences.
3. Adults should be involved in the evaluation of their progress.
4. Experiential techniques work best with adults.
5. Mistakes provide opportunities for adult learning.
6. If the value of past experience is rejected, the adult will feel rejected.
7. Adult readiness to learn is greatest at the point when they recognize that there is a need to know (i.e., in response to a problem).

TABLE 12-2
Obstacles to and Assets for Adult Learning

Obstacles to Learning	Assets for Learning
Institutional barriers.	High self-motivation.
Time.	Self-directed.
Self-confidence.	A proven learner.
Situational obstacles.	Knowledge experience reservoir.
Special individual obstacles.	Special individual assets.

◆ **TABLE 12-3**
Learning Environment of Pedagogy and Androgogy

Pedagogy	Androgogy
The climate is authoritative.	The climate is relaxed and informal.
Competition is encouraged.	Collaboration is encouraged.
Teacher sets goals.	Teacher and class set goals.
Decisions made by teacher.	Decisions by teacher and students.
Lecture by teacher.	Process activities and inquire as to projects by students.
Evaluation by teacher.	Evaluation by teacher, self, and peers.

8. Adults need the opportunity for application very quickly following the learning.
9. Assessment of need is imperative in adult learning.

◆ Needs Assessment for Staff Development

Managers may or may not be involved in the implementation of educational programs, but they are responsible for the identification of learning needs. Often, this function is not performed well.

Organizations often implement training programs because they are faddish and have been well advertised and marketed. Educational programs are costly and should not be undertaken unless a demonstrated need exists and resources used are justifiable. In addition to developing a rationale for educational programs, the use of an assessment plan will be helpful in meeting learner requirements. The following process is useful in needs assessment.

1. Identify the desired knowledge or skills the staff should have.
2. Identify the present level of knowledge or skill.
3. Determine where deficits of desired knowledge and skills exist.
4. Identify the resources available to meet needs.
5. Make maximum use of available resources.
6. After application of resources, evaluate and test conclusions.

◆ Meeting the Educational Needs of a Culturally Diverse Staff

Brink (1994) says that, although meeting the educational needs of a heterogeneous staff may be more time-consuming and beset with communication problems, educational needs must be met. The need for all nurses to work well with a culturally diverse staff is essential. Managers should respect cultural diversity and recognize the desirability of having nurses from numerous cultures on their staff.

Education staff should be aware that learners with diverse learning styles and cultural backgrounds may perceive both the classroom and instruction differently than learners who have never experienced a culture different from that of the mainstream United States. Whether in a classroom or at the bedside teaching, there are several things the staff development personnel can do to facilitate the learning process, such as giving the learner plenty of time to respond to questions and restating things that are not understood.

It is important to remember that non-native speakers of English may have a reticence to participate in small group activities. This reticence may be attributable to insecurity about perceived English proficiency and a general lack of familiarity with group process.

Other staff who may have difficulty with group activities are those who have been educated in a traditional hierarchical system where the instructor is regarded with unquestioned authority. It often difficult for these learners to speak out in the class and give their opinions regarding instruction being discussed. Encouraging participation by drawing reticient members into classroom discussion through requests for their views may be helpful in gaining their involvement.

◆ Evaluation of Staff Development Activities

Because staff development includes participation and involvement from many departments, it is very difficult to effectively monitor this important function. Control becomes extremely difficult when accountability is shared. Because they are often costly, it is important that a means of evaluating staff development activities occur.

Evaluation of staff development consists of more than merely having class participants complete an evaluation form at the end of the class session, signing an employee handbook form, or assigning a preceptor for each new employee. Evaluation should include:

1. the learner's reaction to the process or presentation,
2. the behavior change of the learner (if any) that occurred following the staff development activity,
3. the impact that the activity had on the organization, and
4. the cost effectiveness of the staff development activity.

Heater (1990) found that proper staff development activities could result in decreased medication errors, fewer accidents, increased quality of clinical judgment, reduced turnover, and greater productivity. These are examples of measurements that could be used to determine effectiveness of staff development activities.

Many organizations budget a large amount of money for staff development only to neglect following through appropriately to determine the value of such programs. There is a need to ensure that all such activities be evaluated for quality control, impact on the institution, and cost effectiveness. This is true regardless of whether the educational and training activity is carried out by the manager, the preceptor, the personnel department, or the education department.

◆ Summary

The manager has the responsibility to see that adequate induction, orientation, and socialization is provided for all employees. These activities provide the manager with the opportunity to build loyalty and team spirit and to instill the employee with pride in the organization. This type of affective learning becomes the foundation for subsequent employee satisfaction and motivation.

Although the manager retains ultimate responsibility for unit personnel staff development, and uses appropriate teaching theories to assist with teaching and training staff, there is a shared responsibility. Managers, the personnel department and staff development units work together to assess educational needs, evaluate educational quality, and provide appropriate education and training to ensure that the goals of the organization are met.

◆ References

Alspach JG (1990). Critical care orientation: a discussion of survey results. Crit Care Nurses, 10(6):12–14,16

Asselin ME and Barber ED (1991). Unit orientation for experienced nurses. J Staff Dev 7(3):126–129

Brim OG Jr (1966). Socialization through the life cycle. In Brim OG Jr and Wheeler S (eds): Socialization after Childhood: Two Essays. New York: Wiley

Brooks E, Wilkinson JM, and Popkess-Vawter S (1994). Promoting situational support for nurses in practice. Image: J Nursing Schol, 26(4):305–307

Coudret NA, Fuchs PL, Roberts CS, Suhrheinrich JA, and White A (1994). Role socialization of graduating student nurses: impact of a nursing practicum on professional role conception. J Prof Nurs 10(6):342–349

Gillies DA (1994). Nursing Management: A Systems Approach, 3rd ed. Philadelphia: WB Saunders

Hardy ME and Conway ME (1988). Role Theory: Perspectives for Health Professionals. New York: Apple-Century-Crofts

Heater BS, Olson RK, and Becker AM (1990). Helping patients recover faster. AJN 90(10):19–20

Johnson M (1994). Conflict and nursing professionalization. In McCloskey J and Grace HK (eds): Current Issues in Nursing, 4th ed. St. Louis: CV Mosby

Knowles M (1970). The Modern Practice of Adult Education: Androgogy Versus Pedagogy. New York: Association Press

Kramer M (1974). Reality Shock: Why Nurses Leave Nursing. St. Louis: CV Mosby

Kramer M and Schmalenberg C (1988). Magnet hospitals: Part II. J Nurs Admin 18(2)

Lynn MR, McCain NL, and Boss BJ (1989). Socialization of R.N. to B.S.N. Image: J Nurs Schol, 21(4):232–237

Scalzi CC (1988). Role stress and coping strategies of nurse executives. J Nurs Admin 18(3)

Schumacher KL and Meleis (1994). Transitions: a central concept in nursing. Image: J Nurs Schol, 26(4):119–125

Strader MK and Decker PJ (1995). Role Transition. Norwalk, CT: Appleton & Lange

Sullivan EJ and Decker PJ (1988). Effective Management in Nursing. Menlo Park, CA: Addison-Wesley

Tucker PT (1987). Recruiting nurses with an extern program. Nurs Manage, 18(5):90–94

Verbey MP, Valentine N, and Harrison S (1992). The career development internship program. JONA 22(1):46–49

SAMPLE CASE ANALYSIS

Plan a continuing education program using the following events placed in the proper order. Explain your rationale.

Number	Event
0	Start.
1	Date, time, place established.
2	Program announced.
3	Speaker selected.
4	Audience defined.
5	Evaluation form answered.
6	Topic selected.
7	Program conducted.
8	Objectives formulated.
9	Evaluation form written.
10	Learning needs determined.

Analysis

Beginning with a stated goal will assist in the decision making. An appropriate goal for a continuing education program is, "to increase the knowledge or skills of the staff." Other less appropriate goals would be to: 1) provide an entertaining program for the staff, or 2) meet the requirements specified by the union contract for continuing education.

If the manager wants to increase the knowledge and skills of the staff, then the obvious first choice is to determine the learning needs of the staff. Determining staff learning requirements is frequently referred to as a *needs assessment.* A needs assessment may be accomplished in several ways:

1. By requesting input from the staff.
2. By examining indicators of need; that is, incident reports, number of patient falls, medication errors, patient and/or physician complaints.

3. By the introduction of new procedures, new equipment, or other changes requiring new information.

Many different indicators are used in a thorough needs assessment. It is necessary for the staff to have input into the measurement of their own needs but since staff input has some degree of subjectivity, it should not be the only criteria used in determining educational needs. However, if the continuing educational programs do not satisfy staff needs, attendance will be low unless compulsory.

Not only should general learning needs be determined, but there should be an effort to specify those needs. Here are two examples of general learning needs.

1. The organization wants to begin using nursing diagnosis in nursing records as per a new requirement. The *specific need determination* would include the level of nursing diagnosis expected and determining what knowledge the staff presently has regarding nursing diagnosis.
2. A staff-identified learning need could be a request for an update on new chemotherapy drugs. The *specific need determination* would include what drugs are commonly used, which new drugs have been introduced, what type of pharmacology is appropriate, and the present level of knowledge.

Once staff needs have been clearly identified, a topic from the list of needs must be selected and the audience identified. It is best to recognize the audience prior to writing learning objectives so that they can be specifically written for the target learner.

The speaker needs to be given a copy of the learning objectives so that they can be used in planning the program. If the speaker is selected prior to announcing the date of the program, the program coordinator will be able to arrange the time around the speaker's availability.

The speaker should be announced far enough in advance so that staff can plan their personal time to attend, but not so far in the future that they will forget the date. Some organizations post a 3-month educational calendar followed by reminders at 4- and 2-week intervals.

The evaluation form should be written and duplicated prior to the class, but given out at the conclusion. It is best to collect evaluation forms prior to participants leaving the classroom, as individuals tend to neglect them unless immediate feedback is solicited.

To recap the series of events:

Number	Event	Sequence
0	Start.	0
1	Date, time, place established.	6
2	Program announced.	7
3	Speaker selected.	5
4	Audience defined.	3
5	Evaluation form answered.	10
6	Topic selected.	2
7	Program conducted.	8
8	Objectives formulated.	4
9	Evaluation form written.	9
10	Learning needs determined.	1

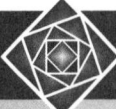

CASES FOR PROBLEM SOLVING

CASE 1

Learning needs and the maturity of those in a class often influence course content and teaching methods used.

Assignment

Recall how your learning needs and maturity level have changed since you were a beginning nursing student. When viewed as a whole, were you and your peers child or adult learners? Compare Knowles' pedagogy and androgogy characteristics to assist in determining this.

If pedagogical teaching strategies are appropriate for beginning nursing students, when does the nursing student make the transition from the child to the adult learner? If you were a first-semester nursing instructor, what teaching modes do you feel would be most conducive to learning? Would this change as students progressed through the nursing program? Support your feelings with rationale.

CASE 2

As a new supervisor of a community health agency one of your goals is to reduce attrition. You plan to do this by increasing employee retention, thus reducing orientation costs. In addition, you feel the increased retention will provide you with a more stable staff.

In studying your notes from exit interviews, it appears that new employees seldom develop a loyalty to the agency, but instead have used it to gain experience for other positions. You believe one difficulty with enculturating new employees is the orientation program in your agency.

Presently the agency allows 2 weeks of orientation time (80 hours) when the new employee is not counted in the nursing-care hours; these are referred to as nonproductive hours and are charged to the education department. Your unit has the following 2-week schedule for new employees:

Week 1: Monday and Tuesday
9 A.M. to 5 P.M.
Classroom
Week 2: Monday and Tuesday
8:30 A.M. to 5:00 P.M.
Assigned to case visits with an employee
Wednesday, Thursday, and Friday
Assigned to primary cases they will be working for orientation, but reviewing visits and patient records with another nurse, both prior to and after home visits.
Weekends are days off.

After this 2-week orientation the new employee is expected to function at 75% productivity for 2–3 weeks followed by full productivity. The exception to

CASE 2 (CONTINUED)

this is the new graduate (RN) orientation. These employees spend one extra week on the day shift and one extra week assigned to a partial case load.

Your nursing administrator has stated that you may alter the orientation program however you wish *as long as:* 1) you do not increase the nonproductive time, and 2) you ensure that the employee receives the information necessary to meet legal requirements and function satisfactorily.

....

Assignment

Is there any way for you to strengthen the new employee orientation to your agency? Outline your plans (if any) and give your rationale for your decision.

CASE 3 ◆

Your unit has decided to assign a preceptor to each new employee and you are serving on a committee that has been given the responsibility to develop a set of criteria that "will ensure an adequate number of qualified personnel to act as preceptors." What should these criteria be?

....

Assignment

Develop at least five criteria for qualifications of preceptors and give rationale for the inclusion of each criterion.

CASE 4 ◆

You are the evening charge nurse for a large surgical unit. Recently your long-time and extremely capable unit clerk retired and the manager of the unit has replaced her with Tran Zang. Ms. Zang is a delightful young Asian woman who speaks English well. She also speaks both Cantonese and Mandarin and you know she will be greatly appreciated on the unit for her ability to translate since your unit has many Chinese patients who do not understand or speak English well.

Ms. Zang received a 2-week unit clerk orientation. This consisted of actual classroom time as well as working directly with the retiring clerk. She has now been functioning on her own for 2 weeks and you realize that her orientation was not sufficient. Last evening, after her tenth mistake transcribing doctor's orders, you became rather sharp, leaving her in tears.

You are very frustrated by this situation. Your unit is extremely busy in the evening with returning surgeries, in addition to surgeons making rounds and leaving a multitude of orders. On the other hand, you believe that Ms. Zang has great potential. You recognize that there is much to learn in this job, and without a hospital background it is very difficult to learn the terminology, the physicians' names, and the unit routine.

CASE 4 (CONTINUED)

You spend time prior to coming to work this evening developing a training plan for Tran.

....

Assignment

Using your knowledge of adult learning theories and cultural diversity, explain your teaching plan and support your plan with appropriate rationale. Was your teaching plan personalized for this individual, and if so how and why was it personalized?

◆ **Bibliography**

The following references will assist you in solving these cases:

Baye AL (1993). Reality shock. Grad Nurse (Fall): 12–17, 71

Blouin AS and Brent NJ (1992). Nurse administrators in job transition: defining the issues. JONA 22(1):10–11

Ceslowitz SB and Loreti ST (1991). Easing the transition from hospital nursing to home care: a research study. Home Healthcare Nurse 9(4):32–35

Dunn SV (1992). Orientation: the transition form novice to competent critical care nurse. Crit Care Nurs Quart 15(10):69–77

Elliott-Burke T (1991). Easing the way for new grads. Clin Manage 11(5):58–60

Hansen HE (1995). A model for collegiality among staff nurses in acute care. JONA 25(12):11–20

Huston CJ and Marquis BL (1987). Use of management and ethical case studies to improve decision-making skills in senior nursing students. J Nurs Educat 26(5)

Jazwiec RM (1991). Learning needs assessment: methods. part 2. J Nurs Staff Dev 7(3):138–144

Lawinger SJ (1991). Competency-based orientation program for a surgical intensive therapy unit. Part I. Crit Care Nurse 11(4):36–44

Morton PG (1991). The 10-minute learning break. J Con Educat Nurs 22(1):39–40

Parrott TE (1994). Humor as a teaching strategy. Nurs Educ 19(3):36–38

Phelps RL (1990). A working model for nursing staff development. J Nurs Staff Dev 6(3):126–130

Seigel H (1991). Innovative approaches to inservice education J Cont Educat Nurs 22(4):147–151

Saarmann L, Freitas L, Rapps J, and Riegel B (1992). The relationship of education to critical thinking ability and values among nurses: socialization into professional nursing. J Prof Nurs, 8(1):26–34

Wolgin FJ (1990). Focus on outcome. J Nurs Staff Dev 6(3):151–152

Zeller C (1995). Cultural vignettes: a multicultural educational teaching strategy. Nurse Educ 20(2):8–9

PERSONAL NOTEBOOK

1. As a learner do you have more characteristics of the adult learner or the child learner?

2. Reflect upon the times in the last 2 years that you felt you were learning. Was this exciting? Did others contribute to your learning or did it come from within yourself?

3. What types of activities are most assistive in your learning, that is, movies, demonstrations, doing it yourself, writing something down, reading a book, hearing a lecture?

4. Describe how you have been socialized to the nursing role. What individuals have been most influential in your socialization?

Staffing and Scheduling

CHAPTER

13

Additional responsibilities in the staffing phase of the management process include ascertaining that there are adequate numbers of personnel available to meet daily unit needs and organizational goals. This frequently embodies all or part of the scheduling duties. The type of scheduling policies developed and staffing patterns implemented are directly related to the management phases of planning and organizing. For example, staffing ratios and the type of patient care delivery system impact heavily on how staffing and scheduling responsibilities are accomplished.

◆ Responsibilities of the Unit Manager in Meeting Staffing Needs

Although many health care organizations employ staffing clerks and/or use computerized staffing, the overall accountability for scheduling continues to be an important function of first- and middle-level management. Each organization has differing expectations regarding the unit manager's responsibilities in long-range human resource planning, and in managing short-range planning of day-to-day staffing.

Some organizations have decentralized staffing, with most staffing decisions being made by the unit manager. Others use centralized staffing, with many of the decisions being made by a central office or staffing center.

In organizations with *decentralized staffing*, the unit manager is often responsible for:

1. covering all scheduled absences,
2. reducing staff during periods of decreased patient census or acuity,
3. adding staff during high patient census or acuity,
4. preparing monthly unit schedules, and
5. preparing holiday and vacation schedules.

Advantages of decentralized staffing are that nurses are more actively involved in planning their own schedules and employees make personal staffing requests directly to their immediate supervisor. Decentralized scheduling and staffing as a means of decreasing nurse attrition has been recommended by Helmer and McKnight (1988). The increased autonomy and flexibility of decentralized staffing is believed to be the reason for increased retention (Marquis, 1988).

Many hospitals are attempting to increase the autonomy of nurses in the work place (Tressner, 1991). One method of achieving this is by using the nurses as partners in the scheduling process. Allowing nurses to trade days off, complete their own schedules, and arrange for illness coverage independently, works best when decentralized staffing is employed by the organization.

The disadvantages of decentralized staffing include the risk that employees may be treated unequally or inconsistently. If this occurs it may result in a negative reaction by the staff. Additionally, the unit manager may be viewed as granting rewards or punishments through the staffing schedule. Last, it is time-consuming for the manager and often promotes more "special pleading" than when staffing is maintained in a centralized manner.

Organizations with *centralized staffing* often use computerized staffing that assumes many of the staffing and scheduling duties of the unit manager. In centralized staffing one individual frequently performs staffing functions for all nursing departments, although the unit manager continues to have the option of making adjustments and providing input. This type of staffing is more equitable to all employees because policies tend to be applied more consistently and impartially. In addition, the first-level manager is left free to complete other management functions, which is more cost effective to the organization.

However, centralized staffing provides limited flexibility for the worker as it is as unable to easily account for the worker's interests or special needs. Another risk in centralized staffing is that managers may develop a habit of neglect toward personnel budget control if they have minimum involvement with staffing.

It is important to remember that the terms centralized and decentralized staffing *are not* synonymous with centralized and decentralized management decision making. For example, one can work as a manager in an organization that promotes centralized staffing, but uses decentralized decision making. Regardless of whether the organization has centralized or decentralized staffing, all managers at the unit level should develop an understanding of the scheduling procedures, the various options for scheduling, and the fiscal responsibilities for personnel staffing.

◆ Staffing and Scheduling Options

The necessity for evening, night, weekend, and holiday work schedules is frequently a source of frustration for nurses (Capuano, Fox, and Green, 1992). Nurses often perceive a lack of control over their work hours. Some studies (Patterson and Goad, 1987; Marquis, 1988) conclude that this lack of control contributes to increased attrition rates and burnout among professional nurses. Therefore, scheduling becomes a major factor in either fostering job dissatisfaction or in promoting job satisfaction and subsequent nurse retention. Managers who strive to develop a perception among staff that they do possess some control over scheduling, shift options, and staffing policies can improve job satisfaction.

It is beyond the scope of this book to provide a complete review of the creative staffing and scheduling options available. As staffing and scheduling influence worker satisfaction, managers should periodically solicit evaluation by their staff of the present system. Because most options consist of both positive and negative aspects, it is important that thorough research be performed prior to introducing staffing and scheduling changes and that adequate input from employees regarding any planned changes be solicited. The following is a partial list of creative staffing and scheduling options aimed at increasing nurse satisfaction that have been successfully implemented.

1. The 10- or 12-hour shift
2. Premium pay for weekend work and shift work
3. A part-time premium-paid supplemental staff pool
4. Cyclical staffing, allowing long-term awareness of future work schedules (Figure 13-1 shows a staffing pattern that repeats every 4 weeks.)
5. Flextime
6. Job sharing
7. Allowing nurses to exchange hours with each other
8. Staff self-scheduling
9. Use of supplemental nursing agencies for weekend coverage

There are advantages as well as disadvantages to each type of scheduling. Some scheduling mandates overtime pay and the subsequent nurse satisfaction must be weighed against the increased cost. Additionally, when long shifts are policy, errors in clinical judgment may occur, as nurses become fatigued. For this reason many organizations limit the number of consecutive days a nurse can work when 12-hour shifts are utilized. Finally, the excessive use of part-time or supplemental nurses, as some creative staffing requires, can result in poor continuity of nursing care.

However, many organizations are making an effort to shift the focus from worker adjustment to the organization to employer adjustment to meet the needs of a diverse work force (Jamieson and O'Mara, 1991). Two staffing options that reflect this shift in focus are the use of flextime and self-scheduling (Wulff, 1994).

Position	Name	Week I S	M	T	W	T	F	S
Full time	RN 1				X			X
Full time	RN 2	X					X	
Full time	RN 3			X				X
Full time	RN 4	X				X		
Full time	RN 5				X			X
Full time	RN 6	X				X		
Full time	RN 7		X					X
Full time	RN 8	X					X	
Part time	8 hrs/wk RN 9	On						
Part time	8 hrs/wk RN 10							On
Part time	8 hrs/wk RN 11	On						
Part time	8 hrs/wk RN 12							On
Total RNs on duty each day		6	7	7	6	6	6	6

Position	Name	Week II S	M	T	W	T	F	S
Full time	RN 1	X					X	
Full time	RN 2				X			X
Full time	RN 3	X				X		
Full time	RN 4			X				X
Full time	RN 5	X					X	
Full time	RN 6		X					X
Full time	RN 7	X				X		
Full time	RN 8				X			X
Part time	8 hrs/wk RN 9							On
Part time	8 hrs/wk RN 10	On						
Part time	8 hrs/wk RN 11							On
Part time	8 hrs/wk RN 12	On						
Total RNs on duty each day		6	7	7	6	6	6	6

Position	Name	Week III S	M	T	W	T	F	S
Full time	RN 1				X			X
Full time	RN 2	X					X	
Full time	RN 3			X				X
Full time	RN 4	X				X		
Full time	RN 5				X			X
Full time	RN 6	X					X	
Full time	RN 7		X					X
Full time	RN 8	X				X		
Part time	8 hrs/wk RN 9	On						
Part time	8 hrs/wk RN 10							On
Part time	8 hrs/wk RN 11	On						
Part time	8 hrs/wk RN 12							On
Total RNs on duty each day		6	7	7	6	6	6	6

Position	Name	Week IV S	M	T	W	T	F	S
Full time	RN 1	X					X	
Full time	RN 2				X			X
Full time	RN 3	X				X		
Full time	RN 4		X					X
Full time	RN 5	X					X	
Full time	RN 6			X				X
Full time	RN 7	X				X		
Full time	RN 8			X				X
Part time	8 hrs/wk RN 9							On
Part time	8 hrs/wk RN 10	On						
Part time	8 hrs/wk RN 11							On
Part time	8 hrs/wk RN 12	On						
Total RNs on duty each day		6	7	6	7	6	6	6

Elements: Every other weekend off
Maximum days worked: 4
Minimum days worked: 2
Number of split days off each period: 2
Operates in multiples of 4, 8, 12...
Schedule repeats itself every 4 weeks

X: Scheduled day off

FIGURE 13-1.
Master time sheet—4 week cycle.

Flextime is a system that allows employees to select time schedules that best meet their personal needs, while still meeting work responsibilities. Flextime works best when used in health care positions where full 24-hour coverage is not required, such as in home health and school nursing. Some hospitals have attempted to use flextime by varying shift start and stop times and using less than an 8-hour work schedule, much like 10- or 12-hour shifts but reducing the time rather than lengthening it. When a hospital uses flextime, employees come and go at varied times. Although this type of staffing creates greater employee choices it could also result in over- or understaffing as it is very difficult to coordinate the staffing requirements.

Self-scheduling is the process that employees use to implement the work schedule collectively. With input from the manager, staff set staffing guidelines that meet fiscal accountability and patient safety and use the guidelines to develop their own work schedules. Although this provides nurses with greater work environment control, it is not an easy concept to implement. Success depends on leadership skills of the manager and on the willingness of all involved to have patience and perseverance (Wulff, 1994).

The use of staffing pools that usually work for premium pay but receive little or no benefits continue to be used in both periods of staffing surpluses and shortages. The supplemental staff may be an internal or an external group of employees. Some managers use these per diem pools to provide more weekends off for their regularly scheduled employees and others use such pools only as an emergency to cover absences of their regular staff. Views among nurse administrators are mixed as to the overall benefits of using such pools (Warren and Rozell, 1995).

Because all scheduling and staffing patterns impact heavily on employees' personal lives, productivity, and budgets, it is wise to have a 6-month trial of any changes. An evaluation at the end of that period should be carried out to determine the impact on financial costs, retention, productivity, risk management, and employee as well as patient satisfaction.

◆ Developing Staffing and Scheduling Policies

Nurses will be more satisfied in the work place if staffing and scheduling policies and procedures are clear. Written policies provide greater consistency and fairness. In addition to being available in written form, policies must be clearly verbalized to all employees. Personnel policies represent the standard of action that is communicated in advance so that employees are not caught unaware regarding personnel decisions (Huston and Marquis, 1989). In addition to being standardized, they should be worded in such a manner as to allow some flexibility.

These policies should be reviewed and updated periodically and when formulating policies, management must examine its own philosophy as well as give consideration to prevailing practices in the community. At the unit level, managers may not be totally involved in designing all personnel policies, but should have some input as they are reviewed. However, there are nursing department as well as unit staffing and scheduling policies that unit supervisors develop and implement themselves. These policies, as shown in Display 13-1, should be formalized by the manager and shared with all personnel.

Unit staffing policies should include adequate input from the staff and be developed in collaboration with personnel and nursing departments (Gillies, 1994). This ensures that personnel policies developed at the unit level will not conflict with those at a higher level. For example, some states have labor laws that restrict 12-hour shifts. Additionally, in organizations with union contracts, many staffing and scheduling policies are incorporated into the union contract. In such cases, staffing alterations may require renegotiation at the time of contract renewal.

DISPLAY 13-1
Unit Checklist of Employee Staffing Policies

1. Name of the individual responsible for the staffing schedule, and the authority of that individual if it is someone other than the immediate supervisor of the employee.
2. Type and length of staffing cycle used.
3. Rotation policies, if shift rotation is used.
4. Request to change fixed shift, if fixed shift is used.
5. Time and location of schedule posting.
6. When shift begins and ends.
7. Day of week that schedule begins.
8. Weekend off policy.
9. Tardiness policy.
10. Low census procedures.
11. Policy for trading days off.
12. Request for days off procedures.
13. Absenteeism policy.
14. Policy regarding rotating to other units.
15. Vacation time request procedures.
16. Holiday time request procedures.
17. Procedures for resolving conflicts regarding requests for days off, holidays, or request time.
18. Emergency time off policies.
19. Policies and procedures regarding request to transfer to other units.

◆ The Impact of Standards for Productivity on Staffing

One of the greatest impacts on staffing is the standard of measurement for productivity that has been adopted by the unit. Standards for productivity, staffing formulas, and staffing terminology were discussed in Chapter 7, which dealt with fiscal planning. Additional staffing formulas are shown in Display 13-2. Standard units for measuring productivity need to be periodically reviewed and adjusted if necessary.

The middle-level manager must be alert to the impact of internal or external forces that may not be reflected in the patient classification system of the organization. Examples of such extraneous circumstances could include a sudden increase in nursing or medical students on the unit, an increase in the number of new graduate nurses, or cultural and language difficulties of recently hired foreign nurses.

The classification system selected may prove to be inaccurate or the hours allotted for each category or classification of patient may be inadequate. This does not imply that managers should be unaccountable for the standard unit of measurement, but rather that they should be cognizant of justifiable reasons that their unit appears over- or understaffed.

Patient classification was defined in Chapter 7 as the grouping of patients according to specific characteristics. The rationale for using patient classification is that the quantity of patients alone has proven to be an inaccurate method for determining nursing care assignments. Because other variables within the system impact on nursing-care hours, it is usually not possible to transfer a patient classification system from one facility to another. Instead, each basic system must be modified to fit a specific institution and a particular setting (Prescott and Soeken, 1996).

Once an organization adopts a suitable system, nursing care hours must be assigned for each classification. An appropriate number of hours of care for each classification is generally suggested by companies marketing such systems. However, each institution makes the final decision regarding the number of care hours allotted for each patient classification. There are many variables in any chosen system; no system is without faults (Prescott, 1991). It is a mistake for managers to believe that patient classification systems will resolve staffing problems. Such systems better define problems, but it is dependent upon the people in the organization to use the information provided to solve the problems at hand. A sample classification system can be found in Chapter 7.

◆ Fiscal and Ethical Accountability for Staffing

Regardless of the difficulties inherent in patient classification systems and in the assignment of nursing care hours, the best method for controlling the staffing function of management has yet to be devised. Assuming that man-

DISPLAY 13-2
Staffing Formulas

- To determine staffing needs:

$$\frac{\text{Patient census}}{\text{Patient/nurse ratio}}$$

- To determine average daily acuity levels (acuity index):

$$\frac{\text{Total acuities in 24 hours}}{\text{Number of patients in 24 hours}}$$

- To determine average monthly patient days:

$$\frac{\text{Average daily census} \times \text{days in calendar year (365)}}{\text{Number of months in a year (12)}}$$

- To determine the actual hours of care being provided a day (NCH/PPD):

$$\frac{\text{Total hours of care in a 24 hour period}}{\text{Number of patients}}$$

- To determine the number of FTEs required:

First: Projected hours of care × average daily census = hours of care/day
Second: Hours of care/day × number of days in year (365) = hours of care/year
Third:

$$\frac{\text{Hours of care needed per year}}{\text{Hours of 1 FTE per year (2080)}}$$

- To estimate percentage of turnover:

$$\frac{\text{Number of employees leaving}}{\text{Total number of employees}} \times 100$$

agers recognize that all systems have weaknesses, and as long as they periodically evaluate the current system, they should be able to initiate change as necessary. It is critical, however, that managers make every effort to use the patient classification system currently authorized by their organization as the basis for unit staffing and scheduling. Nursing care remains labor intensive and the manager is fiscally responsible to the organization for appropriate staffing. Accountability for a prenegotiated budget is a management function.

Fiscal accountability is not incompatible with responsibility to patients or staff. It is possible to stay within a staffing budget and meet the needs of patients and staff. However, it is necessary that managers obtain additional staff when patient acuity increases as well as decrease staffing when acuity is low; to do otherwise is demoralizing to staff.

Some organizations only require that managers end the fiscal year within their budgeted nursing care hours, devoting less attention to daily or weekly nursing care hours. Advantages to scheduling shift staffing based on a patient acuity system include allowing each shift to be adequately staffed and at the same time indicating when there is overstaffing. In addition, this is an equitable method for the allocation of staff.

The disadvantages of shift-based staffing include that it is time-consuming and a great deal of subjectivity exists in any acuity system. The greater the degree of objectivity in any system, the longer the time required to make staffing computations. Perhaps the greatest danger in staffing by acuity is that many organizations are unable to supply the extra staff when the acuity system shows that the unit is understaffed. The same organization may use the acuity-based staffing system as a justification to borrow staff from an overstaffed unit. For this reason, an acuity-based staffing system can be demotivating if not used consistently or correctly.

As employees have the right to assume a reasonable work load, managers must ensure that there is adequate coverage to meet the needs of staff as well as patients. Those who constantly expect employees to work overtime and carry unreasonable patient assignments are not ethically accountable.

However, effective managers do not focus totally on numbers of personnel, but examine all the components of productivity. They examine nursing duties, job descriptions, and patient care organization. Such managers also use every opportunity to build a productive and cohesive team. The authors have witnessed many superhuman efforts on the part of nursing staff during periods of shortages with little complaining, simply because they believed in their supervisor and in the organization. Just as often, though, the opposite has occurred; staff who were only moderately unstaffed wasted an inordinate amount of time and energy complaining of their plight. The difference between the two examples has much to do with trust; trust that such conditions are the exception, not the norm; faith that real solutions and not provisional approaches to problem solving will be used to plan for the future; assurance that the management team will work just as conscientiously as the staff to meet patient needs; and trust that the organization's overriding philosophy is based on patient interest and not financial gain.

◆ Staffing and Absenteeism

Another fiscal goal of the manager that is often related to staffing is the reduction of absenteeism. There is evidence that many things influence absenteeism rates in an organization (Holman, 1995). For instance, one study found that deficient child care is a primary cause of absenteeism among nursing personnel (Miller and Norton, 1986). Therefore, managers who establish staffing policies that allow flexibility and advance notice of scheduling give their employees the opportunity to organize their personal commitments more effectively.

Many organizations closely monitor absenteeism and establish programs to reduce the hours of work lost through employee absence. Studies have shown the most effective method to combat absenteeism is some type of paid bonus plan for employees who do not use their sick time (Holman, 1995).

◆ Summary

The manager has a responsibility to provide adequate staffing to meet patient care needs. Attention must be paid to fluctuations of the patient census so that under- or overstaffing does not occur and to ensure fiscal accountability to the organization and ethical accountability to patients and employees. The prudent manager involves employees in developing unit staffing and scheduling policies and ascertains that adopted policies are not in violation of organizational policies, union contracts, or labor laws.

Unit policies should be reviewed periodically and revised if needed. Additionally, the manager must be alert to factors that impact on the standard for productivity and negotiate for changes when appropriate.

The effective manager attempts to build trust and a team spirit in subordinates to deal with temporary staff shortages and seeks innovative methods to overcome staffing difficulties.

◆ References

Capuano TA, Fox MA, and Green B (1992). Staffing nurses according to episodic census variations. Nursing Manage 23(10):34–37

Gillies DA (1994). Nursing Management: A Systems Approach. Philadelphia: WB Saunders

Helmer FT and McKnight P (1988). One more time: solutions to the nursing shortage. J Nurs Admin 18(11)

Holman DG (1995). Registered nurses' beliefs about absentee-control programs. JONA 25(9):7

Jamieson ML and O'Mara J (1991). Managing Workforce 2000: Gaining the Diversity Advantage. San Franscico: Jossey-Bass

Marquis B (1988). Attrition: the effectiveness of retention activities. J Nurs Admin 18(3):21–24

Marquis B and Huston CJ (1996). Leadership Roles and Management Functions, 2nd ed. Philadelphia: JB Lippincott

Miller D and Norton V (1986). Absenteeism, a chronic disease. J Nurs Admin 16(3):38–42

Prescott PA and Soeken KL (1996). Measuring nursing intensity in ambulatory care. Part I: Approaches to and uses of patient classification systems. Nurs Econ 14(1):14–21,33

Prescott P (1991). Nursing intensity: Needed today for more than staffing. Nurs Econ 9(6):409–414

Patterson SW and Goad S (1987). Incentives for retention. Nurs Manage 18(2)

Tressner M (1991). Controlling the workplace: Total care nurses. Nurs Manage 22(5):88

Warren IB and Rozell BR (1995). Supplemental staffing: nurse mangers views of costs, benefits and quality of care. JONA 25(6):51–57

Wulff KS (1994). Flextime and self-scheduling. In McClosky J and Grace HK (eds): Current Issues in Nursing 4th ed. St. Louis: CV Mosby

SAMPLE CASE ANALYSIS

Your flexible nursing care hours are budgeted at 8.2 hours per patient day (8.2 NCH/PPD). Each day your staffing requirements depend on your patient census and patient acuity. Your acuity index based on the hospital's patient classification system is as follows:

	Days	Evenings	Nights
Classification #1	2.3	2.0	0.5
Classification #2	2.9	2.3	1.0
Classification #3	3.4	2.8	2.0
Classification #4	4.6	3.4	2.8

Note: You must be over- or understaffed by over one-half the total hours a person is working in order to reduce or add staff; that is, if a nurse is working an 8-hour shift you must be over or under 4 hours to delete or add staff.

When you came on duty this morning you had the following patients and classifications:

1 patient in classification #1
2 patients in classification #2
3 patients in classification #3
1 patient in classification #4

SAMPLE CASE ANALYSIS (CONTINUED)

••

Assignment

Calculate your staffing needs. On duty you have one RN and one LVN/LPN in addition to a ward clerk for 4 hours. Are you under- or overstaffed?

You have the same patients and classifications for the P.M. shift and you have two RNs scheduled for duty. Are you under- or overstaffed?

Suppose that instead of shift staffing based on the level of patient acuity, the unit manager need only end the quarterly fiscal period with an *average* 8.2 NCH/PPD. What are the advantages as well as disadvantages of this type of flexible staffing versus an acuity-based system adjusted for each shift?

••

Analysis

Formula: Use the day-budgeted NCH multiplied by the number of patients in each classification.

Day Shift	Needed NCH	Days
1 patient in classification #1	$= 1 \times 2.3$	$= 2.3$
2 patients in classification #2	$= 2 \times 2.9$	$= 5.8$
3 patients in classification #3	$= 3 \times 3.4$	$= 10.2$
1 patient in classification #4	$= 1 \times 4.6$	$= 4.6$

Total NCH needed on day shift = 22.9 hours

Staff	Hours Worked
1 RN	8
1 LVN	8
1 ward clerk	4
	20

22.9 (rounded to 23) hours is needed on the day shift. There is a total number of 20 hours allocated for nursing staff; therefore, there was a shortage of 3 hours but not enough shortage to warrant additional staffing.

Evening Shift	Needed NCH	Days
1 patient in classification #1	$= 1 \times 2.0$	$= 2.0$
2 patients in classification #2	$= 2 \times 2.3$	$= 4.6$
3 patients in classification #3	$= 3 \times 2.8$	$= 8.4$
1 patient in classification #4	$= 1 \times 3.4$	$= 3.4$

Total NCH needed on P.M. shift = 18.4 hours

	Hours Worked
2 RN × 8 hours each =	16 hours

SAMPLE CASE ANALYSIS (CONTINUED)

The evening shift was understaffed by 2.4 hours but not enough to request another staff member.

The advantage of shift staffing based on a patient acuity system is that it allows each shift to be adequately staffed and at the same time indicates to the manager when overstaffing occurs. In addition, this is a fair method of allocation of staff.

An advantage of a fixed number of hours per patient staffing is that it gives the manager more control over under- and overstaffing and allows for more flexibility. Because the staff are less aware of the degree of over- and understaffing in this system, it tends to promote less resentment among the employees.

The greatest disadvantage of the system, however, is that it treats every patient as requiring the exact same number of nursing hours. All nurses are aware that at times their units are extremely busy with relatively few patients and conversely, are relatively quiet with a much higher census. Thus, nursing care hours per patient day not based on an acuity system lacks accuracy in determining staffing needs.

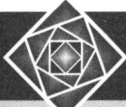 CASES FOR PROBLEM SOLVING

CASE 1

You are the manager of an ICU. Many of the nurses have approached you requesting 12 hour shift assignments. However, others have stated they will transfer out of the unit if 12 hour shifts are implemented.

You are attempting to determine if it is feasible and cost effective to utilize both 8 and 12 hour shifts, so that staff could select which type of scheduling they wanted. You wonder if this will create a scheduling nightmare.

• •

Assignment

List all of the problems you feel might occur as a result of mixing 8 and 12 hour shifts. Share this with other members of your class. What problems did they anticipate that were not included on your list? Be able to demonstrate if this would be cost effective. Assume you have 15 nurses working each 24 hour period (presently 5 each shift). Make a one day schedule with 8 nurses working 8 hour shifts and 7 nurses working 12 hour shifts.

CASE 2

You are a member of a staffing committee on your unit. The function of the committee is to update staffing and scheduling policies and procedures. You represent the night shift. There has been some dissatisfaction with the granting of days off during the holidays. In particular, the night shift is unhappy because many of them are married with small children and believe that this should be a consideration in holiday requests. Others feel that seniority should take precedence when requests are considered.

The unit supervisor has agreed to trial implementation of any policies regarding holiday requests formulated by the committee.

Assignment
Devise staffing policies regarding holiday requests and share them with others for evaluation.

CASE 3

A new rehabilitation unit has been added at Mercy Hospital. You have been given certain constraints in staffing the unit, but other than these restrictions you may choose various staffing modes.
   Your constraints:

1. All-licensed staff.
2. Ratio of LVNs/LPNs to RNs: 1–1.
3. There must always be an RN on duty.
4. Budgeted NCH/PPD is 8.2.
5. You are not included in the NCH/PPD, but ward clerks are counted.
6. Your unit capacity is 7 and you anticipate an average census of 6.
7. You may utilize modular nursing, primary nursing, or total patient care.

   Your patients will be chronic, not acute, but will be admitted for an active 2–12 week program of rehabilitation. The emphasis will be in returning the patient to home with an adequate ability to perform activities of daily living. Other disciplines will be involved, including occupational therapy and physical therapy. It is anticipated that there will be a waiting list for the beds as this has been a needed service in your community. You anticipate that the majority of your patients will be those with: 1) CVAs, 2) spinal cord injuries, 3) other problems with neurological functions, and 4) amputees.
   You have hired four full-time RNs, and two part-time RNs. The part-time RNs desire at least 2 days of work in a 2 week pay period, and in return for this guarantee, have agreed to cover for most of the illnesses and vacations, and some holidays for your regular RN full-time staff.
   You have also hired three full-time LVNs/LPNs and two part-time LVNs/LPNs. However, the part time LVNs/LPNs would like to work at least 3 days per week. You have decided not to hire a ward clerk, but to use the pediatric ward clerk 4 hours each day to assist with various duties. Therefore, you need to calculate her 4 hours each day into the total hours worked.

CASE 3 (CONTINUED)

You have researched various types of patient care delivery and various types of staffing patterns (i.e., 8 hour, 10 hour, 12 hour, etc.). Your newly hired staff is willing to experiment with any type of staffing and patient care management system you select.

• •

Assignment

1. Determine what staffing pattern you will use and explain why it was selected.
2. Show a 24-hour staffing pattern for a 2-week period.

CASE 4

You are serving on an ad hoc committee to examine the pros and cons of changing to rotating shifts instead of fixed shifts that your hospital now has.

• •

Assignment

List five positive and five negative aspects of fixed shifts and five positive and five negative aspects of rotating shifts. If shifts are fixed, what is a fair method for staff to acquire a change of shift? If shifts were changed to rotating, what length of time should be spent on each shift? Should the evening shift be 3:00–11:00 P.M.? Should the night shift be 11:00 P.M.–7:00 A.M.? Could someone request to work only 11:00 P.M.–7:00 A.M. as a permanent shift? Justify your decisions with your rationale.

◆ Bibliography

The following references will assist you in solving these cases:

Brechbiel K (1990). How to justify your staffing. Am J Nurs 20(5):28B

Davis R (1991). The quick fix? . . . traveling nurses to fill the staffing gaps. Am J Nurs 21(4):56

Giovannetti P and Johnson JM (1990). A new generation patient classification system. J Nurs Admin 20(5):33–40

Heater BS, Olson RK, and Becker AM (1990). Helping patients recover faster. Am J Nurs 20(10)

Hogue EE (1991). Inadequate staffing situations: implications for nurses. Pediatric Nurs 17(2):183–184

Houston R (1990). Twelve-hour shifts: answer to job satisfaction? Nurs Manage 21(10):88

Kutash MB (1993). Optimizing the use of nursing pool resources. JONA 23(1):65–68

Ligon R (1990). A blueprint for involving staff in policy development. Nurs Manage 21(7)

Newman KM (1991). Availability of scheduling options important. J Nurs Admin 21(46):49

Nyberg J (1990). The effects of care and economics on nursing practice. J Nurs Admin 20(5):13–18

Parsons ML (1990). A program to manage nurse staffing costs. Nurs Manage 21(10): 42–44

Phillips CY, Castorr A, Prescott PA, and Soeken K (1992). Nursing intensity: going beyond patient classification. J Nurs Admin 22(4):53–57

Prescott PA, Phillips CY, Rayan JW, and Thompson KO (1991). Changing how nurses spend their time. Image 923(1):23–28

Wall J (1990). Patient classification interrater reliability. Nurs Manage 21(11):67–69

PERSONAL NOTEBOOK

1. Have you ever worked a night or evening shift? Did your body adjust to these changes in your sleep patterns?

2. How do you feel about working holidays, weekends, and rotating shifts? What impact do you feel this might have on your life?

3. Take a vote among your friends about the most desirable shift. Also inquire as to how they feel about 8-, 10-, and 12- hour shifts. Is everyone in agreement?

DIRECTING

Seize the opportunity

—*Anne Davis*

In the planning and organizing phases of the management process, the manager provides an environment that is conducive to getting the work done. In directing, the fourth step in the management process, the manager sets those plans into action with the ultimate goal being attainment of organizational goals.

As discussed in Chapter 2, "directing" is the part of the management process that is frequently referred to by a number of terms. Many management experts label this phase "coordinating," whereas others call it "activating." Regardless of the nomenclature used, the learner needs to remember that this is the part of management that requires expert "doing" skills.

In "directing," work is broken down into manageable tasks and, when appropriate, delegated to others. To maximize the work performance of subordinates in meeting organizational goals, the manager must be able to establish a motivating climate, manage time resources efficiently, demonstrate excellent communication skills, manage conflict and facilitate collaboration, negotiate as needed to ensure adequate resources are available for the unit, and work with collective bargaining agents as necessary.

Some employees are more productive than others. This is related in part to their intrinsic motivation, or internal drive to accomplish. It is also, however, related to the level at which the manager is able to extrinsically stimulate or motivate certain behaviors.

Time management is also critical. As managers are able to use time efficiently, they become better able to prioritize the needs for both physical and human resources. In prioritizing time, managers determine what, if any, work should be delegated to subordinates and which subordinate would be best for the job. Given the current movement to replace professional registered nurses with unlicensed assistive personnel, contemporary managers face greater challenges than ever in determining when and to whom delegation is appropriate.

In directing, the manager must also become an expert "people" manager and communicator. Part of being a good communicator lies in understanding how communication occurs within the organization. Intraorganizational communication is as complex as the organization itself. Because this phase of the management process is specifically focused on directing the work of others, managers must be certain they are communicating clearly and assertively to all individuals as needed within the organization, as well as on a one-to-one basis with subordinates.

Since the manager has a broader view of the organization and its needs than subordinates, some interpersonal conflict should be expected in directing the work of individuals who are more self-centered in their approach. Learning to constructively handle conflict to promote win-win outcomes is a critical management skill. Likewise, learning to be an effective negotiator, so that adequate fiscal, technological, and human resources are available, decreases potential conflict within the unit.

If employees in an organization perceive that resources and manpower are being misused or used less effectively than they could be, they may attempt to unionize and force management to listen to their concerns and needs through collective bargaining. As an effective communicator and negotiator, the manager can use these skills in an effort to meet both management and employee needs.

Providing a Motivating Climate

CHAPTER
14

M_otivation_ is the behavior that individuals exhibit to satisfy their needs. Because human beings constantly have needs and wants, individuals are always motivated to some extent. In addition, since all people are unique and have different needs, they are motivated differently.

The amount and quality of work accomplished by managers is a direct reflection of their motivation as well as that of their subordinates. Because motivation comes from within the individual, managers cannot directly motivate their subordinates. The manager can, however, create an environment in which the development of human potential can be maximized. All human beings have needs that motivate them, as does the organization. Therefore, the manager's role is to create an environment that meets both organizational as well as individual needs.

Because motivation is so complex, the manager faces tremendous challenges in accurately identifying individual as well as collective motivators. Even in similar or nearly identical work environments, there are often great variations in individual and group motivation. A great deal of research has been undertaken by behavioral, psychological, and social scientists to develop theories and concepts of motivation. Economists and engineers focused on extrinsic fiscal rewards to improve performance and productivity, whereas human relations scientists stressed intrinsic needs for recognition, self-esteem, and self-actualization. To better understand the current view that both extrinsic and intrinsic rewards are necessary for high productivity and worker satisfaction, it is necessary to look at how motivational theory has evolved over the past century.

◆ Motivational Theory

Chapter 3 introduced traditional management philosophy that emphasized paternalism, worker subordination, and bureaucracy as means of predictable but moderate productivity. High productivity meant greater monetary incentives for workers, who were viewed as being motivated primarily by economic factors. This traditional management philosophy is still in use today. Many factory and assembly line production jobs, and positions that offer production incentive pay, are based on these principles.

The shift from traditional management philosophy to a greater focus on the human element and worker satisfaction as factors in productivity first began during the Human Relations Era (1930–1970). As discussed in Chapter 3, the best known human motivation studies in this era were the Hawthorne Studies conducted by Mayo.

A reinvestigation of human motivation occurred with Maslow's work in the 1950s. Most nurses are familiar with Maslow's hierarchy of needs and his theory of human motivation. Maslow stated that people are motivated to satisfy certain needs ranging from basic survival needs to complex psychological needs and that people seek a higher need only when the lower needs predominantly have been met. Maslow's hierarchy of needs is depicted in Figure 14-1.

Although Maslow's work helped explain personal motivation, his early work was not applied to motivation in the workplace. However, later work offered considerable insight into motivation and worker dissatisfaction. Because of Maslow's work, managers began to recognize that individuals were

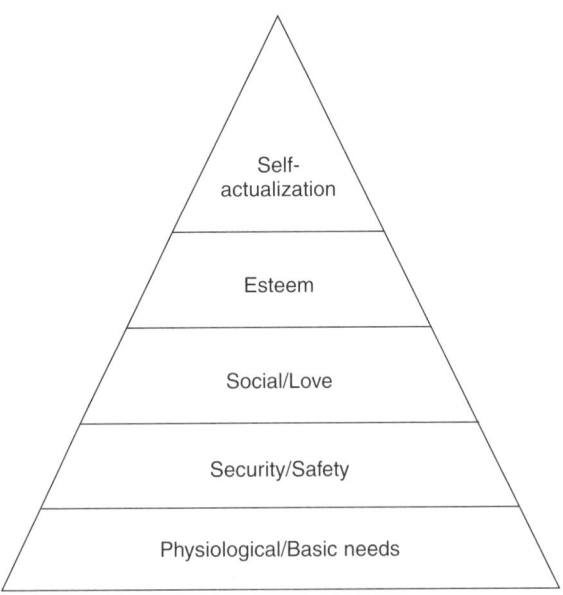

FIGURE 14-1. Maslow's hierarchy of needs.

complex beings, not solely economically driven, and that they had many needs motivating them at any one time. It also became clear that motivation is internalized, and that management must assist individuals in meeting lower level needs before higher level needs can be met if organizational productivity is to increase. This shifting focus in what motivates employees had a tremendous impact on the value organizations place on workers today.

B.F. Skinner was another theorist of this era who contributed to our understanding of motivation, dissatisfaction, and productivity. His research on operant conditioning and behavior modification demonstrated that individuals can be conditioned to behave or not behave in certain ways based on a consistent reward or punishment system. This reinforcement theory postulates that behaviors followed relatively quickly by positive consequences (positive reinforcement) tend to be repeated, whereas negative consequences (punishment) following a certain behavior decrease its occurrence. Skinner's work continues to be reflected today in how many managers view and utilize discipline in the work setting.

Another theorist discussed in Chapter 3 who contributed to our understanding of motivation was Frederick Herzberg. Herzberg believed that the worker could be motivated by the work itself and that there is an internal or personal need to meet organizational goals. He felt that it was possible to separate personal motivators from job dissatisfiers. This distinction between hygiene or maintenance factors and motivating factors was called the *Motivation-Hygiene Theory* or *two-factor theory*. Display 14-1 lists motivator and hygiene factors identified by Herzberg. Herzberg maintained that motivators (also called job satisfiers) are present in work itself and encourage people to want to work and to do that work well.

Hygiene or maintenance factors keep the worker from being dissatisfied or demotivated, but do not act as true motivators. It is important to remember

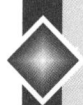

DISPLAY 14-1
Herzberg's Motivator and Hygiene Factors

Motivators	Hygiene Factors
Achievement	Salary
Recognition	Supervision
Work itself	Job security
Responsibility	Positive working conditions
Advancement	Personal life
Possibility for growth	Interpersonal relations/peers
Company policy	
Status	

that the opposite of dissatisfaction may not be satisfaction. When hygiene factors are met, there is a lack of dissatisfaction, but not necessarily an existence of satisfaction. Likewise, the absence of motivators does not necessarily cause dissatisfaction.

For example, salary is a hygiene factor. It does not motivate in itself, although when used in conjunction with other motivators such as recognition or advancement, it can be powerful. If salary is deficient, however, employee dissatisfaction can result. Some individuals argue that money can truly be a motivator and that this is demonstrated by individuals who work insufferable hours at jobs they truly do not enjoy. Most theorists would argue that money (salary) in this case may be taking the place of some other need of which the individual may not be fully conscious.

Some individuals in Herzberg's studies did report job satisfaction solely from hygiene or maintenance factors. Herzberg asserts that such individuals show only a temporary satisfaction when hygiene factors are improved, show little interest in the type and quality of their work, experience little satisfaction from accomplishments, and tend to show chronic dissatisfaction with other hygiene factors such as salary, status, and job security.

As a result of Herzberg's work, managers believe that although hygiene or maintenance factors provide an essential base for the organization to build on, the motivating climate must actively include the worker. The worker must be given greater responsibilities, challenges, and recognition for work well done. The reward system must meet both motivation and hygiene needs and the emphasis given by the manager should vary with the situation and employee involved.

Although hygiene factors in themselves do not motivate the worker, they are necessary to create an environment that encourages the worker to move on to higher level needs. They also keep an employee from being dissatisfied and are useful in recruiting an adequate employee pool (Marquis and Huston, 1996).

Another motivational theorist in the humanistic era was Victor Vroom. He developed an "expectancy model" that looks at motivation in terms of the individual's valence or preferences, based on social values. In contrast to operant conditioning, which focused on observable behaviors, the expectancy model says that people's expectations about their environment or a certain event will influence their behavior. In other words, individuals view all actions as having a cause and effect. The effect may be immediate or delayed, but there is a reward inherent in the behavior that will motivate the individual to undertake such a risk. In a simplification of the expectancy model (see Figure 14-2), people make conscious decisions in anticipation of reward, whereas in operant conditioning, they react in a stimulus-response mode. Managers who attempt to motivate employees using the expectancy model must become personally involved with their employees so they can gain a better understanding of the employee's values, rewards system, strengths, and willingness to take risks.

McClelland also contributed to motivational theory in examining what incentives guide each individual to take action. McClelland stated that people are motivated by three basic needs: *achievement, affiliation,* and *power.* Achievement-

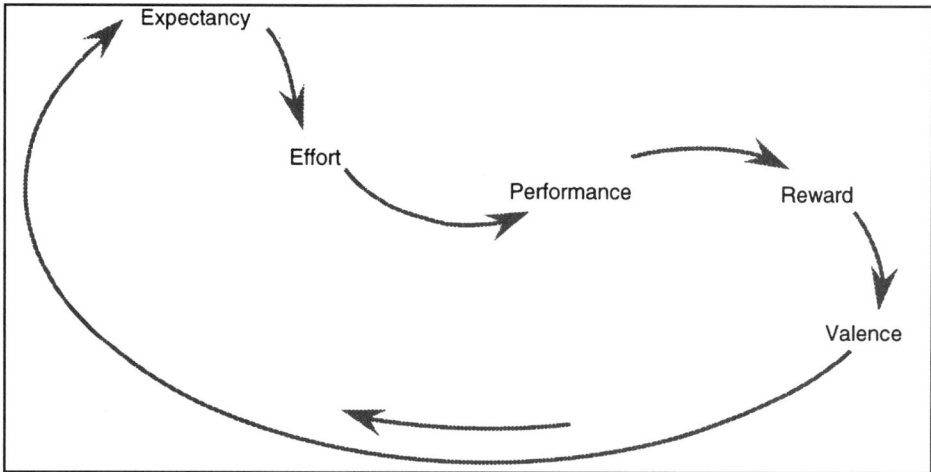

FIGURE 14-2. Vroom's expectancy model.

oriented individuals actively focus their lives on improving what exists. They transform ideas into action, judiciously and wisely, taking risks when necessary.

In contrast, affiliation-oriented individuals focus their energies on families and friends. Their overt productivity may be less as they view their contribution to society in a different light than achievement-oriented individuals. Research has shown that women generally have greater affiliation needs than men and that nurses generally have high affiliation needs.

Power-oriented individuals are motivated by the power that can be gained as a result of a specific action. They want to command attention, get recognition, and control others. McClelland theorized that managers in organizations can identify achievement, affiliation, or power needs of their employees and develop appropriate motivational strategies to meet those needs.

Another humanistic motivational theorist, Gellerman, identified several methods to positively motivate people. One such method is *"stretching."* This involves the assignment of tasks to individuals that are more difficult than what they are used to doing. Stretching must not be a routine or daily activity.

Another method is *"participation,"* or actively drawing employees into decisions affecting their work. Gellerman strongly believed that motivational problems were usually a result of the way the organization managed and not an unwillingness of the staff to work hard. Gellerman stated that most managers in organizations "overmanage," that is, they make the job of the employee too narrow and fail to give the employee any decision-making power.

The work of all these theorists added greatly to our understanding of what motivates individuals, both in and out of the work setting. Their research revealed that motivation is extremely complex and that there are tremendous variations in what motivates different individuals. Therefore, it is important for the manager to understand what can be done at the unit level to create a climate that allows the worker to grow, increases motivation and productivity, and eliminates dissatisfiers that drain energy from employees.

◆ Motivation: Intrinsic and Extrinsic

Motivation requires willingness to put effort into achieving a goal or reward in an attempt to decrease tension. *Intrinsic motivation* is motivation that comes from within individuals and drives them to be productive. To be intrinsically motivated at work, the worker must value job performance and productivity. Hughes, Ginnett, and Curphy (1993), based on findings from diverse work groups, suggest that most people believe they could give as much as 15–20% more effort at work than they do now with no one, including their own bosses, recognizing any difference. Perhaps, even more startling, these workers also believed they could give 15–20% less effort without any one noticing the difference. Hunter, Schmidt, and Judiesch (1990) estimated that the top 15% of the workers for a particular job produced from 20% to 50% more output than the average worker, depending on the complexity of the job. The importance of intrinsic motivation, then, as a component of productivity and outcome cannot be underestimated.

Intrinsic motivation to achieve is directly related to an individual's level of aspiration. Parental and peer influence play a major role in shaping values concerning what individuals want to do and be. Parents who have high but attainable expectations for their children and who provide continuous encouragement in a nonauthoritarian environment tend to impart strong achievement drives in their children.

Even with a strong achievement drive, two other beliefs must be internalized before individuals are intrinsically motivated to behave in a certain way. Individuals must trust that improved performance will lead to a reward they desire and that increased effort will lead to improved performance. Thus, the outcome is worth the energy expenditure.

Extrinsic motivation is motivation enhanced by the job environment or external rewards that occur after the work has been completed. Although all individuals are intrinsically motivated to some degree, it is unrealistic for the organization to assume that all workers possess adequate levels to meet organizational goals. Thus, it must provide a climate that meets both extrinsic and intrinsic worker needs.

◆ The Role of the Manager in Creating a Motivating Climate

The manager plays a vital role in motivating staff to meet organizational goals. To do so, the manager must consider the uniqueness of each staff member and attempt to employ whatever motivational strategy is most appropriate for that employee. Actions the manager can take to create a motivating climate for employees are:

1. Have clear expectations for the workers and communicate these expectations effectively.
2. Be fair and consistent in dealing with all employees.
3. Be a firm decision maker using an appropriate decision-making style.

4. Develop the concept of teamwork.
5. Integrate the needs and wants of the staff with the interests and purposes of the organization.
6. Acknowledge the individuality of each employee and let him or her know that you understand his or her uniqueness.
7. Remove traditional blocks between the employee and the work to be done.
8. Provide experiences that challenge or "stretch" the employee and allow opportunity for growth. Allowing subordinates to produce, create, or excel is a powerful motivational strategy called *empowerment.* Sovie (1987) stated, "Empowerment is absolute recognition of the value of colleagues. It encompasses helping others to become all they are capable of becoming and assists the human assets in the environment to appreciate in value."
9. Request participation and input from subordinates in all appropriate decisions. In *participative management,* managers recognize the power of knowledge and ensure that information flows in every direction so that nurses throughout the organization will be well informed and prepared to engage actively and effectively in organizational decision making. This communication flow guarantees that nurses have the knowledge required to perform effectively in the organization, an important factor in increasing subordinate self-confidence and motivation.

    In participative management, the manager must find a balance between the desire to delegate sufficient authority to empower staff and the need to maintain enough control to ensure goal attainment. This is a difficult balance of often countervailing forces and may require adjustments in organizational structure. This balance is almost always best achieved at the lowest level in the organizational hierarchy (Garner, Smith, and Piland, 1990). Because participative management recognizes the professional nurse's expertise and enhances productivity through a culture of shared ownership, it should be recognized as a powerful motivational strategy (Sovie, 1987).
10. Be sure that employees understand the reason behind decisions and actions.
11. Let employees exercise individual judgment as often as possible.
12. Create a trustful and helping relationship with employees.
13. Let employees exercise as much control as possible over their work environment.
14. Be a role model for employees.
15. Use positive reinforcement whenever possible. This strategy is frequently overlooked or underused (Marquis and Huston, 1996).

◆ Mentoring as a Motivational Tool

Not every manager will be fortunate enough to have a mentor during his or her career. Madison and Huston (1996) define a mentor as a knowledgeable person who chooses to acquaint a novice (mentee) with the customs, resources, and values of the institution. The mentor is a confidante who personalizes role modeling and who freely gives time, energy, and material support to teach, guide, assist, and inspire the mentee.

Mentoring differs from role modeling in several ways. In role modeling the manager's behavior is observed by subordinates who attempt to emulate that behavior. Mentoring, on the other hand, takes more active participation on the part of the manager or mentor. The mentor, usually an older, wiser, and more experienced manager, seeks out potential leaders under his or her supervision, guiding and preparing them for future management roles. The mentor attempts to empower the mentee through various means, such as assignment to committees, introductions to powerful people, or by explanation of the inner political structure of the organization. Display 14-2 identifies some of the roles the mentor may hold in such a relationship.

Men in all levels of management have the opportunity to experience mentoring relationships more frequently than women, and the nursing profession

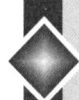

DISPLAY 14-2
Roles of the Mentor

1. *Model:* Someone you admire or want to emulate.
2. *Envisioner:* Someone who can see and communicate a meaning of professional nursing and its potential.
3. *Energizer:* Someone whose dynamism stimulates you to take action.
4. *Investor:* Someone who invests time and energy in your personal and professional growth.
5. *Supporter:* Someone who offers you emotional support and builds self-confidence.
6. *Standard prodder:* Someone who refuses to accept less than standards of excellence.
7. *Teacher-Coach:* Someone who teaches you interpersonal, technical, or political skills essential for advancement.
8. *Feedback giver:* Someone who gives honest positive and negative feedback for growth.
9. *Eye-opener:* Someone who broadens your perspective and gives you new ways of viewing situations.
10. *Door opener:* Someone who, by virtue of his or her position, can provide you with new opportunities or experiences.
11. *Idea bouncer:* Someone who will listen and discuss your ideas.
12. *Problem solver:* Someone who can help you examine problems and identify possible solutions.
13. *Career counselor:* Someone who helps you make short- and long-term career plans.
14. *Challenger:* Someone who encourages you to investigate issues more critically or in greater detail.

(Adapted from Darling, 1984.)

has been especially remiss in providing mentoring relationships for potential leaders and managers (Madison, Knight, and Watson, 1993). Madison further elaborates that the insufficient numbers of mentor–mentee relationships in nursing has resulted in inadequately prepared new managers. Therefore, when a nurse becomes a mentor, it not only creates a motivating climate but produces a greater number of leaders for the nursing profession. Besides serving as a role model for staff, managers should make an effort to enter into a mentoring relationship with novice managers and to encourage mentoring relationships between staff.

◆ Self-Motivation

The manager's own self-motivation is a critical variable in determining motivation at the unit level. Stengrevics and associates (1991) found that both job satisfaction and retention of staff nurses were positively influenced by the motivational level of the nurse manager. Positive outlooks, enthusiasm, productivity, and accomplishment are contagious. The unhappy manager projects unhappiness to subordinates and contributes greatly to low unit morale. The attitude and energy level of managers directly affect the attitude and productivity of employees. A burned-out, tired manager will yield a lethargic and demotivated staff. Therefore, it is essential that managers constantly monitor their own motivational level and do whatever necessary to restore their motivation to be a role model to staff.

Perhaps, then, the greatest challenge for nurse managers is *self-care*. "Self-care is the primary preventive measure against the burnout that inevitably occurs when we put everyone else's needs before our own" (Summers, 1994; 95). To maintain self-care, Summers (1994) suggests:

- finding a counselor or support group that allows you to put your caring for others on hold and listen to your own needs. Motivation is closely tied to support from our peers and significant others. If this support is lacking or is inadequate, the manager may become overwhelmed with responsibilities of the position and become less effective. As a manager it is very important to *network* within a professional support system for the purposes of support, information, and guidance.
- taking time off on a regular basis to detach from the melodrama of caring for others and to move into balance again.
- maintaining proper diet and exercise.
- finding activities or exercises that help you to relax. To do this, it is necessary to give yourself permission to let go of the need to give to somebody else.
- separating work from personal life. Remember that there is life outside of work.
- lowering your expectations of self and others.
- acknowledging your limits.

- recognizing that you are not the only person who can do a job. Learn to appreciate your skills and those of the people you work with.
- saying "no" to just one more thing.
- laughing more and inviting someone else to join you in a few hours of sustenance and renewal.
- reacquainting yourself with your heart. Why did you choose to serve others?

Perhaps Felder (1991) said it best in the following quote:

"What you do to assist another human being is extremely worthwhile. Now if you can just remember to take good care of yourself too, you'll do an even better job. Good luck!"

◆ Summary

Most human behavior is driven by something—usually by a goal we wish to achieve. Identifying those goals in employees and fostering their attainment allows managers to motivate their employees to not only reach personal, but organizational goals. The motivational strategy used by the manager in doing so will vary with the situation and the employee involved. The success of any motivational strategy, however, can be measured by the increased productivity and benefit to the organization, as well as the growth in the individual, which motivates them to accomplish again.

◆ References

Darling LA (1984). What do nurses want in a mentor? J Nurs Admin 14(10):42–44

Felder L (1991). When a Loved One Is Ill: How to Take Better Care of Your Loved One, Your Family, and Yourself. New York: Penguin Books

Garner JF, Smith HL, and Piland NF (1990). Strategic Nursing Management: Power and Responsibility in a New Era. Gaithersburg, MD: Aspen

Hughes RL, Ginnett RC, and Curphy GJ (1993). Understanding and influencing follower motivation, in Wren JT (ed.) (1995). The Leader's Companion. New York: The Free Press

Hunter JE, Schmidt FL, and Judiesch MK (1990). Individual differences in output variability as a function of job complexity. J Appl Psychol 74:28–42

Madison J, Knight BA, and Watson K (1993). Mentoring amongst academics in Australia: a case study. Australian Educ Res 20(1):18–32

Madison J and Huston C (1996). A comparative study of faculty–faculty mentoring relationships in an American and Australian university. Nat Assoc Stud Pers Admin 33(4):316–330

Marquis B and Huston C (1996). Leadership Roles and Management Functions: Theory and Application, 2nd ed. Philadelphia: JB Lippincott

Sovie MD (1987). Exceptional executive leadership shapes nursing's future. Nurs Econom 5(1), 13–20, 31

Stengrevics SS, Kirby KK, and Ollis ER (1991). Nurse manager job satisfaction: the Massachusetts perspective. Nurs Manage 22(4):60–64

Summers C (1994). Self-care: the greatest challenge for nurses. Rev J Nurse Empow 4(3):92–96

SAMPLE CASE ANALYSIS

THE CASE ◆

You have been a community health nurse for 3 years. Prior to this, you worked for 3 years in a hospital following your graduation from State College. At the hospital, you were a staff nurse for 18 months and then spent 18 months as the evening charge nurse on a surgical floor.

Recently you seem to have lost your "drive" and motivation for your present position. When you first became a public health nurse you had a high level of drive and energy and your supervisor complimented you on your strong motivation. Now you realize that you constantly become fatigued and irritable. You have been discouraged over the lack of self-initiative in some of your clients. You feel you are not performing at your best and have begun to have an ambivalent attitude.

You decide to go camping this weekend to reflect on what is happening and to attempt to discover a way to recapture your lost motivation.

....

Assignment

What are some steps you can take to become remotivated? Identify some specific steps that would assist you in solving this burnout problem.

....

Analysis

We do not know the cause of the lack of motivation of this nurse. It could be changing or unfulfilled needs, job dissatisfaction caused by a lack of maintenance factors, or it could be the type of burnout that results from constant job stress. However, this nurse is very fortunate in recognizing the increasing lack of motivation and has taken steps to determine the cause. Unfortunately, most individuals do not acknowledge when they are experiencing a lack of motivation and are often unable to take concrete action.

Since motivation is behind the action one takes in response to individual needs, the first goal must be to identify "wants or needs." Apparently these needs have changed, so that the present job is no longer supplying the personal needs required, resulting in demotivation. The weekend can best be spent outlining present personal needs.

Often changes occur in the life of an individual that alter one's needs. Perhaps this nurse has gotten married, become a parent, or experienced other changes that have made her priorities different. If the motivating factor 2 years ago was the stimulation of a new job, perhaps this position is no longer challenging. Thus, the need is for a more challenging position. Or, it may be that just the opposite is true; perhaps the job has been so formidable that the present most pressing need is to find a less challenging position or to go on vacation to refuel.

Another possibility in this situation is that the nurse might be highly motivated to learn. If education is a high-priority need, the answer may be to become more actively involved in the learning process by attending a course, returning to school for an additional degree, or learning something in a field outside of nursing.

Once personal needs have been identified, it is important to examine the present job situation. Is there anything about the position itself that is creating dissatisfaction that results in decreasing motivation? At this point, it is often a good idea to fantasize about the job. The nurse needs to visualize being highly moti-vated at work, and to simulate what that feels like. Then, the ideal should be compared with the real world to see if something is amiss; that is, inadequate salary, a difficult coworker, a demanding boss, too heavy a client load.

The third action this nurse must take is to evaluate what can be changed about the dissatisfying aspects and decide if there is a way to meet the presently identified needs. If the present situation cannot be altered, the nurse must deter-mine if the unchangeable can be acceptable. If it is impossible to either alter or totally accept the present situation, then a final area to examine is the possibil-ity for support, networking, and/or counseling. The flow sheet shown in Figure 14-3 is of value when an individual becomes cognizant that he or she is no longer motivated in some aspect of life.

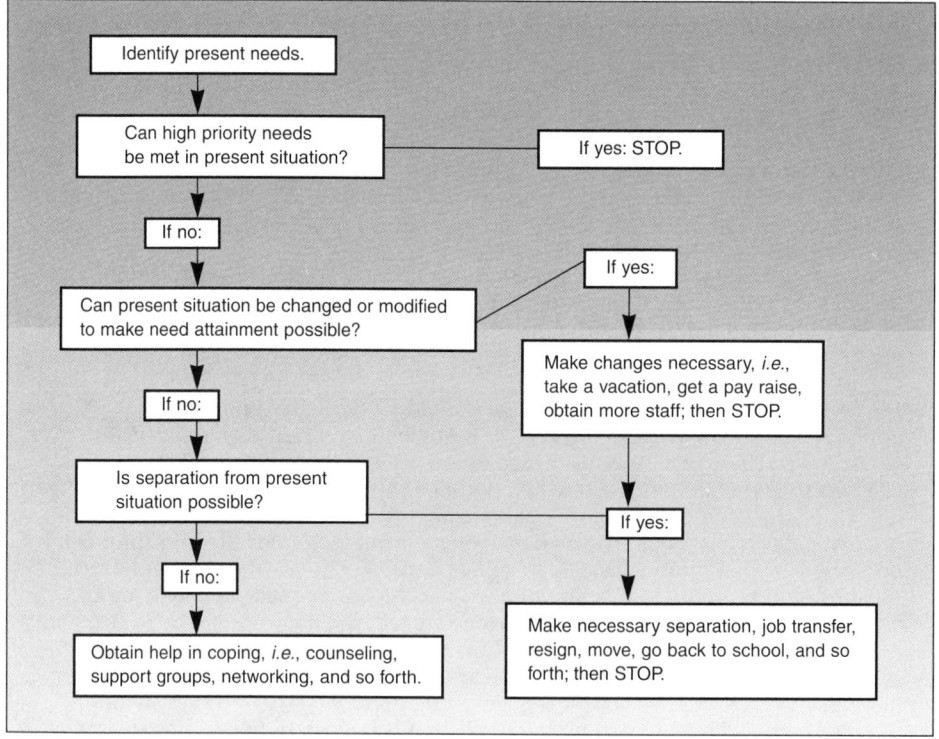

FIGURE 14-3. Flowsheets to help an individual evaluate what can be changed to meet present needs in life.

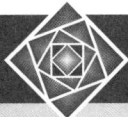 **CASES FOR PROBLEM SOLVING**

CASE 1

You are the 3:00 P.M.–11:00 P.M. charge nurse on the surgical unit and have become increasingly concerned regarding the behavior of one of the new RNs assigned to your unit. This new nurse, a recent graduate of a local BSN program, is named Barbara Brown. She came to work at Lakeside Hospital immediately on her graduation. She was assigned to work 7:00 A.M.–3:00 P.M. for 2 months and appeared to be extremely hard working, knowledgeable, well liked, and highly motivated. After her 2-month day shift orientation she was assigned to a permanent P.M. shift, where she has been working for the last 4 months. Approximately 7 weeks ago several small incidents happened to Ms. Brown. One of the physicians became very angry with her over a minor medication error she had made, and she was already feeling badly about the error.

Following this episode, the husband of a patient took a dislike to Ms. Brown (for no discernable reason) and refused to allow her to care for his wife. Then, 2 weeks ago, a patient died suddenly and although no one was to blame, Ms. Brown apparently believed that if she had been more observant and skilled in her assessment she would have picked up the subtle changes in the patient's condition sooner. Although you have been supportive of Ms. Brown, you recognize that she is in danger of becoming demotivated. Her once flawless appearance has been replaced by wrinkled uniforms; she is frequently absent from work; and her once pleasant personality has been exchanged by withdrawal from her coworkers.

Assignment

Using your knowledge of new role identification and assimilation, as well as motivation theory, develop a plan to assist this young nurse. What can you do to provide a climate that will remotivate her and decrease her job dissatisfaction? Explain what you believe is happening to this nurse and the rationale behind your plan. Your plan should be realistic in terms of the time and energy you may spend on one employee and should include the responsibilities of the employee.

CASE 2 (Marquis and Huston, 1996)

You are the Chief Nursing Officer at Shady Knoll Hospital. Dr. Smith, a cardiologist, has approached you regarding having an ICU-CCU nurse make rounds with him every morning, visiting all the patients in the hospital with a cardiac-related diagnosis. He feels this will probably represent a 90-minute commitment of nursing time daily. He is vague about the nurse's exact role or purpose, but you believe there is great potential for better and more consistent patient education and care planning. Beth Simpson, one of your finest ICU-CCU nurses, agrees to assist Dr. Smith. The other ICU-CCU staff agree to cover her patients while she is gone, although it is obviously an extension of an already full patient load.

After 3 weeks of making rounds with Dr. Smith, Ms. Simpson comes to your office. She tearfully reports that making rounds frequently takes from 2 to 3

CASE 2 (CONTINUED)

hours, and that doing so with Dr. Smith amounts to little more than "carrying his charts, picking up his pages, and being a personal handmaiden." She also maintains that she has assertively stated her beliefs and has attempted to demonstrate to Dr. Smith how their collaboration could result in improved patient care. She states that she has not been allowed any input into patient decisions and is frequently reminded of "her position" and his ability to "have her removed from her job if she does not like being told what to do." She is demoralized and demotivated. In addition, she believes that her peers resent having to cover her workload since it is obvious that her role is superficial at best.

You call Dr. Smith and he agrees to meet with you at your office when he completes rounds the following morning. At this visit, Dr. Smith confirms Ms. Simpson's description of her role, but justifies his desire for the role to continue by saying, "I bring millions of dollars of business to this hospital every year in cardiology procedures. The least you can do is provide the nursing assistance I am asking for. If you are unable to meet this small request, I will be forced to consider taking my practice to a competing hospital."

Assignment

Do you meet Dr. Smith's request? Does it make any difference whether Ms. Simpson is the nurse or can it be someone else? Does the revenue Dr. Smith generates supersede the value of professional nursing practice? Should you try and talk Ms. Simpson into continuing in the position for a while longer? While trying to reach a goal, people must sometimes endure a difficult path, but at what point do the means not justify the end? Be realistic about what you would do in this situation. What do you perceive to be the greatest obstacles in implementing your decision?

CASE 3 ◆▶

You are the supervisor of a medical unit. At the department head meeting today, the CEO stated that the cost of contracted dialysis services would be increased by 30% in 3 months. At present, all dialysis is performed by outside contractors. The CEO has asked you to develop a proposal comparing the cost of developing in-house dialysis services to that of contracting for such services. Because establishing an in-house dialysis service would take at least 3 to 4 months, you have been asked to have the report in 2 weeks.

You have never worked as a dialysis nurse and have very limited knowledge regarding the extent of what would be required to establish an in-house program. You could, however, gather the information with the help of some networking contacts you have in nephrology nursing.

You also have a nurse on your staff with 10 years of experience as both a manager and clinician in a dialysis clinic. She has the knowledge needed to complete such an analysis and prepare the report. She is, however, not one of your most motivated workers, and in the past has assumed responsibility for projects with poor follow through. You feel that the completion of this project could be used as a motivational strategy to empower this employee, but

CASE 3 (CONTINUED)

are concerned that the time frame is short and that it would be necessary for you to maintain some control regarding goal attainment.

••
Assignment

Will you elect to prepare the report yourself or will you attempt to empower the employee with the project? Give the rationale for your choice. If you have chosen to delegate the project to the employee, what, if any, controlling safeguards have you built into your plan? Is it possible that the delegation of such a project could demotivate the employee as well as motivate?

CASE 4

You are a critical care nurse in a busy trauma unit. Your unit is understaffed, as are many critical care units across the nation owing to a nursing shortage. Although hospital recruitment efforts have been extremely active, there is little chance of resolution in the near future. The unit supervisor is extremely supportive of the staff's efforts, but can do little to ease the actual staffing shortage other than to refuse patients or close the unit, and this is the only facility for a 100-mile radius providing trauma care. As a result, all the nurses on the unit have been working at least 40 hours per week during the last 6 months, with many working several double shifts each pay period, as well as putting in many hours of overtime.

Morale is deteriorating and the staff have begun to complain. Many of the staff have started refusing to work extra shifts or to do overtime. Because you feel a responsibility to the patients, the community, and the organization, you have continued to work the extra hours. As others refuse to work more, your extra hours have increased accordingly. You are exhausted and have had little time with your family in the last several months.

Today is your first evening off in 6 days. At 2:00 P.M., the phone rings and you suspect it is the hospital calling you to come in to work. You delay answering while you decide what to do. Your answering machine turns on and you hear the voice of your unit supervisor. She says they are "desperate." There were two new admits during the day from an auto accident and the unit is full. She says "she really appreciates all the hours you have been working and asks if you would come in and work at least a 4-hr shift this evening, although she is unable to give you a day off tomorrow in compensation."

••
Assignment

Although you do not have formal plans for the evening, you really feel as if you need a day off, especially if you must work tomorrow as well. You feel conflicting loyalties to the unit, patients, supervisor, and yourself. Decide what you will do. Will you agree to work? Will you return your supervisor's phone call or pretend you are not home? When do your loyalties to your patients and the organization end and your loyalties to yourself begin? Is the unit supervisor taking advantage of you? Are the other staff being irresponsible? What values have played a part in your decision making?

CASE 5

Given rising costs and shrinking reimbursement, more and more hospitals are *downsizing* in an effort to shrink personnel costs. Registered nurses (RNs) as a group have been hit hard with downsizing and many experienced, qualified nurses have found themselves, for the first time in their lives, unemployed. The threat of termination, rapid organizational changes, and the unpredictability inherent in a rapidly changing health care market have all contributed to work-related stress, lowered self-esteem, and burnout for registered nurses.

Assume that you are a middle level manager in an acute care hospital. In a recent department head's meeting, the Chief Officer for Nursing Operations announced that personnel cutbacks in the coming 6 months were probable. The degree of the cutback, although unknown, should not be large, but it does appear that the expected attrition/turnover rates in the next 6 months will be inadequate to eliminate the need for some terminations.

The news travels rapidly through the hospital grapevine. Semihysteria prevails, with many personnel consulting you regarding whether their position is in jeopardy and what they can to do to increase the likelihood of their retention. Morale is rapidly plummeting and staff relationships are becoming increasingly competitive rather than cooperative.

Assignment

Determine how you will handle this situation. What strategies might you implement to reduce the immediate anxiety level? What advice can you give to staff who may face layoffs within the next few months? Is it possible to preserve the morale of your employees in an uncertain situation such as this?

◆ Bibliography

The following is a list of references to help you solve these cases.

Austin BA (1990). The art of motivation. Today's OR Nurse 12(12):3

Baard PP and Neville SM (1996). The intrinsically motivated nurse: help and hindrance from evaluation feedback. J Nurs Admin 26(7/8):19–26

Bass LS (1991). Motivation strategies: a new twist. Nurs Manage 22(2):24–26

Brito H and Hernandez-Piloto (1992). Nurses in action—an innovative approach to mentoring. J Nurs Admin 22(5):23–28

Burke R, McKeen C, and McKenna C (1994). Benefits of mentoring in organisations. J Manag Psychol 9(3):23–32

Carey SJ and Campbell ST (1994). Preceptor, mentor, and sponsor roles: creative strategies for nurse retention. J Nurs Admin 24(12):39–48

Hegge M (1990). What keeps nurses in nursing? Nurs Manage 21(11):65

Keyes MA (1994). Recognition and reward: a unit-based program. Nurs Manage 25(2):52–54

Kinsey DC (1990). Mentorship and influence in nursing. Nurs Manage 21(5):45–46

McGrail GR (1990). Motivation of healthcare workers. Hosp Topics 68(2):24–26

Moore S, Kuhrik M, Kuhrik N, and Katz B (1996). Coping with downsizing. Nurs Manage 27(3):28–32

Russ AM (1994). Downsizing: a survival kit for employees. Nurs Manage 25(8):66–68

Smith L (1994). Burned out bosses. Fortune 130(2)(July 25):44–52

Tschudin V (1990). Essentials of management: motivate yourself. Nurs Times 86(11)(Mar 14–20):29–30

Tumulty G, Jernigan IE, and Kohut G (1995). Reconceptualizing organizational committment. J Nurs Admin 25(1):61–65

Vincent A and Seymour J (1994). Mentoring among female executives. Women Manage Rev 9(7):15–20

Yearta SK, Maitis S, and Briner RB (1995). An exploratory study of goal setting in theory and practice: a motivational technique that works? J Occup Org Psychol 68:237–252

PERSONAL NOTEBOOK

1. At this point in your life, what are your five greatest desires? Where would they fall in Maslow's hierarchy?

2. Think back to when you were a child. What rewards did your parents use to promote good behavior? Was your behavior more intrinsically or extrinsically motivated? Were high levels of achievement encouraged and supported by your family?

3. What do you feel is the most rewarding aspect of nursing?

4. Identify the greatest motivator in your life at this time. Has it always been the strongest motivator? Could you list the strongest motivator for others who are significant in your life? If so, have you ever used this awareness to motivate those individuals to do something specific?

Time Management

In order for managers to effectively direct employees, they must first be able to find the time to do so. *Time management* is making optimal use of what time you have. Although some individuals appear to naturally manage their time more wisely than others, it is a learned skill that improves with practice. Time management can be summarized in three basic steps, as shown in Figure 15-1. In the first step, time is allowed for planning and establishing priorities. The second step entails completing the highest priority task (as determined in step 1) whenever possible and finishing one task before beginning another. In the final step, the individual must reprioritize based on new information that may have been received. Because this is a cyclic process, all three steps must be approached sequentially.

Because time is a scarce and valuable resource for the manager, learning to use it wisely is essential to effective management. It is critical that managers be able to manage time in three different areas: 1) personal organization, 2) organizing work, and 3) delegation and supervision. Personal organization and organizing work are discussed in this chapter. Chapter 16 is devoted to delegation and supervision.

◆ Personal Organization

Personal organization refers to "the knowing of self." Managing time is difficult if one is unsure of priorities, including personal short-, intermediate-, and long-term goals. These goals give structure to what should be accomplished today, tomorrow, and in the future. By setting goals, one decides how to allot time. If

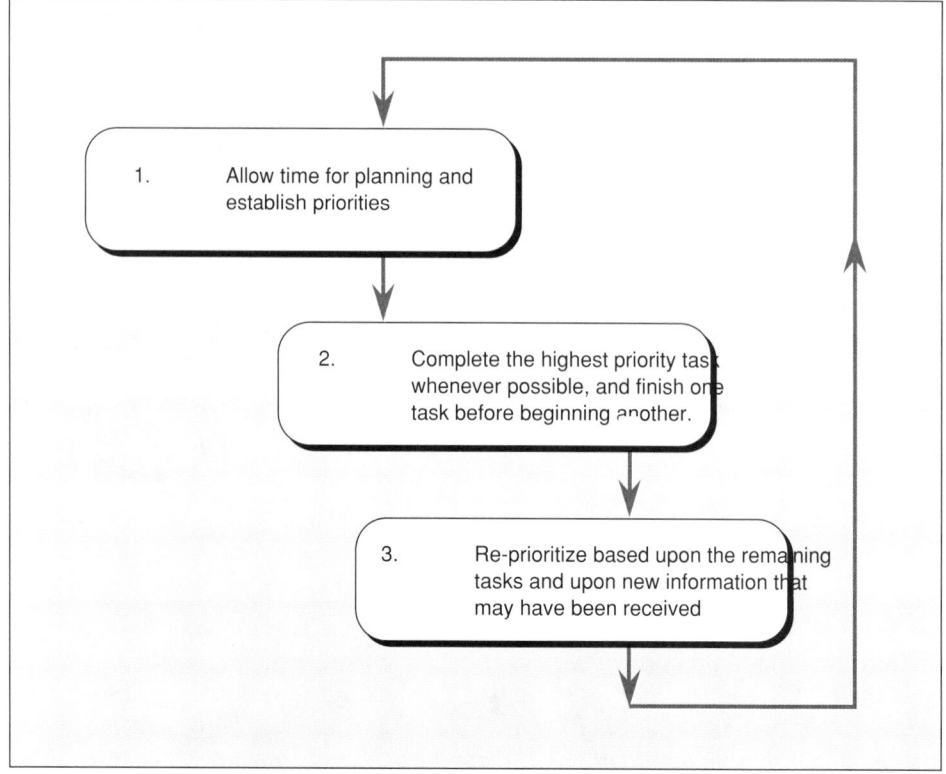

FIGURE 15-1. The three basic steps in time management.

goals are not set, others often end up deciding how a person should spend his or her life or time, and all too often, irrelevant decisions and insignificant activities take priority over real purposes.

Catalano (1996) concurs, suggesting that the key to time management is setting priorities. "In the world of nursing and client care, some activities are essential to the safety and well-being of clients. These include getting medications to clients on time, meeting their comfort needs, and preventing accidental injuries. Beyond these actions, nurses really have a great deal of discretion in what they can do when providing care to clients" (Catalano, 1996; 153).

A study by Hendrickson, Doddato, and Kovner (1990) showed that within a typical 8-hour shift, nurses in six specialty units averaged only 31% (2.5 hours) of their time with patients—an average of 25–30 minutes per shift with each patient. This occurred despite an average of one nurse for every 4.8 patients during day shift and one nurse for every 6.9 patients on evening shift.

Likewise, a study by Prescott and colleagues (1991) showed that hospital nurses inappropriately used their time doing the work of other departments, such as dietary, housekeeping, transportation, and pharmacy. They also were required to do the work of lesser trained personnel such as vocational nurses, aides, orderlies, unit clerks, and secretaries.

In addition, Bassler and Goedde (1993) found that more than 30 hours each week of managerial time were spent on clerical work. Clearly, work redesign might alleviate some of these problems. Sometimes, there is simply an overwhelming amount of work to be accomplished. However, it is also clear that unclear values and priorities contribute to the problem. Professional nurses who are self-aware and have clearly identified personal and professional goals and priorities have greater control over how they expend their energy and over what they subsequently accomplish (Marquis and Huston, 1996).

Robbins (1991) suggests that if you work very hard, complete every single thing on your to-do list, and still feel unfulfilled at the end of the day, you probably took care of urgent items that demanded your immediate attention, but didn't do what was important—the things that would make a long-term difference. "The only way to master your time is to organize your schedule each day to spend the majority of time doing things that are important rather than urgent" (Robbins, 1991; 479).

Another strategy to mastering personal organization is increasing your self-awareness regarding how you personally waste time. All people have set patterns of what types of work they avoid or how they go about wasting time. Likewise, each individual works better at certain times of the day or for certain lengths of time. Display 15-1 identifies some personal or internal time wasters.

◆ The Relationship Between Planning and Organizing

Many individual nurses appear disorganized in their effort to accomplish patient care. Usually this disorganization results from poor planning rather than poor organization. The ability to be organized develops from good planning. As planning occurs there is a need to pause and decide how people, activities, and materials are going to be put together in order to carry out plans.

A mistake common to novice managers is not allowing adequate time for planning. Without sufficient planning, the manager experiences difficulty in getting started and begins to manage by crisis. Setting aside time at the beginning of each day to plan allows the manager to spend time on high-priority tasks. During this scheduling, the manager should review short-, immediate-, and long-term goals and determine what progress should be made on these goals.

Sometimes, the new manager does allow time for planning, but has problems accurately predicting the length of time it will take to complete a given activity. This ability is a management skill that is acquired with experience (Bernhard and Walsh, 1990).

It is important, however, that the manager remember that no amount of planning can prevent periodic crises and therefore, as in all planning, daily planning must be flexible. If a crisis does occur, the manager should resort to *crisis control,* as described by Grohar-Murray and DiCroce (1992). In crisis con-

DISPLAY 15-1
Internal Time Wasters

1. Procrastination
2. Poor planning
3. Failure to establish goals
4. Failure to set objectives
5. Inability to delegate
6. Inability to say no
7. Management by crisis
8. Haste
9. Indecisiveness
10. Open-door policy

(From Lancaster, 1984.)

trol, the manager sets aside the original priorities established for the day, and reorganizes, communicates, and delegates a new plan reflecting the new priorities associated with the unexpected and untoward event causing the crisis.

◆ Organizing Work To Be Accomplished

Being overwhelmed by work and time constraints leads to an increase in errors, the omission of important tasks, and generalized feelings of stress and ineffectiveness (Tappen, 1995). Because most managers have more than enough work to accomplish, learning to manage time at work is essential.

In organizing patient care delivery, expert nurses reduce travel to and from activities by gathering all the supplies they will need before they start. They also group activities together that are in the same location. If a nurse must walk a long distance down a hallway, he or she should attempt to do several things there before going back to the nurse's station.

Expert nurses also use time estimates to help organize their work. For example, if the nurse knows an intermittent intravenous medication (IV piggyback) will take 30 minutes to finish, then he or she must be careful not to begin any activity that will take longer than 30 minutes to complete.

As an administrator, the unit manager also needs to structure how other duties will be performed on the unit and to devise methods to make work simpler and more efficient. Often this includes simple tasks, such as specifying how supplies are stored or determining the most efficient lunch and break schedules for staff. The goal in organizing work and activities is to facilitate greater productivity and worker satisfaction.

Swansburg (1990) suggests that the unit manager use the following day-to-day planning actions to promote time efficiency:

1. At the beginning of the day, make a list of all tasks to be accomplished for the day.
2. Plan ahead for meetings, preparing and distributing agendas in advance.
3. Identify growing problems and put them in the appropriate portion of the unit's short- or long-term plans.
4. On a regular basis, review the short-, intermediate-, and long-term plans of the unit, including how they will affect colleagues and subordinates.

◆ Setting Priorities

Because managers are inundated with many requests for their time and energy, the next step in time management is prioritizing. It is important to develop a systematic means of determining which items are to be accomplished by whom. One simple method is to divide all such requests into three categories: 1) "don't do," 2) "do later," and 3) "do now." The "don't do" items probably reflect problems that will take care of themselves, are already outdated, or that are better accomplished by someone else. In any case, the manager either discards the unnecessary information or passes it on to the appropriate person in a timely fashion. In either case, the manager removes unneeded clutter from the work area.

"Do later" items may reflect problems that are trivial or that do not have immediate time constraints. Although it is appropriate for managers to selectively procrastinate, procrastination is not appropriate just because a task is overwhelming or unpleasant. Before setting "do later" items aside, the manager must be certain that large projects have been broken down into smaller projects and that a specific time frame and plan for implementation is in place. This plan should include short-term, intermediate, and final deadlines. Likewise, items without immediate time limits cannot be ignored indefinitely, and the manager must make a definitive time commitment in the near future to address these requests.

The "do now" requests most commonly reflect day-to-day operational needs at the unit level. These requests may include daily staffing needs, dealing with equipment shortages, meeting deadlines, hiring interviews, performance appraisals, and so on. "Do now" requests may also represent items that had been put off at an earlier date.

◆ Making Written Lists

In prioritizing all the "do now" items, the manager may find it helpful to prepare a written list. Although the manager may use monthly or weekly lists, the daily list is a helpful tool in coordinating day-to-day unit operation. This list, however, should not include more than what can be realistically accomplished in one day, otherwise, it demotivates instead of assisting the manager. In addition, although the manager must be cognizant and plan for routine daily tasks, it is not always necessary to list them, as they only serve to distract the manager from priority tasks for the day. Lists should allow adequate time for each item and blocks of time must be built in for the unexpected.

Periodically, the manager should examine lists from prior days to review what was not accomplished or completed. If an item appears for several successive days, the manager must reexamine it and assess why it was not accomplished. Some projects need to be removed from lists. Often, the reason a project has not been accomplished is that it was not divided into manageable tasks. For example, many well-meaning individuals begin thinking about completing their tax returns in early January, but feel overwhelmed by a project that cannot be accomplished in a single day. If they do not break the work of preparing their tax return down into several smaller tasks, with intermediate deadlines, it may be delayed indefinitely.

It is important that the manager remember that a list is a planning tool and there must be some flexibility in its implementation. In fact, the last step in time management is reprioritizing. Often, the manager's priorities (and list) will change during the course of a day, week, or longer, because new information is received. If the manager does not take time to reprioritize after each major task is accomplished, other priorities set earlier may no longer be accurate.

◆ External Time Wasters

Managers also need to become skillful at preventing interruptions that keep them from managing time effectively. First- and middle-level managers are at greater risk for interruptions in their work than are high-level managers because first- and middle-level managers are more involved in day-to-day planning than high-level managers, and thus directly interact with a greater number of subordinates on a daily basis. In addition, many low-level managers do not have offices that provide a quiet work space, or clerical help to filter interruptions. Frequent work interruptions result in situational stress and lowered job satisfaction.

Interruptions that keep managers from accomplishing their "do now" and "do later" lists include ten external time wasters identified by Lancaster (1984). These external time wasters are listed in Display 15-2. There are several ways that individuals can be discouraged from consuming your time with idle chatter. Among them are the following.

1. Make yourself less accessible and make it easy for people to ignore you. If you have charting to do, sit with your back to others. If you have an office, close the door. Both behaviors will discourage casual conversation.
2. Interrupt. When someone is rambling, break in and gently say, "Excuse me—I'm not getting your message. What exactly are you saying?"
3. Avoid promoting socializing. Having several comfortable chairs in your office, a full candy dish, and posters on your walls that invite comments lead to the use of your office as a social gathering place.

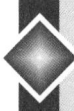

DISPLAY 15-2
External Time Wasters

1. Telephone interruptions
2. Socializing
3. Meetings
4. Lack of information
5. Poor communication
6. Lack of feedback
7. Lack of or unclear policies and procedures
8. Incompetent coworkers
9. Poor filing system
10. Paperwork

(From Lancaster, 1984.)

4. Be brief. Gauge your own long-winded comments and stand when you are finished. This will signal an end to the conversation.
5. Limit long-winded pests to scheduled visits. If a physician or employee has a pattern of lengthy chatter and manages to corner you on rounds, or at the nurse's station, say, "Not now, but I'm going to have some free time at 11:00 A.M., why don't you see me then?" Unless the meeting is important, an individual without a specific agenda will not bother to make a formal appointment.

An adequate filing system is also invaluable in handling the external time waster of "paper overload." Keeping correspondence organized in easily retrievable files rather than disorganized stacks saves time when managers need to find specific information. Unsorted papers should not be allowed to accumulate on the manager's desk or critical, time-sensitive correspondence may be missed (Tappen, 1995).

◆ Summary

Time management begins with the individual taking stock of him- or herself and developing an awareness of whether he or she personally manages time poorly or well. Managers must have an understanding of their own values system, which influences how they use time and how they expect subordinates to, as well.

Wise managers know that structuring time carefully will increase their personal productivity and value. Because time is a finite and valuable resource, managers with well-developed time management skills are more likely to accomplish unit goals in a timely and appropriate manner.

◆ References

Bassler S and Goedde L (1993). Clerical activities and the nurse manager. Nurs Manage 24(1):63–64

Bernhard LA and Walsh M (1990). Leadership—The Key to the Professionalization of Nursing, 2nd ed. St. Louis: CV Mosby

Catalano JT (1996). Contemporary Professional Nursing. Philadelphia: FA Davis

Grohar-Murray ME and DiCroce HR (1992). Leadership and Management in Nursing. Norwalk, CT: Appleton and Lange

Hendrickson G, Doddato TM, and Kovner CT (1990). How do nurses use their time? J Nurs Admin 20(3):31–37

Lancaster J (1984). Making the most of every minute: reminders for nursing leaders. In Berger MS, Elhart D, Firsich S, Jordan S, and Stone S (eds): Management for Nurses. St. Louis: CV Mosby

Marquis B and Huston C (1996). Leadership Roles and Management Functions: Theory and Application, 2nd ed. Philadelphia: JB Lippincott

Prescott PA, Phillips CY, Ryan JW, and Thompson KO (1991). Changing how nurses spend their time. Image 23(1):23–27

Robbins A (1991). Awaken the Giant Within. New York: Simon & Schuster

Swansburg RC (1990). Management and Leadership for Nurse Managers. Boston: Jones and Bartlett

Tappen RM (1995). Nursing Leadership and Management: Concepts and Practice, 3rd ed. Philadelphia: FA Davis

SAMPLE CASE ANALYSIS

THE CASE ◆

You are employed at a Native American health agency where it is the policy for some public health nurses to be available in the office every day. This morning is your turn to provide such coverage. In the afternoon, from 1:00 to 5:00 P.M., you will be the public health nurse at the scheduled immunization clinic. However, you hope to be able to spend some time today finishing your end-of-month reports, which are due at 5:00 P.M. The office remains open during lunch and you have a luncheon meeting with a cancer society group from noon to 1:00 P.M. today.

The RN in the office is to serve as a resource person to the receptionist and handle client phone calls as well as drop-ins. In addition to the receptionist, you may appropriately delegate to a clerical worker. However, the clerical worker also serves the other public health nurses in the clinic and is usually fairly busy.

While you are in the office today trying to finish your reports, the following interruptions occur:

SAMPLE CASE ANALYSIS (CONTINUED)

8:30 A.M.   Supervisor comes in and wants you to give her the number of diabetic and hypertensive clients you have.

9:00 A.M.   A client is waiting to see you regarding her daughter, who has just found out she is pregnant. The mother is upset.

9:00 A.M.   Three drop-in clients are waiting to be interviewed for possible referral to the chest clinic.

9:30 A.M.   The public health physician calls you needing someone to contact a family regarding a child's immunization.

9:30 A.M.   The dental department drops off 20 referrals for which you must pull charts.

10:00 A.M.   You receive a call from a client concerned about bills he has received. Client sounds extremely confused regarding what to do.

10:45 A.M.   Six families are waiting to be enrolled for food vouchers. They have been waiting since 8:30 A.M.

11:45 A.M.   Call comes in from client regarding the fact that she has been using drugs and is unsure what to do. Has heard about Narcotics Anonymous and would like more information *now*.

••

Assignment

How would you handle each interruption? Justify your decisions. Be sure to include lunch for yourself and the two office workers.

Time	Task	Rationale
ANALYSIS		
8:00 A.M.	Assign lunch breaks	Since you have a luncheon engagement at noon, make sure other employees know when their lunch times are.
11:30 A.M.–12:30 P.M.	Receptionist	
12:30 P.M.–1:30 P.M.	Clerical worker	
12:00 M.–1:00 P.M.	Personal time	
	Finish reports	Since reports are due at 5:00 P.M., this would be the immediate task to be pursued. Plan to finish these by 9:00 A.M.
8:30 A.M.	Supervisor's request	Ask when the information is needed and state that an estimation using primary diagnosis is available now, but an accurate figure (including secondary diagnoses) will have to wait until you have the time to examine your 150 family case files, which will be next week.

S A M P L E   C A S E   A N A L Y S I S   (C O N T I N U E D)

Time	Task	Rationale
9:00 A.M.	Client with pregnant daughter/chest clinic	This takes priority over chest clinic drop-ins. Have the receptionist and drop-ins start paperwork while you spend 30 minutes with the mother.
9:30 A.M.	Phone call	Delegate this to the receptionist.
9:30 A.M.	Dental clinic referral	Delegate this to the clerical worker.
10:00 A.M.	Client call	Since this person is confused and you do not have the necessary information available, request that he come in at 10:00 A.M. tomorrow with his bills.
10:45 A.M.	Food voucher families	Ask the receptionist to finish paperwork and interviews with the families. Then, quickly review information and sign vouchers. As these families should not have had such a long wait, make a note to find out what happened, and later counsel office staff as necessary regarding the delay.
11:45 A.M.	Drug abuse call	Speak with client. Make a referral to a local drug clinic and arrange appointment for the part-time psychiatrist at Native American clinic. Do not get extensively involved on the phone with the client. It is better to make appropriate referrals.

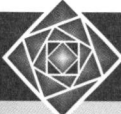

C A S E S   F O R   P R O B L E M   S O L V I N G

CASE 1 ◆ (Marquis and Huston, 1996)

You are an RN providing total patient care to four patients on an orthopedic unit during the 7:00 A.M.–3:00 P.M. shift. Given the following patient information, prioritize your activities for the shift into eight 1-hour blocks of time. Be sure to include time for reports, planning your day's activities, breaks, and lunch. Be realistic about what you can accomplish. What activities will you delegate to the next shift? What overall goals have guided your time management? What personal values or priorities played a factor in setting these goals?

•••

Patient Information

101 A: Mrs. Riley, 84 years old. Fractured left hip secondary to fall at home. Disoriented since admission, especially at night. Soft restraints in use. Moans fre-

CASE 1 (CONTINUED)

quently, being given IV pain medication every 2 hours prn. Vital signs and checks for circulation, feeling, and movement in toes ordered every 2 hours. Scheduled for surgery at 1030. Preoperative medications scheduled for 0930 and 1000. Consent yet to be signed. Family members will arrive at 0800 and have expressed questions about the surgery and the recovery period. Patient to return from surgery at approximately 1430. Will require postop vitals every 15 minutes.

101 B: Ms. Wilkins, 26 years old. Compound fracture of the femur with postop fat emboli, now resolved. 10 lb. Buck's Traction. Has been in the hospital 3 weeks. Very bored and frustrated with prolonged hospitalization. Upset about "roommate who calls out all night and keeps her from sleeping." Wishes to be moved to new room. Has also requested to have hair washed during bath today. Has IV running at 100 cc/hr. IV antibiotic piggybacks at 0800 and 1200. Oral medications at 0800, 0900, and 1200.

102 A: Mr. Jenkins, 47 years old. T-6 quadriplegic due to diving accident 14 years ago. 2 days postop above knee amputation owing to osteomyelitis. Cultures have shown Methicillin Resistant Staph Aureus. Strict wound isolation. Has been hospitalized for 2 weeks. Expressing great deal of anger and frustration to anyone who enters room. IV site red and puffy—IV needs to be restarted. Dressing change of operative site ordered daily. Heat lamp treatments ordered bid to small pressure sores on coccyx. IV antibiotic piggybacks at 0800, 1000, 1200, and 1400. Primary IV bag to run out at 1000. 0600 labwork results to be called in to physician this morning. Needs total assistance in performing ADLs (activities of daily living, such as bathing, feeding self, etc.).

103 A: Mr. Novak, 19 years old. Severe tear of rotator cuff in left shoulder while playing football. One day postop rotator cuff repair; very quiet and withdrawn. Refusing pain medication, which has been ordered every 2 hours prn. Says "he can handle it and does not want to mess up his body with drugs." Wants to be "recruited into the pros after this semester." Nonverbals of grimacing, moaning, and inability to sleep suggest moderate pain is present. Physician states that likelihood of Mr. Novak ever playing football again is very low, but has not yet told patient. Girlfriend frequently in room at patient's bedside. IV infusing at 150 cc/hr. IV antibiotics at 0800 and 1400. Has not had a bath since admission 2 days ago.

CASE 2

It is October of your second year as the Coordinator of Nursing for the surgical department. Attached is a copy of your appointment calendar for Monday, 27 October.

APPOINTMENT CALENDAR FOR MONDAY, 27 OCTOBER

8:00 A.M.	Arrive at work.
8:15 A.M.	Daily rounds with each head nurse in your area.
8:30 A.M.	Continuation of daily rounds with head nurses.
9:00 A.M.	Open.
9:30 A.M.	Open.

CASE 2 (CONTINUED)

APPOINTMENT CALENDAR FOR MONDAY, 27 OCTOBER

10:00 A.M.	Department heads meeting.
10:30 A.M.	United Givers Committee meeting.
11:00 A.M.	United Givers Committee (continued).
11:30 A.M.	Open.
12:00 M.	Lunch.
12:30 P.M.	Lunch.
1:00 P.M.	Weekly meeting with administrator—budget and annual report due.
1:30 P.M.	Open.
2:00 P.M.	Infection Control Committee meeting.
2:30 P.M.	Infection Control meeting (continued).
3:00 P.M.	Fire drill and critique of drill.
3:30 P.M.	Fire drill and critique (continued).
4:00 P.M.	Open.
4:30 P.M.	Open.
5:00 P.M.	Off duty.

Assignment

You will review your unfinished business from the preceding Friday and look at the new items that have arrived on your desk this morning (items 1–13, pages 268–271).

1. Assign a priority to each item, with 1 being the most important and 5 having the least priority.
2. Decide when you will pursue each item, being careful not to schedule more time than you have open on your calendar.
3. If the problem is to be dealt with immediately, explain how you will do this (e.g., by delegation, phone call, etc.).
4. The unit ward clerk is usually free in the afternoon to provide you with an hour of clerical assistance, plus you have a charge nurse on each shift to whom you may delegate appropriate duties.
5. You will need to explain the rationale for your decisions.

Item 1

From the Desk of M. Hardy, Personnel Manager
October 24
Dear Joan,
I am sending you the names of two new graduate nurses who have expressed an interest in working in your area. I have processed their applications and they

CASE 2 (CONTINUED)

seem well-qualified. Could you try to see them as early as possible in the week? I would hate to lose these prospective employees and they are most anxious to obtain definite confirmation of employment.

••••••••••••••••••••••
Item 2

From the Desk of Jerome Brown, Purchasing Agent
October 23
Joan,
We really must get together this week and devise an inventory method to control supplies. Your area has used three times as many thermometer covers as any other area. Are you taking that many more temperatures? This is just one of the supplies used in an excessive amount in your area. I'm open to suggestions.

••••••••••••••••••••••
Item 3

Roger Johnson, M.D.
Chief of Surgical Department
October 24,
Ms. Kerr,
I know you have your budget ready to submit, but I just remembered this week that I forgot to include an arterial pressure monitor. Is there something else we can leave out? I'll drop by Monday morning and we'll discuss this further.

••••••••••••••••••••••
Item 4

October 23
Ms. Kerr,
The following personnel are due for merit raises and I must have their completed and signed evaluations by Tuesday afternoon.

1. Lucy Rocas
2. Jim Newman
3. Marge Newfield

M. Hardy, Personnel Manager

••••••••••••••••••••••
Item 5

Roger Johnson, M.D.
Chief of Surgical Department
October 23
Ms. Kerr,
The physicians are complaining regarding the availability of nurses to accompany them on rounds. I believe we need to sit down with the doctors and head nurses to discuss this recurring problem. I am available part of Monday afternoon.

CASE 2 (CONTINUED)

••••••••••••••••••••••

Item 6

5:00 A.M.
Joan,
Meg Knight (your regular night RN) requested a leave of absence due to her
mother's illness. I told her it would be OK to take the next three nights off. She
is flying out of town on the 9:00 A.M. commuter flight to San Francisco—phone
her right away if you don't want her to go. (I felt I had no choice but to say yes.)

Jennifer Wheeler
Night Supervisor

P.S. You'll need to find a replacement for her for the next 3 nights.

••

Item 7

To: Ms. Kerr
From: Administrator
Re: Patient Complaint
Date: October 23
Please investigate the attached patient complaint. I would like a report on this
matter this afternoon.
Dear Sir:
My mother, Gertrude Boswich, was a patient in your hospital and I just want to
tell you that no member of my family will ever go there again.
She had an operation on Monday and was not given a bath for 3 days. Besides
that, she didn't get anything to eat for 2 days, not even water. What kind of a
hospital do you run anyway?

Edward Boswich
4832 Crabtree St.

••

Item 8

To: Joan Kerr
From: Alice Newton, R.N., Head Nurse
Re: Problems with X-Ray Dept.
Date: October 23
We have been having problems getting diagnostic X-ray procedures scheduled
for patients. Many times, patients have had to stay an extra day to get X-ray
tests done. I have spoken with the radiology chief several times, but the situa-
tion has not improved. Can you do something about this?

••

Item 9

To: All Department Heads
From: Storeroom
Re: Supplies
Date: October 23

CASE 2 (CONTINUED)

The storeroom is out of the following items:

toilet tissue
pencils
paper clips
disposable diapers

We are expecting a shipment next week.

. . . .

Telephone Messages

. . . .

Item 10

Phil Connors, Superior Surgical Supplies, Inc., returned your call at 7:50 A.M. on October 27. He will be at the hospital this afternoon, re: problems with defective equipment received.

. . . .

Item 11

Donald Haden, Channel 32 TV, called at 8:10 A.M., October 27, to say he will be here at 11:30 A.M. to do a feature story on the open-heart-surgery unit.

. . . .

Item 12

Lila Green, Director of Nurses at St. Joan Hospital, called at 8:05 A.M. October 24, regarding phone reference on Jane Walker, RN. Ms. Walker has applied for a job there. Isn't that the one we fired last year? Please call collect.

. . . .

Item 13

Betty Woods, Bluebird Troop 35, called at 8:00 A.M. October 27, regarding Bluebird troop visit to patients on Halloween with trick-or-treat candy. She will call again.

CASE 3 (adapted from Marquis and Huston, 1996)

. . . .

Assignment

Using the following time inventory, identify your activities for a 24-hour period. Record your activities on the time inventory on a regular basis. Be specific and do not trust your memory. Star the periods when you were most productive. Circle periods of time you were least productive. (Do not include sleep time.) Put an asterisk beside those activities that moved you closer to completion of intermediate and long-term goals. Place a checkmark beside those activities that you completed as a result of someone else's priorities rather than your own. Was this a typical day for you? Could you have modified your activity during the least productive time periods? How?

◆ Bibliography

The following is a list of references to help you solve these cases:

Augustine NR (1995). Managing the crisis you tried to prevent. Harvard Bus Rev Nov/Dec, 147–158

Brunsman R (1993). Time control—a waste of life. Life Assoc News. 88(Nov):114–117

Carter S (1993). Working harder and getting nowhere—no wonder you are stressed. Nurs Admin Quart 18(1):51–56

Chaleff I (1993). Overload can be overcome. Ind Week. 242(June 7):44–48

Comstock LG and Moff TE (1991). Cost-effective time—efficient charting. Nurs Manage 22(7):44–48

Grainger RD (1991). What does time mean to you? Amer J Nurs 91(7):13

Hayes PM (1994). Non-nursing functions: time for them to go. Nursing Econ 12(3):12–125

Haynes ME (1991). Practical Time Management. Los Altos: Crisp Publications

Josephs R (1992). How to Gain an Extra Hour Every Day: More Than 500 Time Saving Tips. New York: Penguin

Lee C, Ashford SJ, and Jamieson LF (1993). The effects of type A behavior dimensions and optimism on coping strategy, health, and performance. J Organ Behav 14(2):143–158

Lynch M (1991). P-A-C-E yourself: tips on time management. Nursing 91(3),21(3): 104,106,108

McFarlane M (1991). It's time to manage your time. Dermatol Nurs 3(3)June:172,182

Moshovitz R (1993). How to Organize Your Work and Your Life. New York: Doubleday

Oncken W Jr and Wass DL (1990). Management time: who's got the monkey? J Nurs Admin 20(12):6–9

Short B, Woodburne C, and Sumner S (1990). Making the most of your time ... by involving others. Nursing 20(1):99–100,102,104

Singhvi SS (1993). Time management can boost white-collar productivity. Natl Product Rev 12(Autumn):463–469

Storlie F and Leon J (1990). Making the most of your time ... by trusting yourself. Nursing 90 20(3):124,127–128,130+

Webb DM (1991). Interruptions and crises. Hosp Topics 69(1):43–44

Wilkinson R (1991). Forget that meeting. Nurs Manage 22(12):42+

Williamson D (1994). Automation at the point of care. Nurs Manage 35(7):32–35

PERSONAL NOTEBOOK

1. Think of the last major paper you were assigned to write for a class. Did you set short-term and intermediate deadlines? Did you break the task down into smaller tasks to eliminate a last-minute crisis? What short-term and intermediate deadlines have you set to accomplish major projects assigned to you this quarter or semester?

2. What personal "time wasters" pose the greatest difficulty for you?

3. Are lists a helpful way for you to organize your time? Why or why not?

4. Do you feel most comfortable with the organizing skills you use in your personal life or work (school or employment)? Is there a difference? If so, why?

CHAPTER 16

Delegation and Supervision

Managers can learn to control both personal and external time wasters to increase their productivity. However, even with minimal time wasted, there is frequently too much work to be accomplished by any one person. In those situations, delegation, or sharing work and responsibility with other persons is indicated. Delegation can be defined as getting work done through others. It can also be defined as directing the performance of one or more individuals to accomplish organizational goals (Marquis and Huston, 1996). Delegation is not an option for the manager—it is a necessity.

Delegation need not limit the manager's control, prestige, and power; rather, delegation can extend the manager's influence and capability by increasing what can be accomplished. The right to delegate and the ability to provide formal rewards for successful completion of delegated tasks are a reflection of the legitimate authority inherent in the management role. In addition to increased productivity, delegation can provide the opportunity for subordinates to experience feelings of accomplishment and enrichment. Much of the work achieved by managers reflects not only their efforts, but those of their subordinates.

◆ Errors in Delegating

Delegation is a learned skill and new managers with little experience in its use frequently make mistakes. Some of the errors made in delegating include:

> *1. Under-delegating.* In under-delegating, the manager becomes overworked and overwhelmed. This frequently comes from his or her false assump-

tion that delegation may be interpreted as a lack of ability on his or her part to do a correct or complete job.

Another frequent cause of under-delegating is the manager's desire to "do the whole job myself" (lack of trust in the subordinates) because of the belief that he or she needs the experience, or the belief that he or she can do it better and faster than anyone else. It is important to remember that time spent in training another individual to do a job for you may be repaid tenfold in the future.

An additional cause of under-delegation is the fear that subordinates will not "like you" or will resent the work delegated to them. Generally, the opposite is true. Subordinates who are not delegated enough responsibility will become bored, lazy, and ineffective (Bernhard and Walsh, 1990). Properly delegated work can increase employee satisfaction and foster a cooperative working relationship between managers and their subordinates.

2. *Over-delegation.* Some managers over-delegate as they are poor monitors of time and spend most of their time just trying to get organized. Others over-delegate because they feel insecure in their ability to perform a task.

3. *Improper delegation.* Improper delegation includes such things as delegating at the wrong time, to the wrong person, or for the wrong reason. It may also include assigning tasks and responsibilities that are beyond the capability of the person being delegated to, or that should be done by the manager.

Managers should use the following steps to ensure effective delegation:

1. Plan ahead in identifying tasks to be accomplished.
2. Identify the skill and educational level necessary to complete the job.
3. Single out the individual best able to complete the job in terms of capability as well as availability.
4. Clearly communicate exactly what is to be done, including the purpose for doing so. Include any limitations or qualifications that have been imposed. Although managers should specify the end product desired, it is important to allow the subordinate feedback and an appropriate degree of autonomy in deciding exactly how the work can be accomplished. Delegation is useless if the manager is unwilling to allow divergence in problem solving and subsequently redoes all work that has been assigned to others. Some managers delegate, but then oversupervise the employee in the completion of the task. To give too much supervision to a competent professional leads to interpersonal conflict, as well as to poor management of time (Grohar-Murray and DiCroce, 1992).
5. The manager must be sure to delegate the authority, as well as the responsibility, necessary to complete the task. Employees should be encouraged to attempt to solve problems themselves before coming to the manager, but should be permitted to ask questions about the delegated task or to seek clarification of the desired outcome at any time prior to completion.

6. Set timeframes and monitor how the task is being accomplished. This may be done through informal but regularly scheduled meetings. This shows an interest on the part of the manager, provides for a periodic review of progress, and allows ongoing communication to clarify any questions or misconceptions that may have come up. In addition, it keeps the delegated task in view of both the subordinate and the manager, who share accountability for the completion of the delegated task.

7. If the subordinate is having difficulty carrying out the delegated task, the manager should be available as a role model and resource in helping the subordinate identify other alternative solutions. Taking the delegated task back should be a last resort as it fosters a sense of failure in the employee and demotivates rather than motivates. However, it may also be necessary for the manager to reclaim work previously assigned to this individual so that he or she has time to devote to a newly assigned task.

8. Evaluate the performance of the subordinate after the task has been completed. Include both positive and negative aspects of how the subordinate has completed the task. Be sure to appropriately reward the individual who has successfully completed a delegated task. Delegation is a high-level skill essential to the manager. As managers gain the maturity and self-confidence needed to delegate wisely, they can increase their impact and power both within and outside the organization. Subordinates gain self-esteem and increased job satisfaction because of the responsibility and authority given to them and the organization itself moves a step closer toward achieving its goals.

◆ Delegating to Unlicensed Assistive Personnel

In an effort to contain spiraling health care costs, many health care providers have chosen to replace licensed professional nurses with unlicensed assistive personnel (UAP). The A.N.A. (1992) defines UAP as unlicensed individuals who are trained to function in an assistive role to the licensed RN in the provision of patient/client activities as delegated by the nurse. This term includes, but is not limited to, nurses aides, orderlies, assistants, attendants, and technicians.

Blegen, Gardner, and McCloskey (1992) found that 80% of the RNs in acute care institutions and 98% of RNs working in long-term care facilities are currently involved in some capacity with the assignment, delegation, and supervision of UAP in the delivery of nursing care. Ninety-seven percent of the hospitals surveyed by the American Hospital Association (A.J.N., 1991) and 85% of hospitals surveyed by the A.N.A. and the American Organization of Nurse Executives (A.O.N.E) indicated they had begun nurse extender programs (1992).

The primary argument for utilizing UAP in acute care settings is cost: UAP can free professional nurses from tasks and assignments (specifically, non-nursing functions) that can be completed by less well-trained personnel at a lower cost (Huston, 1996). Some experts argue, however, that the RN, although well-trained in the role of direct care provider, is often inadequately prepared for the roles of delegator and supervisor of UAP (Lengacher and colleagues, 1993; Crawley and colleagues, 1993; Jung and colleagues, 1994). Many RNs who supervise UAP, especially those who entered practice in the 1980s, have experienced only total RN staffing or primary nursing systems of care delivery. Thus, they have received little or no instruction in personnel supervision and delegation principles.

With the restructuring of care delivery models, RNs are increasingly being expected to make assignments for and supervise the work of different levels of employees. RNs asked to assume the role of supervisor and delegator need preparation to assume these leadership tasks. Lengacher and colleagues (1993), and Crawley, Marshall, and Till (1993) suggest that repeated education programs on delegation principles and role clarity are necessary for RNs to demonstrate consistency in delegating appropriate role activities to UAP and to begin to feel confident in delegating. Abts, Hofer, and Leafgreen (1994), however, found that a lack of registered nurse skill to empower others persisted even after a delegation class was held. Findings by Jung, Pearcey, and Phillips (1994) were similar, suggesting that a large percentage of RNs continued to feel uncomfortable supervising UAP even after inservice programs designed to help them in these new roles were held.

◆ The Liability of Supervision

Assuming the role of delegator and supervisor to UAP also increases the scope of liability for the RN. Although nurses are not automatically held liable for all acts of negligence on the part of those they supervise, they may be held liable if they were negligent in the supervision of those employees at the time they committed the negligent acts. Liability is based on a supervisor's failure to determine which patient needs could safely be assigned to a subordinate or for failing to closely monitor a subordinate who requires such supervision.

In assigning tasks to UAP, then, the RN must be aware of the UAP job description, knowledge base, and demonstrated skills of each individual. It is important that the registered nurse remember that although the Omnibus Budget Reconciliation Act of 1987 established regulations for the education and certification of "nurse aides" (minimum of 75 hours of theory and practice and successful completion of an examination in both areas), no federal or community standards have been established for training the more broadly defined UAP (Huston, 1996).

In a study of 102 hospitals by Barter, McLaughlin, and Thomas (1994), only 20% required a high school diploma for UAP, 26% preferred previous clinical bedside experience, and 29% preferred certification as a nursing assistant. A number of the hospitals did not have a standardized hiring requirement and provided only a minimal amount of training and orientation; 80% provided newly hired UAP with less than 40 hours of classroom instruction, and 99% provided less than 120 hours of on-the-job training.

This does not imply that all UAP are uneducated and unprepared for the roles they have been asked to fill. It merely suggests that the registered nurse, in delegating to UAP, must carefully assess what skills and knowledge each individual UAP has, or risk increased personal liability for the failure to do so.

Cronenwett (1995) developed a strategy assessment guide to assist nurses in determining situations where UAP should be used to assist or substitute for licensed nurses (see Display 16-1). When scores are low, delegation to UAP can more likely be carried out in a safe manner. As scores rise, the use of and delegation to UAP become more inappropriate.

Dietz (1994) suggests that decisions to use or not use UAP should not be made on a blanket yes or no basis, but rather on four factors.

1) *Is the complete nursing process, or are the more complex portions of the nursing process, to be utilized?* If the task is simple and the needs of the nursing process are data gathering or basic assessment, a UAP may be an appropriate delegate. If complex, multiple dimensions or complex areas of nursing process are needed, then UAPs should not be used.

2) *Is the task or service involved of a repetitive nature?* If so, UAP should be considered appropriate for performance of the task.

3) *What is the patient's condition and has the task or procedure already been performed on the patient by a licensed provider?* If the task has already been performed by a licensed provider and the patient is stable, the UAP may be able to complete the task the next time. If the task is complex, multidimensional, or represents the first time it is being performed on a specific patient, that use of UAP is probably not appropriate.

4) *Does the environment specifically mandate a particular level of task implementation?* (e.g., Intensive Care Unit (ICU), Emergency Room (ER), or Critical Care Unit (CCU)?) The more the environmental mandates, the less likely that UAP will be the appropriate person to deliver the care.

Dietz (1994) also suggests that the decision to use or not use UAP should represent the following four control mechanisms.

1) The delegated skills must consist of highly proscribed activities that do not require nursing judgment. There should be no room for independent nursing judgment by the UAP.

2) The UAP must have the specific competency or certification and have received the appropriate training for the implementation of the delegated tasks.

3) There must be a process in place for evaluating and monitoring the implementation of the task.

4) The registered nurse must consider the severity of the patient care task and the overall physical and psychological stability of the patient.

◆ Subordinate Resistance to Delegation

One of the most common causes of subordinate resistance to, or refusal of, delegated tasks is the failure of the delegator to see the subordinate's perspective. Workloads assigned to UAP are generally highly challenging, both physically

DISPLAY 16-1
Strategy Assessment Guide for Nursing's Response to the Use of Unlicensed Assistive Personnel

How complex is (are) the task(s) involved?	Very simple 1	2	3	4	Very complex 5
What is the potential for harm to clients?	Very low 1	2	3	4	Very high 5
How predictable are client responses to the interventions/tasks?	Very predictable 1	2	3	4	Very unpredictable 5
How stable are the conditions of the clients involved?	Very stable 1	2	3	4	Very unstable 5
To what extent is problem solving and judgment required during the intervention or task?	Never required 1	2	3	4	Always required 5
To what extent are clients monitored by other societal or family agents so that untoward outcomes would be observed?	Continuously 1	2	3	4	Very sporadically 5
To what extent would a registered nurse be held liable for an untoward outcome?	Never 1	2	3	4	Always 5
How soon could the unlicensed assistive personnel or client be in contact with a professional healthcare provider if needed?	Very soon (min) 1	2	3	4	Very long time (hrs) 5
How certain can society be that the unlicensed assistive personnel being considered will have the necessary competencies to perform the tasks/judgments required?	Very certain 1	2	3	4	Very uncertain 5
If the client were your family member, how comfortable would you be with the proposal for unlicensed assistive personnel care?	Very comfortable 1	2	3	4	Very uncomfort-able 5
How willing are you, as a member of society, to commit fiscal resources to ensure that a registered nurse could be available to cover every person who needed the proposed interventions?	Very unwilling 1	2	3	4	Very willing 5

Source: Cronenwett LR (1995). The use of unlicensed assistive personnel: when to support, oppose, or be neutral. J Nur Admin 25(6):11–12; with permission.

and mentally. In addition, the UAP frequently must adapt rapidly to changing priorities, priorities often imposed on them by more than one delegator.

Johnson (1994) suggests that one of the best ways to avoid getting a "no" from nursing assistants is to show them respect and to consult them whenever possible in decisions related to their role. The registered nurse should also try to mix the assistants' more routine, boring tasks with more challenging, and rewarding, assignments. An additional strategy is to provide the subordinate with consistent, constructive feedback, both positive and negative, to foster growth and self-esteem.

◆ Summary

Delegation provides a means of increasing unit productivity. It is also a managerial tool for subordinate accomplishment and enrichment. Delegation, however, is not easy; it is a high-level management skill. Novice managers often make delegation errors such as delegating too late, not delegating enough, delegating to the wrong person or for the wrong reason, and failing to provide appropriate supervision and guidance of delegated tasks.

With the increased use of unlicensed assistive personnel in patient care, the need for nurses to have highly developed delegation skills has never been greater. The ability to appropriately use delegation skills will help to reduce the personal liability associated with supervising and delegating to unlicensed assistive personnel. It will also assure that client needs are met and their safety is not jeopardized.

◆ References

Abts D, Hofer M, and Leafgreen PK (1994). Redesigning care delivery: a modular system. Nurs Manage 25(2):40–46

AJN (1991). Nurse extenders now found in 97% of hospitals: AHA prepares to fight regulation of new workers. Am J Nurs 91(8):88–90

American Hospital Association (AHA) and the American Organization of Nurse Executives (AONE) (1991). Joint Position Statement on Differentiated Practice, AHA

American Nurses Association (ANA) (1992). Progress Report on Unlicensed Assistive Personnel: Informational Report. Report: CNP-CNE-B. Washington, DC

Barter M, McLaughlin FE, and Thomas SA (1994). Use of unlicensed assistive personnel by hospitals. Nurs Econ 12(2):82–87

Bernhard LA and Walsh M (1990). Leadership—The Key to the Professionalization of Nursing, 2nd ed. St. Louis: CV Mosby

Blegen MA, Gardner DL, and McCloskey JC (1992). Who helps you with your work? Am J Nurs 92(1):26–31

Crawley WD, Marshall RS, and Till AH (1993). Use of unlicensed assistive staff. Orthop Nurs 12(6):47–53

Cronenwett LR (1995). The use of unlicensed assistive personnel: when to support, oppose, or be neutral. J Nurs Admin 25(6):11–12

Dietz E (1994). Should nurses use assistants? In McCloskey JM and Grace HK (eds). Current Issues in Nursing, 4th ed. St. Louis: Mosby-Year Book

Grohar-Murray ME and DiCroce HR (1992). Leadership and Management in Nursing. Norwalk, CT: Appleton and Lange

Huston C (1996). Unlicensed assistive personnel: a solution to dwindling health care resources or the precursor to the apocalypse of registered nursing. Nurs Outlook 44(2):67–73

Johnson SH (1994). How to avoid getting a no from a nursing assistant: tips for improving your delegation strategy. Nursing 94 24(12):66–68

Jung FD, Pearcey LG, and Phillips JL (1994). Evaluation of a program to improve nursing assistant use. J Nurs Admin 24(3):42–47

Lengacher CA, Mabe PR, Bowling CD, Heinemann D, Kent K, and Cott ML (1993). Redesigning nursing practice. J Nurs Admin 23(12):31–37

Marquis B and Huston C (1996). Leadership Roles and Management Functions: Theory and Application, 2nd ed. Philadelphia: JB Lippincott

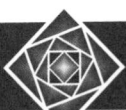 **CASES FOR PROBLEM SOLVING**

CASE 1

You are the charge nurse on the 3:00–11:00 P.M. shift on a medical-surgical unit. On returning from dinner you are greeted by several personnel, who relate the following information:

1. Mrs. Murphy's IV has infiltrated, she is behind on her IV fluids, and she has missed her 6 P.M. antibiotic.
2. A visitor has fainted.
3. The public toilet is overflowing and waste is pouring out rapidly.
4. Three patients have not received their dinner trays and it is now 7 P.M.
5. The OR has just called and they are on their way up to take Mr. Smith for a cardiac catheterization. His preoperative medication has not been given.
6. Dr. Russo is waiting to discuss a medication error that was made 2 weeks ago.

Assignment
The other RNs are all very busy with their patients, but you do have the following people you may delegate to: yourself, a ward clerk, and an IV-certified LVN/LPN. Decide who should assume what responsibilities and list in order of priority. Justify your decision.

CASE 2

You are a staff nurse who functions as a modular leader on a general medical-surgical unit. The group for which you are responsible is assigned patients in rooms 401 through 409, with a maximum capacity of 13 patients.

CASE 2 (CONTINUED)

In your unit a modular type of patient care organization is employed, using a combination of licensed and unlicensed staff. Each module consists of one RN, one LVN/LPN, and one UAP. The LVN/LPN is IV-certified and can maintain and start IVs, but cannot hang piggybacks or give IV push medications. The LVN/LPN may give all other medications except IV medications. The RN gives all IV medications. The UAP, with the assistance of his or her modular team members, generally bathes and feeds patients, and provides other care that does not require a license.

The RN, as modular leader, divides up the workload at the beginning of the shift, between the three modular team members. In addition, he or she acts as a teacher and resource person for the other members of the module. Today is Wednesday. You have one LVN/LPN and one UAP assigned to work with you, LVN Franklin, and UAP Martinez.

LVN Franklin is 26 years old and the mother of four preschool children. Her husband is a city bus driver. UAP Martinez is 53 years old and a grandmother with no children living at home. Her husband died 2 years ago. She says that work keeps her "happy." The patient roster this morning is as follows.

Room	Patient Acuity level	Age	Diagnosis	Condition	
401	Mrs. Jones	33	Mastectomy for CA breast	2 days postop/fair	II
402	Mrs. Redford	55	Back pain	Pelvic TX/good	I
403	Mrs. Worley	46	Cholecystectomy	2 days postop/good	III
404-1	Mrs. Smith	83	Parkinsons, CVD, hypertension	Fair	II
404-2	Mrs. Dewey	26	PID	Good—home today	I
405-1	Mr. Arthur	71	Metastatic CA	Poor—semicomatose/IV therapy	IV
405-2	Mr. Vines	34	Possible peptic ulcer	Good—UGI today	II
406-1	Vacant				
406-2	Miss Brown	24	Dilation and curettage	To OR this A.M.	III
407-1	Mrs. West	41	Myocardial infarction	Fair/from ICU yesterday	III
				Heparin lock/telemetry	
408-1	Mr. Niles	21	Open reduction femur (MVA)	Fair/3 days postop	III
408-2	Mr. Ford	44	Gastrectomy	Fair/1 day postop/IV therapy	III
409	Mrs. Land	42	Depression	Fair/BA enema today	III

CASE 2 (CONTINUED)

Additional information about patients:

408-1	Mr. Niles is depressed because he feels his football career is over.
408-2	There have been problems with Mr. Ford's IV and his nasogastric tube. Both will need to be replaced today.
403	Mrs. Worley requires frequent changes (every 2–3 hours) of her laparoscopic site dressings owing to a high volume of serous drainage.
401-1	Mrs. Jones will need instructions regarding her postoperative activities and has begun to talk about her prognosis.
409-1	Mrs. Land began yesterday to talk with you about her husband's recent death.
	The prep for the barium enema will result in Mrs. Land having frequent toileting needs today.
404-1	Mrs. Smith requires assistance with feeding at mealtime.
405-1	Mr. Arthur is no longer able to turn himself in bed.
405-2	Mr. Vines states that being in the same room with a critically ill patient makes him upset and he has asked to move to a new room.

••

Assignment

How will you make out your assignments this morning? Assign these patients to the LVN/LPN, UAP, and yourself. Be sure to include assessments, procedures, and basic care needs. What will you do if a patient is admitted to your team? Explain your rationale for all your patient assignments. Sample acuity levels are provided to assist in determining patient needs and staffing (see Display 16-2).

CASE 3

••

Assignment

Interview a middle- or top-level manager of a local health care agency. Ascertain the staffing mix. Are there minimum hiring criteria for UAP? Are there written guidelines for determining tasks appropriate for UAP delegation? What educational or training opportunities on delegation are made available to staff who must delegate work assignments on a regular basis?

On the basis of your interview results, write an essay evaluating whether you feel there are adequate safeguards in place at that agency to protect the licensed staff, unlicensed staff, and clients. Would you feel comfortable working in such a facility?

CASE 4 ◆

You are a home-health nurse who makes in-home visits to a moribund elderly man with advanced cancer. He is now confined to bed and his major care needs are comfort-based. In addition to directly providing pain medication to this gen-

DISPLAY 16-2
Sample Patient Dependency Categorization Guidelines

Area of Care	Category I	Category II	Category III	Category IV
Eating	Feeds self or needs little food for eating	Needs some help in preparing. May need encouragement	Cannot feed self but is able to chew and swallow	Cannot feed self and may have difficulty swallowing
Grooming	Almost entirely self-sufficient	Needs some help in bathing oral hygiene, hair combing, and so forth	Unable to do much for self	Completely dependent
Excretion	Up and to the bathroom alone or almost alone	Needs some help in getting up to the bathroom or using a urinal	In bed needing bedpan or urinal placed. May be able to partially turn or lift self	Completely dependent
Comfort	Self-sufficient	Needs some help with adjustment of position or bed (tubes, IVs, and so forth)	Cannot turn without help, get drink, adjust position of extremities, and so forth	Completely dependent
General health	Good—in for diagnostic procedure, simple treatment, or surgical procedure (D&C, biopsy, minor fracture)	Mild symptoms—more than one mild illness, mild debility, mild emotional reaction, mild incontinence (not more than once per shift)	Acute symptoms—severe emotional reaction to illness or surgery, more than one acute medical or surgical problem, severe or frequent incontinence	Critically ill—may have severe emotional reaction

continued

Area of Care	Category I	Category II	Category III	Category IV
Treatments	Simple—supervised ambulation, dangle, simple dressing, test procedure preparation not requiring medication, reinforcement of surgical dressing, X-pad, vital signs once per shift	Any category-I treatment more than once per shift, Foley cath care, I & O, bladder irrigations, sitz bath, compresses, test procedures requiring medications or follow-ups, simple enema for evacuation, vital signs every 4 hours	Any treatment more than twice per shift, medicated IVs, complicated dressings, sterile procedures, care of tracheostomy, Harris flush, suctioning, tube feeding, vital signs more often than every 4 hours	Any elaborate or delicate procedure or procedure requiring two nurses, vital signs more often than every 2 hours
Medications	Simple, routine, not needing pre- or post-evaluation, PRN medications no more than once per shift	Diabetic, cardiac, hypotensive, hypertensive, diuretic, anticoagulant medications, PRN medications, more than once per shift, medications needing pre- or post-evaluation	Unusual amount of category-II medications, control of refractory diabetics (need to be monitored more than every 4 hours)	More intensive category-III medications, IVs with frequent, close observation and regulation
Teaching and emotional support	Routine follow-up teaching, patients with no unusual or adverse emotional reactions	Initial teaching of care of ostomies, new diabetics, tubes that will be in place for periods of time, conditions requiring major change in eating, living or excretory practices. Patients with mild adverse reactions to their illness (depression, overly demanding, and so forth)	More intensive category-II items, teaching of apprehensive or mildly resistive patients, care of moderately upset or apprehensive patients, confused or disoriented patients	Teaching of resistive patients, care, and support of patients with severe emotional reaction

CASE 4 (CONTINUED)

tleman, you, as a case manager, are responsible for overseeing other personnel who assist in caring for him. These personnel include rotating health aides who are responsible for bathing the patient, preparing his meals, and providing other basic care not requiring a professional license. The patient's family generally stays with him at night.

At times, during your in-home visits, you have noticed food crumbs in the bed, that the patient's hair is uncombed, that his teeth have not been brushed, and you suspect that he has not been recently bathed.

You decide to confront the health aides as a group regarding your concerns. During that meeting, you clarify their job assignments and the expected outcomes. The health aides listen attentively, but offer no insight or suggestions as to why the problem is occurring. No one health aide acknowledges the problem as his or her own.

Assignment

Despite your confrontation, the problem continues to persist. Determine how you will proceed next. What are possible causes of the health aides' resistance to your delegation? Which of the causes you identified are controllable? How much supervision or guidance can you realistically give to these health aides to ascertain that they are completing the delegated work at a satisfactory level?

CASE 5   (Marquis and Huston, 1996)

You are the team leader for 10 patients. An experienced LVN and nurse's aide also are assigned to the team. It is an extremely busy day and there is a great deal of work to be done. Several times today, you have found the LVN taking long breaks in the lounge or chatting socially at the front desk, despite the unmet needs of many patients. On those occasions, you have clearly delegated work tasks and timelines to her. Several hours later you follow up on the delegated tasks and find that they were not completed. When you seek out the LVN, you find that she went to lunch, without telling you or the aide. You are furious at her apparent disregard of your authority.

Assignment

What are possible causes of the LVN's failure to follow up on delegated tasks? How will you deal with this LVN? What goal serves as the basis for your actions? Justify your choice with rationale.

◆ Bibliography

The following is a list of references to help you solve these cases:

American Association of Colleges of Nursing (AACN), American Nurses Association, American Organization of Nurse Executives, and the National League for Nursing (1990). Statement on Assistive Personnel to the Registered Nurse. Chicago: National League for Nursing

American Nurses Association (ANA) (1994). A.N.A. to blue-ribbon panel: R.N. restructuring puts patient care and safety at risk. Revolution J Nurse Empower 4(4):17–18

Blouin AS and Brent NJ (1995). Unlicensed assistive personnel: legal considerations. J Nurs Admin 25(11):7–8

Buresh B (1994). PCAs and CTAs: are they the beginning of the end for nursing? Revolution J Nurse Empower 4(2):8–11

California Nurse's Association (1994). California Nurse on RNs and Health Care Restructuring

Fralic MF (1995). Into the future: new models, new methods. Nurs Leader Manage 3(1):9

Gollard LT and Soo Hoo WE (1993). Maximizing limited resources through TEAMCARE. Nurs Manage 24(11):36–45

Hasten RI (1991). Delegation: learning when and how to let go. Nursing 91 21:126

Hasten R and Washburn M (1992). What do you say when you delegate work to others AJN 92 (7):48

Hasten R and Washburn M (1992). How to plan what you delegate. AJN 92 (4):71

Hayes PM (1994). Non-nursing functions: time for them to go. Nurs Econ 12(3):120–125

Herrick K, Hansten R, O'Neil L, Hayes P, and Washburn M (1994). My license is not on the line: the art of delegation. Nurs Manage 25(2):4850

Jung FD (1991). Teaching registered nurses how to supervise nursing assistants. J Nurs Admin 21(4):32–36

Kostovich CT, Mahneke SM, Meyer PA, and Healy C (1994). The clinical technician as a member of the patient-focused healthcare delivery team. J Nurs Admin 24(12):32–38

Krapohl GL and Larson E (1996). The impact of unlicensed assistive personnel on nursing care delivery. Nurs Econ 14(2):99–110

McLaughlin FE, Thomas SA, and Barter M (1995). Changes related to care delivery patterns. J Nurs Admin 25(5):35–46

Neidlinger SH, Bostrom J, Stricker A, Hild J, and Zhang JQ (1993). Incorporating nursing assistive personnel into a nursing professional practice model. J Nurs Admin 23(3):29–37

O'Brien YM and Stepura BA (1992). Designing roles for assistive personnel in a rural hospital. J Nurs Admin 22(10):34–37

Parkman CA (1996). Delegation: are you doing it right? Am J Nurs 96(9):42–48

Schmieding N (1992). The complexity of an authority role. Nurs Manage 23(1):57–58

PERSONAL NOTEBOOK

1. Is it difficult for you to delegate to others? If so, do you know why?

2. Are you more prone to under-delegating, over-delegating, or improper delegation? What safeguards can you build in to decrease this delegation error?

3. Do you work with UAP in your role as student nurse or registered nurse? How comfortable do you feel with your ability to assess each UAP's knowledge and/or qualification level?

4. When someone refuses to accept a task you have delegated, how does it make you feel? Do you tend to take the refusal personally or are you generally able to view the decision more objectively?

Organizational, Interpersonal, and Group Communication

Although some management functions can be reasonably isolated, such as planning, organizing, and controlling, communication forms the core of the manager's activities and cuts across all phases of the management process. Kotter (1990) suggests that a central feature of modern organizations is interdependence, where no one has complete autonomy, and where most employees are tied to many others through their work, technology, management systems, and hierarchy. Highly developed managerial communication skills encourage and support organizational interdependence.

Depending on the manager's position in the organizational hierarchy, more than 80% of managerial time may be spent in some type of organizational communication. Sixteen percent of this time represents reading, 9% writing, 30% speaking, and 45% listening (Swansburg, 1990). Developing expertise in all aspects of communications is critical to managerial success.

Because so much of managerial communication time is spent speaking and listening, it is clear that the manager must also have excellent interpersonal communication skills. The manager communicates with patients, colleagues, superiors, and subordinates. In addition, because nursing practice tends to be group oriented, interpersonal communication between group members is ongoing and necessary for productivity. If group members are to work cohesively in meeting organizational goals, the manager must explicitly express issues and concerns so workers will not become confused about priorities. Hackman and Johnson (1991) suggest that successful leaders use communication as a tool to reach their ends; they match their behavior with their goals. When leaders understand what communication skills are needed to meet their goals, they are better able to put those behaviors into action.

◆ The Communication Process

Tappen (1995) defines communication as the sharing of thoughts, feelings, and ideas and suggests that whenever two or more people are working together, some kind of communication occurs, even if they are working in silence. Huber (1996) states that communication is the art of being able to structure and transmit a message in a way that another can easily understand and/or accept. These definitions impart a sense of the complexity involved in communication. For example, what if the verbal and nonverbal messages are incongruent? What if one of the parties involved in the communication interprets a message differently than the intent of the sender? Does communication occur if an idea is transmitted but not translated into action?

Because communication is so complex, many models exist to explain how organizations and individuals communicate. Basic elements common to most models are shown in Figure 17-1. In all communication, there is at least one sender, one receiver, and one message. There is also a mode through which the message is sent, such as verbal, written, or nonverbal.

There is also an internal and external "climate" in which the communication takes place. The internal climate includes the values, beliefs, temperament, and stress levels of the sender as well as the receiver. Weather conditions, temperature, power factors, and timing are examples of external climate factors. Organizational culture, as discussed in Chapter 8, also affects the external climate. Both the sender and the receiver must be sensitive to the internal and external climates, as the perception of the message is greatly altered depending on the climate that existed at the time the message was sent and received.

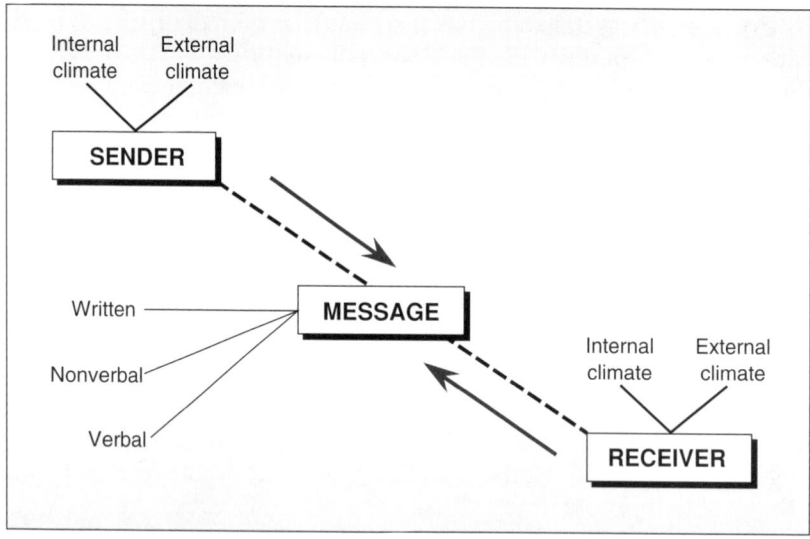

FIGURE 17-1. The communication process.

◆ Barriers to Organizational Communication

Although organizational communication is particularly complex in large-scale organizations, the manager can take several steps to increase the likelihood that it is clear and complete.

1. Managers must understand the structure of their organization, including an understanding of who will be affected by any decisions that are made. Both formal and informal communication networks need to be considered.
2. Communication is not a one-way channel. If other departments or disciplines will be affected by the communication, the manager must consult with those areas for feedback prior to communicating any changes.
3. The communication must be clear, simple, and precise. It is the responsibility of the manager (sender) to ensure that the message is understood. The clarity of the message is directly influenced by the mode of communication used. A telephone call is rapid, allowing the receiver to clarify the message at the time it is given. It does not, however, give the receiver any nonverbal cues or allow any reference for subsequent questions or follow-up. Written messages allow for documentation, but may be open to various interpretations and generally are more time-consuming. Verbal communication is rapid but may result in fewer people receiving the information than is necessary. In general, the more direct the communication, the greater the probability that it will be clear. The more people involved in filtering messages, the greater the chance of distortion. The manager must evaluate each circumstance individually to determine which mode or combinations thereof are optimum for that situation.
4. The manager should seek feedback regarding whether the communication was accurately received. One way to do this is to ask the receiver to repeat the message or instructions. In addition, the sender should continue to follow up any communication in an effort to determine if the communicated task is being carried out.
5. Becoming a good listener is a vital component of the communication process for the manager. There is an art to active listening. One must employ nonverbal cues to assure others that they are really being heard. Often, employees do not expect managers to resolve all the organization's problems, but they do expect management to listen.

◆ Channels of Communication

Because large organizations are so complex, communication channels used by the manager may be upward, downward, horizontal, diagonal, or through the informal grapevine.

In *upward* communication, the manager is a subordinate to higher management. Needs and wants are communicated upward to the next level in the hierarchy. Individuals at this level hold the responsibility for decision making for a greater portion of the organization than the manager.

In *downward* communication, the manager relays information to subordinates. This is a traditional form of communication in organizations and helps coordinate the activities of various levels within the structural hierarchy.

In *horizontal* communication, the manager interacts with managers of other departments in the organization. The need for horizontal communication increases as interdepartmental dependence increases.

In *diagonal* communication, the manager interfaces with the personnel and managers of other departments, and groups such as physicians, who are not on the same level of the organizational hierarchy. Although these individuals have no formal authority over the manager, this communication is vital to the functioning of the organization. Diagonal communication tends to be less formal than other types of communication.

The most informal communication network is called the *grapevine,* from which information flows haphazardly between individuals on all levels of the hierarchy, usually involving three to four at one time. Communication that occurs through the grapevine is subject to error and distortion because of the speed with which it is passed and because the sender has little formal accountability for the message. Once managers have knowledge of how information flows within their organization, they can use that knowledge to best promote both clear and efficient communications within the organization.

◆ Modes of Communication

The manager is involved in the following types of communication:

1. Written communication: Written communication is necessary for any large organization. In order to reach all the individuals, most organizations have developed certain methods of formal downward communication. These might include company publications, letters to employees' homes, pay-envelope inserts, formal memos, and bulletin boards. Depending upon the level of his or her position, the manager may be involved with few or many of these written communications to subordinates.

However, all managers are involved with some written communications. These might take the forms of budget requests, performance appraisals, letters of reference for former employees, or annual reports. Written communication, by virtue of its nature, suggests attention and deliberation on the part of the sender and gives receivers a record for reference and review. There is, however, great danger in written communication because usually there is no feedback mechanism available for the sender of the message to clarify the intent. The manager needs to be able to write clearly, using language that is understood. Having others read a sensitive communication before it is distributed can often prevent the manager from having misunderstood communication with subordinates.

Health Care Education Associates (1988) suggest the following guidelines for writing good letters and memos:

1. Know what you want to say before you start writing; this requires that you think clearly before you begin to write.
2. Put people into your writing; when you write about a subject, discuss it in terms of those affected by it. Avoid words such as administration, authorization, and implementation, as they are abstract and impersonal.
3. Use action words; action verbs have a stronger impact.
4. Write simply; use familiar, specific, and concrete words. Simple writing is more easily understood and thus is more apt to be read.
5. Use as few words as possible; find one good way to make your point and trust that your reader will understand it.
6. Keep sentences under 20 words and include only one idea per sentence. Make positive statements that clearly outline your position on an issue. State the pertinent facts first.
7. Give the reader direction; be consistent in the tone of the message to help establish a clear point of view.
8. Arrange the material logically; an orderly presentation of facts increases the reliability the reader places in the writer. The material may be organized deductively, inductively, by order of importance, from the familiar to the unfamiliar, chronologically, by close relationship, or by proximity.
9. Use paragraphs to lead readers; they should not exceed eight to ten lines in a memo, or five to six lines in a letter.
10. Connect your thoughts; to achieve this, you must add enough details, use repetition to tie thoughts together, and employ transitional words to tell the reader when you are moving to a new thought.
11. Be clear; be certain your pronouns are clearly defined.
12. Express similar thoughts in similar ways.

2. Face-to-face communication: Managers communicate verbally upward and downward, both formally and informally. They also communicate verbally in formal meetings, with individuals in peer work groups, and in making formal presentations.

One goal in face-to-face communication is assertiveness. Assertive behavior is a way of communicating that allows individuals to express themselves in direct, honest, and appropriate ways that do not infringe upon another person's rights. The position of the individual is expressed clearly and firmly using first-person or "I" statements. In addition, assertive communication always requires that verbal and nonverbal messages be congruent. To be successful in the directing phase of management, one must have well-developed skills in assertive communication.

There are many misconceptions about assertive communication. The first misconception is that any given communication is either assertive or passive. Actually, there are at least four possibilities:

1. passive,
2. aggressive,
3. indirectly aggressive (often called passive–aggressive), and
4. assertive.

Passive communication occurs when one individual suffers in silence, although he or she may feel strongly about the issue at hand. Aggressive individuals express themselves in a direct and often hostile manner that *does* infringe on another person's rights. This behavior is generally oriented toward "winning at all costs" or demonstrating one's own superiority. Passive aggressive communication is aggressive communication presented in a passive way. It generally involves a limited verbal exchange (with incongruent nonverbal behavior) by an individual who feels strongly about a situation. For example, an individual may feign withdrawal in an effort to manipulate the situation.

A frequently heard misconception is that assertive and aggressive are synonymous. In fact, to be assertive is to not be aggressive. Even when faced with someone else's aggression, the assertive communicator remains assertive and does not become aggressive. An individual can remain assertive when under attack by an aggressive person by doing several things:

1. *Reflection:* Repeat to the speaker what he or she is saying.
2. *Repeated assertion:* Continue to repeat the original assertive message.
3. *Point out the implicit assumptions:* This involves listening closely and letting the aggressor know that you have heard him or her.
4. *Restating:* By using assertive language to rephrase the aggressor's language, one can defuse the aggression.
5. *Questioning:* When the aggressor uses nonverbal cues to be aggressive, the assertive person should confront this behavior in the form of a question.

Another common misconception about assertiveness is that assertiveness is unfeminine. Although the role of women in society has undergone tremendous change in the last century, nursing as a female profession has had great difficulty in accepting the role of the nurse as an assertive, active, decision maker. All nurses, and nurse managers especially, are being urged to develop more effective personal communications skills. One means of doing this is by teaching assertive communication skills as part of nursing school curriculum. A study by Kruse (1992) found that the higher the educational level, the greater the degree of assertiveness on the part of nurses. Display 17-1 shows a list of the rights and responsibilities of the assertive individual.

3. Nonverbal communication: Nonverbal communication includes facial expression, body movements, and cues or gestures and is commonly referred to as body language. Because nonverbal communication includes the emotional component of the message, it is generally considered more reliable than verbal communication (Arnold and Boggs, 1989). However, there is a significant danger in the misinterpretation of nonverbal messages if they are not assessed in context with the verbal message. Nonverbal communication occurs anytime managers are seen. A message is transmitted by managers to subordinates not only while communicating verbally, but simply by walking down the hallway.

Because the potential for misinterpretation of nonverbal communication is even greater than verbal communication, it should be examined in context with the verbal content expressed. Generally, if verbal and nonverbal messages are

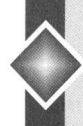

DISPLAY 17-1
Rights and Responsibilities of the Assertive Individual

Rights	Responsibilities
To speak up	To listen
To take	To give
To have problems	To find solutions
To be comforted	To comfort others
To work	To do your best
To make mistakes	To correct your mistakes
To laugh	To make others happy
To have friends	To be a friend
To criticize	To praise
To have your efforts rewarded	To reward other's efforts
To independence	To be dependable
To cry	To dry tears
To be loved	To love others

(Chenevert, 1988)

incongruent, the receiver will believe the nonverbal message. Also, because nonverbal behavior can be and frequently is misinterpreted, it is important for receivers to validate perceptions with senders. The incongruency between verbal and nonverbal messages is the most significant difficulty in effective interpersonal communication (Sullivan and Decker, 1988).

The following is a partial list of nonverbal cues that can occur with or without verbal communication:

- *Environment:* The area where the communication takes place is an important part of the communication process. Communication that takes place in a superior's office is often given more credence than communication that occurs in the cafeteria.
- *Outward appearance:* Much is communicated via our clothing, hairstyles, use of cosmetics, and relative attractiveness. The term "dressing for success" appropriately defines the impact of dress and appearance upon role perception and power.
- *Eye contact:* This nonverbal cue is often associated with sincerity. Richmond and associates (1987) stated that eye contact constitutes an invitation or readiness to interact. Likewise, breaking of eye contact nonverbally indicates that the interaction is about to cease.
- *Body posture:* The weight of a message is increased if the sender stands and faces the person or sits appropriately close and leans toward the receiver with the head erect.

- *Gestures:* A message accented with appropriate gestures takes on added emphasis. However, overemphasis is distracting. For example, hand movements can either punctuate or distract from the message.
- *Facial expressions:* Effective communication requires facial expressions that agree with your message.
- *Timing:* Hesitation often diminishes the effect of your statement or implies untruthfulness.
- *Vocal cues—tone, volume, and reflection:* These add to the message being transmitted.

Effective managers are congruent in their verbal and nonverbal communication, so subordinates are clear about the messages they receive (Marquis and Huston, 1996). Likewise, managers are sensitive to nonverbal as well as verbal messages from subordinates, and look for inconsistencies that may indicate unresolved problems or needs. Often, organizational difficulties can be prevented when managers recognize the nonverbal communication of subordinates and take timely appropriate action.

4. Verbal communication (telephone): Since managers today are quite reliant on the telephone, it has become an important communications tool. With call forwarding, telephone voice mail, and remote access message retrieval, managers today have the opportunity to be promptly responsive to the telephone messages of others, even when the manager is not on site. It is important, however, that prerecorded voicemail messages be kept as short as possible and that the complexity of leaving a message is not so great that it discourages callers from doing so.

Most important, all managers and their support staff must be polite and show respect to all callers. When it is absolutely necessary to place callers on hold, the hold period should be brief or arrangements should be made to return the call at the earliest possible opportunity. Placing callers on hold for long periods of time conveys a message that their time is not valuable.

◆ Listening Skills

It has been shown that most individuals hear or actually retain only a small amount of the information given to them. Although the average person spends 70% of his or her time listening, only one-third of the messages sent are retained. Listening is an active process, and is as important, if not more so, than speaking for the leader.

To become a better listener, the leader must first become aware of how past experiences, values, attitudes, and biases affect the way messages are received and in turn, perceived. The leader must also overcome the information and communication overload inherent to the middle-management role. It is very possible for overwhelmed managers to stop actively listening to the many subordinates who simultaneously need and demand their time.

Last, the leader must continually work to be a better listener, as active listening is an interpersonal communications skill that improves with practice.

The leader who actively listens gives genuine time and attention to the sender, interpreting both verbal and nonverbal communication. As a receiver, the primary purpose is to receive the message being sent, rather than form a response before the transmission of the message is complete.

◆ Group Communication

Managers must communicate with large and small groups, as well as with individual employees. Because a group takes on an entirely different form of communication than do individuals, it is essential that the manager have an understanding of group dynamics, including the sequence each group must proceed through before work can be accomplished. Tuckman and Jensen (1977) labeled these stages forming, storming, norming, and performing (see Table 17-1).

When individuals are first introduced, they must go through a process of meeting each other: the forming stage. They then progress through a stage where there is much competition and attempts at the establishment of individual identities: the storming stage. Next the group begins to establish rules and

◆ TABLE 17-1
Stages of Group Process

Group Development Stage	Group Process	Task Process
Forming	Testing to identify boundaries of interpersonal behaviors; establishing dependent relationships with leaders and other members; and determining what is acceptable behavior.	Testing to identify the tasks, appropriate rules, and methods suited to the performance of the task.
Storming	Resistance to group influence shown as members polarize into subgroups; conflict ensues and members rebel against demands imposed by the leader.	Resistance to task requirements and the differences regarding demands imposed by the task.
Norming	Consensus evolves as group cohesion develops; norms develop; conflict and resistance are overcome.	Cooperation advances as differences are expressed and resolved.
Performing	Interpersonal structure focuses on the task and its completion; roles become flexible and functional; energies are directed toward task performance.	Problems are solved as the task performance improves; constructive efforts to complete task; more of group energies available for the task.

(Condensed from Tuckman and Jensen, 1977.)

design the work to be done, the norming stage. Finally, during the performing stage, the work actually gets done.

Some experts suggest there is a another stage: termination or closure. In this phase, the manager guides members to summarize, express feelings, and come to closure. A celebration at the end of group work is a good way to terminate a project.

Because groups become more effective over time, the addition of new members to a group slows productivity. It takes some time for new members to be accepted, and often, some of the developmental stages of the group will be performed again, or be delayed if several new members join. Therefore, it is important when forming groups to select those who can remain members until the work is finished, or until their appointment is over.

The manager must also be alert to and assess the significance of the formation of subgroups within the larger group. Generally this occurs in response to a sense of powerlessness (Miller, 1991). The manager then must measure the power distribution within the group, and encourage the use of democratic rather than autocratic decision-making styles by the informal group leaders.

◆ Group Dynamics

In addition to forming, storming, and norming, two other functions of groups are necessary. One has to do with the *task* or the purpose of the group and the other has to do with *maintenance* of the group or support functions. Managers should understand how groups carry out their specific tasks and roles.

◆ Task Roles of Groups

There are 11 tasks that each group performs. A member of a group may perform more than one task, but all tasks will be carried out either by the members or by the leader. These roles are as follows.

1. *Initiator:* Contributor who proposes or suggests group goals or redefines the problem. There may be more than one initiator during the lifetime of the group.
2. *Information seeker:* Seeks a factual basis for the work.
3. *Information giver:* Gives an opinion regarding what the pertinent values should be.
4. *Opinion seeker:* Seeks opinions that clarify or reflect the value of other members' suggestions.
5. *Elaborator:* Gives examples or extends the meanings of suggestions given and how they could succeed.
6. *Coordinator:* Clarifies and coordinates ideas, suggestions, and activities.
7. *Orienter:* Summarizes decisions and actions and identifies and questions discrepancies from prestated goals.

8. *Evaluator:* Questions group accomplishments and compares them to a standard.
9. *Energizer:* Stimulates and prods the group to act and raises the level of their actions.
10. *Procedural Technician:* Facilitates group action by arranging the environment.
11. *Recorder:* Records all activities and accomplishments.

◆ Group Building and Maintenance Roles

The group task roles contribute to the work to be done. The group building roles provide for the care and maintenance of the group. Examples of group building roles include:

1. *Encourager:* Accepts and praises contributions, viewpoints, and ideas from all members with warmth and solidarity.
2. *Harmonizer:* Mediates, harmonizes, and resolves conflict.
3. *Gatekeeper:* Promotes open communication and facilitates participation so all members are involved.
4. *Standard setter:* Expresses or evaluates standards of group process.
5. *Compromiser:* Yields his or her own position in a conflict situation.
6. *Group commentator:* Provides feedback to the group.
7. *Follower:* Accepts collective ideas and listens to discussions and decisions.

Individuals may carry out one or more roles in a group, but they often perform the same role in each group they are in.

Managers must recognize the importance of both task and maintenance roles and appoint individuals to accomplish both roles on committee assignments (Marquis and Huston, 1996). In order for the work of a committee to be accomplished, there must be individuals who can carry out the task roles. But in order for the committee to develop a spirit that will endure, there must be individuals who can perform maintenance roles. Simply stated, someone must make the group laugh while someone must move the agenda along; both are necessary.

The manager can also assist groups to increase productivity by adequately preparing prior to meetings. This includes selecting an appropriate site and time, and outlining an agenda. This program and any necessary accompanying material should be sent to all members prior to the meeting. At meeting time the manager should begin promptly, follow the agenda, assign tasks appropriately and clearly, and conclude expeditiously. Later, the manager should disseminate the minutes and follow up on the progress of assigned tasks.

◆ Cultural Diversity: A Challenge to Organizational Communication

The workforce in contemporary organizations continues to be increasingly culturally diverse in terms of race, ethnicity, and gender. Dicken and Blomberg

(1991) note that between the years 1991 and 2000, immigrants will represent the largest share of increase in the U.S. population and workforce since World War I. In addition, 85% of new workers will be composed of U.S.-born white females (42%), immigrants (23%), and minorities (20%). This cultural diversity will pose significant challenges for organizations in both creating a shared organizational culture and in communicating effectively.

A lack of sensitivity to cultural diversity may result in messages not being received or being misinterpreted. For example, one nonverbal cue that plays a role in interpersonal communication and may be affected by cultural diversity, is space. The space between the sender and receiver of the message often influences what is communicated. In American culture, distance implies a lack of trust or warmth; however, inadequate space, as defined by other cultural norms, may make individuals feel threatened or intimidated. Generally, North American, Indian, African, Pakistani, and Asian cultures require greater space between sender and receiver than Latinos and southern Europeans (Richmond, McCroskey, and Payne, 1987). Davis (1990) states "Arabians like to conduct business discussions within spitting distance—literally. They bathe in each other's breath as part of building the relationship. That is why there is no word for privacy in Arab cultures."

Davis (1990) states:

> We each wear a zone of privacy like a hoop skirt, inviting others in or keeping them out with body language—by how closely we approach, the angle at which we face them, the speed with which we break a gaze. It's a subtle code, but one we use and interpret easily, indeed automatically, having absorbed the vocabulary from infancy. At least we *assume* we're reading it right. But from culture to culture, from group to group within a single country, even between the sexes, the language of space has distinctive accents, confusing umlauts. This leaves tremendous room for misinterpretation.

Managers then, must be sensitive to the needs of the individual for personal space. Likewise, interpretation of the subtle code of body language should be approached with caution.

As with space, the presence or absence of eye contact is strongly influenced by cultural standards. Hall stated, "Americans frequently make their business counterparts in Japan uncomfortable with the kind of direct eye contact that's normal here. Not only do most Japanese businessmen not look at you, they almost always keep their eyes down" (Davis, 1990).

Virtually every type of organizational communication—verbal, nonverbal, or written—may be influenced by work force diversity. Differences in communication modes, communication styles, frequency of communication, and directness of communication should be expected when there is diversity in gender, race, and ethnicity. It is imperative then that managers be perceptive of cultural factors that may influence interpersonal and organizational communication. Managers also must be open to using multiple, different means of communication to assure that everyone in the organization receives the messages that are being sent.

◆ The Impact of Technology on Organizational Communication

Telecommunication technology has been and will continue to proliferate at a rapid rate as we enter the 21st century. Warminger (1990) suggests that this advancing technology may help to balance the constraints being placed on other resources. For example, Spurck and colleagues (1995) describe the implementation of a wireless telecommunication system (staff nurses carrying portable phones) that dramatically reduces nurse waiting time at the station, clerical time to locate nurses, and time callers spent on "hold."

Other telecommunication technology, such as electronic mail, faxes, teleconferences, and CD-ROM, are quickly becoming an integral part of organizational communication systems. The use of hospital information system (HIS) configurations, such as stand alone systems, on-line interactive systems, networked systems, and integrative systems, has also increased. Computerized patient records (CPR) have been mandated by the federal government and many healthcare organizations are expected to adopt this technology by the year 2000 (Yoder-Wise, 1995). Physiological monitoring systems will become even more refined. The nursing minimum data set (NMDS), which has been used to standardize the collection of nursing data, has been suggested by many authors as an appropriate tool in the future to develop nursing information systems and to structure nursing documentation.

The communication challenges managers will face in such a rapidly evolving technological society will be threefold:

1. to determine which technological advances can and should be used at each level of the organizational hierarchy to promote efficiency and effectiveness of communication;
2. to provide workers with adequate training to appropriately and fully utilize the technological communication tools that may become available to them; and
3. to find a balance between the technological communication option and the need for human touch, caring, and one-on-one face-to-face interaction.

◆ Summary

Communication is as important in management as it is in the personal life of an individual. Indeed, communication may be the most critical management skill as it cuts across all phases of the management process. Although managers communicate in many ways, written, face-to-face, nonverbal, and telephone communication are most common. Developing skill in all four areas is essential for the manager. Because so much organizational communication occurs in groups, the manager must also have an understanding of group dynamics.

The large size of some organizations makes adequate communication difficult, as does power, status, and authority. Cultural diversity and rapidly flourishing communication technologies also add to the complexity of organizational communication.

Perhaps, however, the most critical communication skill is listening. Managers can easily become overwhelmed by many people wanting to communicate with them at the same time. Although some communication filters are appropriate, the manager must be very careful not to stop listening closely and attentively to subordinates. A failure to do so will rapidly result in increasing unit unrest and decreased worker morale.

◆ References

Arnold E and Boggs K (1989). Interpersonal Relationships: Professional Communication Skills for Nurses. Philadelphia: WB Saunders

Chenevert M (1988). Pro-Nurse Handbook, 3rd ed. St. Louis: CV Mosby

Davis L (1990). Where do we stand? Health 4(5)Sept/Oct:34–36

Dicken B and Blomberg R (1991). Immigrants—can they provide the future work force? Public Pers Manage 20(1):91–100

Hackman MZ and Johnson CE (1991). Leadership: A Communication Perspective. Prospect Heights IL: Waveland Press

Health Care Education Associates (1988). Professional Writing Skills for Health Care Managers: A Practical Guide. St. Louis: CV Mosby

Huber D (1996). Leadership and Nursing Care Management. Philadelphia: WB Saunders

Kotter JP (1990). What leaders really do. Harvard Bus Rev 68(3) May/June: 103–111

Kruse JM (1992). What kinds of nurses most assert themselves? Nurs Manage 23(3):66–67

Marquis B and Huston C (1996). Leadership Roles and Management Functions: Theory and Application, 2nd ed. Philadelphia: JB Lippincott

Miller D (1991). Group dynamics: Handling subgroups. Nurs Manage 22(12):33–35

Richmond V, McCroskey J, and Payne S (1987). Nonverbal Behavior in Interpersonal Relations. Englewood Cliffs, NJ: Prentice-Hall

Spurck PA, Mohr ML, Seroka AM, and Stoner M (1995). The impact of a wireless telecommunication system on time efficiency. J Nurs Admin 25(6):21–26

Sullivan EJ and Decker PJ (1988). Effective Management in Nursing, 3rd ed. Menlo Park, CA: Addison-Wesley

Swansburg RC (1990). Management and Leadership for Nurse Managers. Boston: Jones and Bartlett

Tappen RM (1995). Nursing Leadership and Management, 3rd ed. Philadelphia: FA Davis

Tuckman BW and Jensen MAC (1977). Stages of small group development revisited. Group Organ Stud 2(4):419

Warminger P (1990). Staff and patient communications—trends and technologies. Health Estate J 44 (6):2–8

Yoder-Wise PS (1995). Leading and Managing In Nursing. St. Louis: Mosby

S A M P L E   C A S E   A N A L Y S I S

THE CASE ◆

As the 3:00–11:00 P.M. charge nurse on a surgical unit, you routinely have a short, weekly educational conference letting each staff member take turns presenting a 15-minute summary of a topic of their choice. You also have two short weekly staff meetings, one for general sharing and one for patient care conferences. Lately, you have found that the meetings are not going well because one member of the group (Ms. Morgan) tends to monopolize all of the meeting time, except when someone is making a formal presentation. You have spoken privately to her about this and although apologetic, her behavior has continued. In all other respects, Ms. Morgan is an excellent nurse and a good employee.

Assignment

Using your knowledge of group dynamics and communication, outline what steps you would take to facilitate more group participation.

Analysis

You have already met with the nurse and made her aware of her behavior. This is a good first step. However, individuals who monopolize groups often have difficulty controlling this behavior and need some assistance from the group itself. Remember that immediate feedback is the most effective way to change behavior.

Your goal here is to extinguish the behavior, without humiliating or embarrassing the employee. Often, group members take their cue from the group facilitator, so you need to act as an appropriate role model for the group. Roles you need to assume include gatekeeper and group commentator. The following might be appropriate methods of dealing with Ms. Morgan.

1. Ask specific employees in the group, by name, for input into the item under discussion.
2. If Ms. Morgan begins to answer, interrupt by saying, "Let's hear from John now, Ms. Morgan."
3. If she persists, say, "Please don't interrupt, Ms. Morgan."
4. If her comments are rambling, state that you don't see the point and feel that her points are irrelevant to the topic under discussion.
5. Should Ms. Morgan continue, state in front of the group "I am frustrated that other members of the group do not have a chance to share their ideas and feelings as well."

Eventually the group will take over the task of monitoring her behavior. Make sure that this modification is only of her group behavior. Ms. Morgan might be somewhat hurt by the actions of you and the group and may verbally withdraw. This behavior is usually only temporary and she should eventually become a participant in the group again. Do not encourage her to participate during her withdrawn state. This would be giving a mixed message.

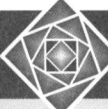

CASES FOR PROBLEM SOLVING

CASE 1

Assignment

Decide if the following responses are assertive, aggressive, or passive. Change aggressive or passive responses into assertive responses.

Situation	Response
1. A coworker withdraws instead of saying what is on his mind. You say:	"I guess you are uncomfortable talking about what's bothering you. It would be better if you talked to me."
2. This is the third time in two weeks that your coworker has asked for a ride home because her car is not working. You say:	"You're taking advantage of me and I won't stand for it. It's your responsibility to get your car fixed."
3. An attendant at the gas station you frequent neglected to replace your gas cap. You notice this and return to inquire about it and you say:	"One of the guys here forgot to put my gas cap back on! I want it found now or you'll buy me a new one."
4. You would like to have a turn at being in charge on your shift and you say to your head nurse:	"Do you think that you could see your way clear to letting me be in charge once in a while?"
5. A committee meeting is being established. The time is convenient for other people but not for you. The schedule is such that it will be next to impossible for you to attend regularly. When you asked about the time, you said:	"Well, I guess it's OK. I'm not going to be able to attend very much, but it fits into everyone else's schedule."
6. In a conversation, a doctor suddenly says, "What do you women libbers want anyway?" You respond:	"Fairness and equality."
7. An employee makes a lot of mistakes in his work. You say:	"You're a lazy and sloppy worker!"
8. You are at a meeting of seven men and one woman. At the beginning of the meeting, the chairman asks you to be the secretary. You respond:	"No, I'm sick and tired of being the secretary just because I'm the only woman in the group."
9. A physician asks you to borrow your stethoscope. You say:	"Well, I guess so. One of you doctors walked off with mine last week and this new one cost me $35. Be sure you return it, okay?"
10. You are interpreting the intake and output sheet for a physician and he interrupts you. You say:	"You could understand this if you'd stop interrupting me and listen."

CASE 2   (Marquis and Huston, 1996)

Assume that you are the project director of the small North Hills Family Planning Clinic. You have just received word that your federal and state fund-

CASE 2 (CONTINUED)

ing have been slashed and that the clinic will probably close in about 3 months. There is a chance that an additional funding source will be found, but it is improbable this will occur within the next 3 months. The Board of Directors informed you that this knowledge is not to be made public at this time. You have five full-time employees working at the clinic. Two of these employees are close friends and you are experiencing some conflict about withholding this information from them. You are aware that another clinic in town currently has job openings, and that the positions are generally filled quickly.

••

Assignment

It is important that you continue to be able to staff the clinic for the next 3 months. Determine when you will notify the staff of the clinic's intent to close. Will you communicate the closing to all at the same time? Will you use downward communication? Should the grapevine be used to "leak" news to employees? When is it appropriate for the manager to use the grapevine to pass on information?

CASE 3 ◆

Mrs. White is the coordinator for the multidisciplinary mental health outpatient services of a 150-bed psychiatric facility. She has been very frustrated because the hospital is very centralized; she feels this keeps the hospital therapists and nurse managers from being as effective as they could if they had more authority. Therefore, she has worked out a plan to decentralize her department, giving the therapists and nurse managers more control and new titles.

She sent her new plan to Mr. Short, the CEO, and has just received this memo in return:

Dear Mrs. White:

The Board of Directors and I met to review your plan and think it is a good one. In fact, we have been thinking along the same lines for quite some time now. I'm sure you must have heard of our plans. Since we have recently contracted with a physician's group to cover our crisis center, we feel this would be a good time to decentralize in other ways. We suggest that your new Substance Abuse Coordinator report directly to the new Chief of Mental Health. In addition, we feel your new Director of the Suicide Prevention Center should report directly to the Chief of Mental Health. He will then report to me.

I am pleased that we are both moving in the same direction and have the same goals. We will be setting up meetings in the future to iron out the small details.

Sincerely,
Joseph Short, CEO

CASE 3 (CONTINUED)

••

Assignment

1. How and why did Mrs. White's plan go astray? Could it have been prevented?
2. What communications mode would have been most appropriate for her to share her plan with Mr. Short?
3. What should be her plan now? Outline what you would do now if you were Mrs. White. Explain your rationale.

CASE 4 (Marquis and Huston, 1996)

You are a school nurse for kindergarten through grade 6 in a primarily affluent, small, community. The school board trustees who set policy are outspoken and conservative in their views. Recently, a policy was established regarding the education of children known to be HIV positive. This policy allows children who have tested positive for the virus to attend school, although physical segregation in the classroom is mandatory for children under the age of 7. This policy is based on the belief that children under the age of 7 could inadvertently transmit body fluids in the course of spitting, drooling, urination, and so on. The policy also requires that all school personnel involved with the child be aware of the child's health care status. This mandate has yet to be tested in the classroom. Although you are glad to see the district establish policy in this area, you feel that the current policy holds great potential for the discrimination and isolation of HIV-positive children.

Recently, a new kindergarten student entered your district. He is a 5-year-old, known hemophiliac whose parents recently completed and returned his health screening history. At that time, they requested a copy of the current HIV policy for the district, which you sent to them.

One week later, you completed an initial screening visit with the child as part of the registration process. The child appeared to be pale and thin, and was easily fatigued. On direct confrontation, the parents admitted that their son was HIV positive, but implored you not to place this on his record. They have not yet discussed the presence of HIV with their son, as they feel he is not old enough to understand the ramifications. They feel the current policy is discriminatory and that their son would be physically and socially ostracized from the other children. They also feel the community in general is conservative and would be unaccepting of both their son and themselves.

••

Assignment

Who has a right to information in this case? To whom will you relate this information? In what communication mode? How will you control the dissemination of that information? Can this communication be limited to the formal network? What safeguards can you build into your communication to protect all the individuals who might be affected by this situation?

CASE 5

You are a unit manager at a long-term care facility. Your personnel expenses, as a result of overtime, have exceeded the budget for 10 of the last 12 months. On discussing the problem with your charge nurses, they report that most of the overtime is in response to the need to complete extensive handwritten charting and they suggest that computerized charting might be both a more rapid and effective means of accomplishing this task. Although there is capital equipment money in the budget to purchase the computer hardware necessary to implement such a plan, you have some reservations about the resources that would need to be directed for ongoing training of the staff for computerized charting, the potential for even greater overtime during the period the staff would first be using the new system, and the risk of confidentiality breaks inherent in any computerized data base. However, you also recognize that computerized charting is likely to be mandated within the next 5 years and you are reluctant to not take advantage of your staff's readiness to make the change.

··

Assignment

1. Using Lewin's force field analysis, identify the driving and restraining forces for making such a change.
2. If you decide that such a change is indicated, identify what steps you would take to initiate the change. If you determine not to make a change, identify other options you may have to address the problem.

◆ Bibliography

The following is a list of references to help you solve these cases:

Anthonypillai F (1993). Cross-cultural communication in an intensive therapy unit. Int Crit Care Nurse 9(Dec):263–267

Armstrong MA and Kelly AE (1993). Enhancing staff nurses' interpersonal skills: theory to practice. Clin Nurse Special 7(Nov):313–317

Arrow H and McGrath JE (1995). Membership dynamics in groups at work: a theoretical framework. Res Organ Behav 17:373–411

Axtell RE (1991). Gestures: the do's and taboos of body language around the world. New York: Wiley

Borisoff D and Merill L (1992). The Power to Communicate: Gender Differences as Barriers, 2nd ed. Prospect Heights, IL: Waveland

Brown SJ (1994). Communication strategies used by an expert nurse. Clin Nurs Res 3(Feb):43–56

Chu L-MK and Chu G SF (1991). Feedback and efficiency: a staff development model. Nurs Manage 22(2):28–31

Conrad C (1990). Strategic Organizational Communication. Fort Worth, TX: Holt, Rinehart, and Winston

Cornell D (1993). Say the words: communication techniques. Nurs Manage 24(3):42–44

Felts A (1992). Organizational communication: a critical perspective. Admin Soc 23(4): 495–513

Fiesta J (1994). Communication: are you listening? Nurs Manage 25(9):15–16

Goodall R (1993). Assert yourself: effective communication for nurses. AORN J 57(4):894, 896–899

Griffin C (1993). Women as Communicators. Communication, Monographs 60(2):158–77

Hansten R and Washburn M (1992). What's your feedback style? Am J Nurs 92(12):56–61

Harri-Augstein S and Thomas LF (1991). Learning Conversations. The Self-Organised Learning Way to Personal and Organisational Growth. London: Routledge

Hollingshead AB, McGrath JE, and O'Connor KM (1993). Group task performance and communication technology: a longitudinal study of computer-mediated versus face-to-face work groups. Small Group Res 24(3):307–333

Hon J (1994). Bad news, I'm afraid ... communication skills of doctors. Nurs Stand 8(32):52–53

Hull C (1994). Communication and effective learning: communication and the learning environment. Nurs Times 90(10):i–viii

Johnson D and Martin K (1996). Preparing for electronic documentation. Nurs Manage 27(7):43–44

Kennedy C, Camden C, and Timmerman G (1990). Relationships among perceived supervisor communication, nurse morale, and sociocultural variables. Nurs Admin Quart 14(4):38–46

Laing M (1993). Gossip: does it play a role in the socialization of nurses? Image 25(Spring):37–43

Lloyd A (1991). Stop, look, and listen. Nurs Times 87(12):30–32

Manss VC (1994). Effective communication: gender issues. Nurs Manage 25(6):79–80

Mathias JM (1992). Nurses need good communication skills. OR Manage 8(4):19

Parry Bush AM and Ebel CA (1996). Testing an electronic documentation system. Nurs Manage 27(7):40–42

Peloqion SM (1995). The issue is: communication skills: why not turn to a skills training model? Am J Occupat Ther 49(7):721–723

Rondeau KV (1992). Effective communication means really listening. Can J Med Technol 54(2):78–80

Rothenburger RL (1990). Transcultural nursing: overcoming obstacles to effective communication. AORN J 51(5)P:1349–1350, 1352, 1354

Sellers S (1991). Language and Sexual Difference. London: Macmillan.

Sheafor M (1991). Productive work groups in complex patient units. J Nurs Admin 21(5):25–30

Simpson R (1994). Ensuring patient data, privacy, confidentiality and security. Nurs Manage 25(7):18–20

PERSONAL NOTEBOOK

1. Which modes of communicating do you find the most effective? Which modes are most difficult for you?

2. Do you *most frequently* use the informal grapevine or formal channels of communication?

3. Think back to the last communication you had with someone that was greatly affected by either the internal or external climate. Describe this situation in writing. Were you aware of the climate at the time? What, if any, steps did you take to modify the impact of the climate on the message? Were you successful?

4. Which of the group building and maintenance roles do you assume most often? Which of the task roles? Which roles are most difficult for you to assume?

CHAPTER 18

Conflict, Collaboration, and Negotiation

Conflict can be defined as the internal or external discord that occurs as a result of differences in ideas, values, or beliefs of two or more people. Littlefield (1995) suggests that conflict can be considered either an incident or a process. As an incident, conflict occurs as a disagreement between two persons or parties in which one perceives the act of the other to be detrimental to his or her interests or actions. As a process, conflict is manifested in a series of actions by two persons or groups in which each person or group tries to thwart the other's purposes or prevent satisfaction of the other's interests.

An important factor in conflict is the number of opportunities individuals have within the organization to interact with each other. Because managers have a variety of interpersonal relationships with individuals having different values, beliefs, backgrounds, and goals, conflict is an expected outcome. A developmental study of two psychiatric hospitals found that there was more conflict among individuals, regardless of their professional status, at a structurally more complex hospital than at a less complex hospital (Erwin, 1992). Possible sources of conflict found in all complex organizations include power divisions, communications, personal and organizational goals and values, resource allocation, competing attitudes and personalities, and role confusion (Huber, 1996).

Conflict can be destructive and demoralizing. It is always energy intensive. However, it can also be a positive and dynamic force in the organization, preventing stagnation, stimulating curiosity and interest, and serving as a medium for airing problems. Regarded and managed with such a viewpoint, conflicts can actually serve to hold organizations together. Brett, Goldberg, and Ury (1990) suggest that managers must make two fundamental assumptions about conflict: 1) that conflict is inevitable in an organization, and 2) if successfully managed, conflict can produce high quality, creative solutions that lead to innovation and progress.

The manager's role in the organization then is to create a work environment that uses conflict constructively as a conduit for growth, innovation, and productivity. When organizational conflict leads to dysfunction, the manager must recognize its early stages and actively intervene so that subordinate motivation and organizational productivity are not adversely affected. Learning to handle conflict constructively to yield a win–win outcome is a critical management skill.

◆ The History of Conflict Management

The open acknowledgment of conflict as a naturally occurring and expected phenomenon in organizations reflects a tremendous shift from how sociologists viewed conflict one hundred years ago. Early in the 20th century, conflict was considered to be an indication of poor organizational management and was avoided at all costs. Organizational harmony was expected and conflict always deemed destructive. When conflict occurred, it was either ignored, denied, or immediate adjustment demanded. It was believed that conflict could be avoided if employees were taught the one "right way" to do things and if employee dissatisfaction was expressed, it was met with swift disapproval. Termed *restrictive conflict* management, this approach emphasized organizational values and limited individual initiative (Erwin, 1992).

In the mid-1900s, when worker satisfaction and feedback became paramount, conflict was accepted passively and perceived as a normal and expected outcome in organizations. Attention centered on teaching managers how to resolve conflict rather than trying to prevent it. Although it was considered to be primarily dysfunctional, it was felt that conflict and cooperation could occur simultaneously.

The interactionist theorists of the 1970s recognized conflict as an "absolute necessity" and actively encouraged organizations to promote conflict as a means of producing growth. This view has since been tempered by the realization that conflict in itself is neither good nor bad and that it can produce growth or destruction depending upon how it is managed. Greenhalgh (1986) states that because conflict is inevitable in the organization, it should be considered managed when it does not interfere with ongoing functional relationships.

Some level of conflict appears desirable, although the optimum level for any individual or unit at a given time is difficult to determine. Too little conflict results in organizational stasis, although too much conflict reduces the effectiveness of the organization and eventually immobilizes its employees. Until there is a sophisticated measuring instrument for assessing whether a given conflict level is functional or dysfunctional, it will continue to be the manager's responsibility to determine appropriate levels of conflict in a unit.

Conflict can be qualitative as well as quantitative. Although conflict produces distress at the time it occurs, it can lead to growth, energy, and creativity by the generation of new ideas and solutions. *Constructive conflict management* creates an environment conducive to discussions characterized by a proper focus on issues, open communication, and the mutual sharing of responsibilities for resolving differences (Erwin, 1992).

If conflict is handled inappropriately, it can lead to demoralization, decreased motivation, and lowered productivity. For conflict to produce growth, managers must understand the categories of conflict, the conflict process itself, and be able to apply appropriate conflict resolution strategies.

◆ Categories of Conflict

There are three primary types of conflict: 1) intrapersonal, 2) interpersonal, and 3) intergroup. *Intra*personal conflict refers to conflict that occurs within an individual. It is an internal struggle to clarify conflicting values or wants. It is often manifested as a result of competing roles (Huber, 1996). For example, the manager may feel an intrapersonal conflict between loyalty to the profession, loyalty to the employer, and loyalty to patients. Being self-aware and conscientiously working to resolve intrapersonal conflict as soon as it is first felt is essential to the physical and mental health of the manager.

*Inter*personal conflict is conflict between two or more individuals whose values, goals, and beliefs are considered to be incompatible. This is the most frequent type of conflict because people are constantly interacting and therefore differing (Bernhard and Walsh, 1990). The manager may experience conflict in upward, downward, horizontal, or diagonal communication.

Intergroup conflict occurs between two or more groups of people, departments, or organizations. Sources of intergroup conflict include struggles for power and authority, opposing goals, territoriality, and scarcity of resources. An example of intergroup conflict might be two religious affiliations with widely differing or contradictory beliefs.

Regardless of the size of the groups involved, intergroup conflict has certain predictable consequences. Within each group, cohesiveness increases, but members become more task-oriented and less concerned with the needs of the individual members. Each group tends to recognize only its own positive aspects and only the negative aspects of the other group. Negative stereotypes begin to form and, as hostility increases, and communication between groups decreases, it is easy to perpetuate the stereotypes. If the groups are required to meet, they will see and hear only those aspects of the other group that will support their opinions (Bernhard and Walsh, 1990).

Organizational conflict can reflect intrapersonal, interpersonal, and intergroup conflict. Typically, however, organizational conflict is viewed as being either vertical or horizontal (Marquis and Huston, 1996). Vertical conflict occurs between superiors and subordinates or management and employees and frequently concerns policy, power, and status. Horizontal conflict occurs between line-staff positions and between individuals with similar power and status in the organizational hierarchy. Horizontal conflict typically involves authority, expertise, or practice.

◆ The Conflict Process

Before managers can or should attempt to intervene in conflict, they must be able to accurately assess its current stage. The first stage in the conflict process is called *latent* conflict, which implies the existence of *antecedent conditions.* Conditions such as short staffing and rapid change are examples of antecedent conditions. In latent conflict, the conditions are ripe for conflict, although no conflict has actually occurred and may never occur.

If the conflict progresses, it may become *perceived* conflict. Also called substantive conflict, this form is intellectualized and often involves issues and roles. It is recognized logically and impersonally by the individual as occurring. Sometimes an individual can resolve conflict at this stage before it is internalized or felt.

Felt conflict is emotionalized and these emotions include hostility, fear, mistrust, and anger. This is also referred to as affective conflict. It is possible for an individual to perceive conflict and not feel it; that is, there is no emotion attached to the conflict, and the individual views it only as a problem to be solved. Also possible is for someone to feel the conflict, but not perceive the problem; that is, they are unable to identify the cause of the felt conflict.

In *manifest* conflict, action is taken. The action may be to withdraw, compete, debate, or seek conflict resolution. Many individuals unconsciously learn to use competition, dominance, and aggression to resolve conflict as they are growing up. Conflict resolution or problem solving, on the other hand, appears to be learned less frequently through developmental experiences and a conscious effort generally is required to develop and learn those skills. It is through conscientious effort and practice that managers become adept at conflict resolution.

Conflict resolution implies a solution that satisfies all parties involved in the conflict. The optimal goal, then, in conflict resolution is to create a win–win solution for everyone involved. This is not possible in every instance and often the manager's goal is limited to lessening the perceptual differences that exist between the clashing parties in conflict.

The final stage in the conflict process is *conflict aftermath.* This aftermath may be more significant than the original conflict if the conflict has not been handled in a constructive manner. Figure 18-1 shows a schematic of this conflict process. It is important to note that there is a feedback loop between conflict aftermath and latent conflict. In other words, the resolution of one conflict may become the antecedent condition for the next conflict.

◆ Conflict Resolution Strategies

It is important for the manager to distinguish which situations can or cannot result in a win–win solution, and to implement the conflict resolution strategy most appropriate for each situation. Six common conflict resolution strategies are shown in Display 18-1.

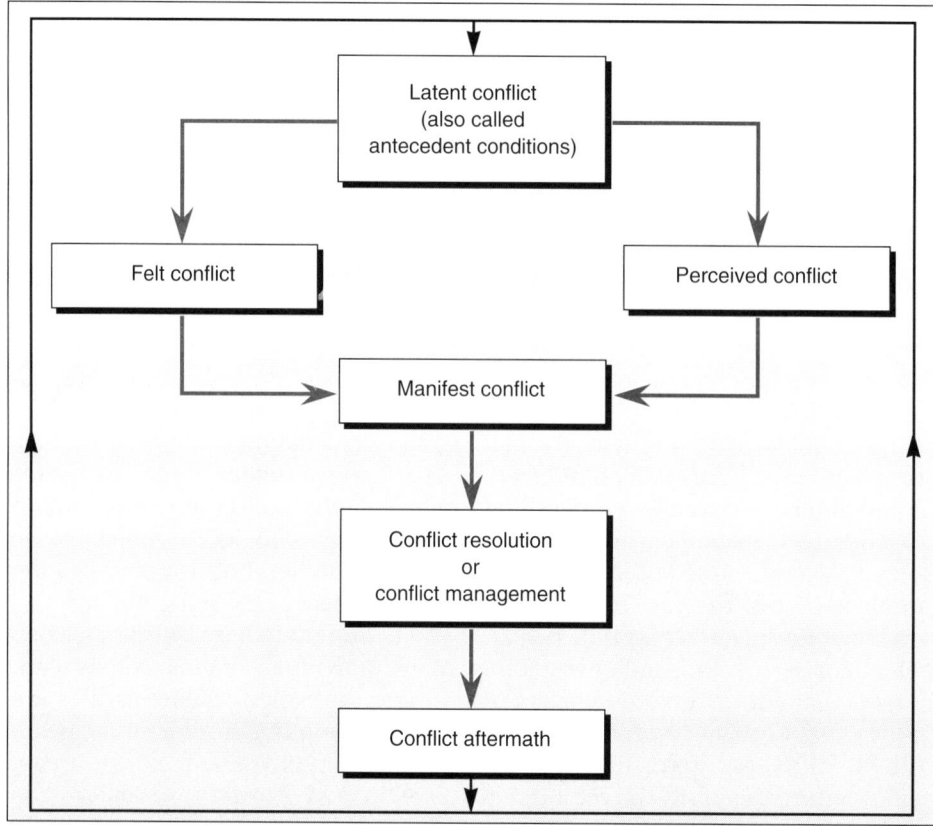

FIGURE 18-1. The conflict process.

In using *compromise* or *negotiation* as an approach to conflict resolution, parties of equal power give up something that they want. Although many individuals view compromise as an acceptable conflict resolution strategy, this antagonistic cooperation frequently results in a *lose–lose* situation, because either or both parties perceive they have given up more than the other. Both feel defeated as a result of the lose–lose compromise. It is possible for compromising not to result in such a situation, but this can only be achieved if both parties cooperate and give up something of equal value. Barton (1991) found compromising to be the most frequently used conflict resolution strategy by middle- and top-level nursing administrators.

The *competing* approach to conflict resolution is used when one party pursues what they want at the expense of the other party(ies). Only one party wins and seeks the victory regardless of the cost to others. Win–lose conflict resolution strategies leave the loser filled with anger, frustration, and a desire to "get even" in the future. This competing approach may be used by managers when a quick or unpopular decision needs to be made. It may also be used when one party has more information or knowledge about a certain situation than the other.

DISPLAY 18-1
Six Common Conflict Resolution Strategies

Compromising–Negotiating

Competing

Accommodating

Smoothing

Avoiding

Collaborating

Accommodating is the opposite of competing. In accommodating, one individual sacrifices his or her beliefs and wants in an effort to allow the other party to win. The actual problem is usually not solved in this win–lose situation. Cooperation is another term that may be used for this strategy. The person cooperating or accommodating often collects IOUs from the other party for use at a later date. Cooperating and accommodating are appropriate political strategies if the issue in debate is not of high value to the person doing the accommodating.

Smoothing is a type of conflict resolution used to reduce the emotional component of the conflict. In smoothing, one party attempts to compliment the other party or to focus on areas of agreement rather than on differences. Smoothing may be appropriate for minor disagreements, but rarely results in resolution of the actual conflict.

The manager may also use *avoiding* as a conflict resolution strategy. In avoiding, the parties involved are aware of a problem but choose not to acknowledge that conflict or attempt to resolve it. Avoidance may be indicated in situations where the disagreement is trivial, the cost of dealing with the conflict exceeds the benefits of solving it, when the problem should be solved by other people than yourself, and when the problem will eventually solve itself.

In Barton's study (1991), first- and middle-level nursing managers ranked avoiding as their third most commonly used conflict resolution strategy behind compromise and collaboration. This may be because first- and middle-level managers frequently find themselves in situations where they perceive themselves as less powerful, as in disagreements with physicians, top-level nursing administrators, and other managers.

Collaboration is an assertive and cooperative means of conflict resolution that results in a win–win solution. In collaboration, both parties set aside their original goals and work together to establish a *supraordinate* or common goal. Because both parties have identified the joint goal, each believes they have achieved their goal and an acceptable solution. The focus throughout collaboration remains on problem solving, and not on defeating the other party.

Collaboration will not work if competitive incentives are part of the situation, the parties involved have poor problem-solving skills, and neither party trusts each other (Bowditch and Buono, 1994).

◆ Collaborative Relationships in Organizations

Only a small percentage of managerial time is spent in true collaboration. Many individuals think of collaboration as a form of cooperation, but this is not an accurate definition. In collaboration there is a joint effort toward problem solving. There can be no superior–subordinate, order-giving–order-taking relationships in collaboration.

Collaboration has been called the most effective strategy for managing conflict to achieve long-range benefits (Huber, 1996) and is fashionable in current literature, but because it involves others the manager has no control over and because it is a lengthy process, it may not be the best approach for all situations. Bowditch and Buono (1994) suggest that that time frame is one of the most critical variables that must be considered in determining whether to use collaboration. When dealing with short-term goals, competition or compromise may be a more pragmatic way to deal with the conflict. However, with long-term goals, collaboration remains the best alternative for complex problem solving involving many others.

Collaboration is especially critical in *team building*. In team building, members share a common goal, interdependence, cooperation, coordination of activities, task specialization, division of effort, and mutual respect (Neubauer, 1993).

Managers who model collaboration maintain mutual respect as the expected standard of behavior. They communicate honestly, face-to-face. They uncover and define common goals through discussion. They visibly share decision making and carefully negotiate for mutually acceptable goals (Erwin, 1992).

◆ Managing Unit Conflict

In addition to their own interpersonal conflicts, managers also have a responsibility to occasionally facilitate conflict resolution between others. This requires the manager to recognize the situational variables, including the values and motivation of each party, their attitudes and beliefs about one another, and the nature of the issue underlying the conflict (Erwin, 1992). The manager must also consider the social environment, possible consequences of the conflict, and the strategy and tactics that conflicting parties have employed thus far.

A conflict resolution model proposed by Brett, Goldberg, and Ury (1990) suggests that there are three basic principles to dispute resolution. The first principle is an assumption that resolving the dispute will not alter the underlying conflict of interests that generated the dispute. In other words, the potential for future disputes will exist as long as the original conflict of interests remains. The second principle is the proposition that from the long-term perspective of the organization, reconciling conflicting interests is generally a less costly way to resolve disputes than determining who is right or more powerful. Tradeoffs and reconciling interests on low priority interests (called bridging) are strategies used to accomplish this goal. The third principle is an observation that dispute resolution procedures differentially focus parties on reconciling interest versus determining who is right or more powerful. With this principle, mediation and the use of neutral third parties would be advocated over proxy fights, elections, strikes, and wars.

It is critical that the manager be sensitive to conflict between employees before it becomes dysfunctional. The manager can then assist employees to consider many possible alternatives to resolving their conflict. Through coaching, the manager can help employees with conflicts to select an appropriate conflict resolution strategy or behavior.

Other strategies the manager may employ in assisting subordinates to resolve interpersonal conflicts are as follows:

1. *Urge confrontation:* Often subordinates approach the manager expecting the manager to solve their interpersonal conflicts before they make any attempt to do it themselves. It is inappropriate for managers to intervene in this situation; instead, they should urge the complaining individual(s) to attempt to handle their own problems.

2. *Third party consultation:* Sometimes managers can be used as a neutral party to help others resolve conflicts in a constructive manner. This should be done only if both parties are motivated to solve the problem, and if there is not a difference in status or power being used by either party. In third-party consultation, the manager may act as a buffer and use procedures or physical space to decrease abrasive interactions among the individuals in the conflict (Erwin, 1992).

3. *Behavior change:* This is reserved for serious cases of dysfunctional conflict. Use of educational modes, training development, or sensitivity training can be effective in resolving conflict by developing self-awareness and promoting a behavior change in the involved parties.

4. *Responsibility charting:* When ambiguity occurs over unclear or new roles, it is often necessary to have those involved cooperate in defining the respective functions and responsibilities attached to those roles. If there are areas of joint responsibility, the manager must clearly outline such things as ultimate responsibility, approval mechanisms, support services, and responsibility for informing. This is a useful technique for elementary jurisdictional conflicts.

5. *Structure change:* Sometimes managers need to intervene in unit conflict by the transfer or discharge of individuals. Other structural changes may include moving a department under another manager, adding an ombudsman, or instituting a grievance procedure. Often, increasing the boundaries of authority for one member of the conflict will act as an effective structural change in resolving unit conflict. Changing titles and/or creating policies are also effective techniques.

6. *Soothing one party:* This is a temporary solution that should only be used in situations where there is not sufficient time to handle the conflict effectively. The manager temporarily soothes one party so that cooperation will occur until the crisis has subsided. The manager then must address the underlying problem or this technique will lead to dysfunction.

7. *Foster self-awareness:* The manager may attempt to foster greater insight by guiding individuals involved in a conflict to better understand their own behavior—to gain a new perspective on an old situation. This strategy is not appropriate if the parties are already enraged.

◆ Negotiation

Negotiation in its most creative form is similar to collaboration and in its most poorly managed form may resemble a competing approach (Marquis and Huston, 1996). Negotiation frequently resembles compromise when it is used as a conflict resolution strategy. During negotiation, each party gives up something, and the emphasis is on accommodating differences between the parties.

Smeltzer (1991) identified two basic types of negotiation: *cooperative* (everybody wins) and *competitive* (only one party wins). A basic principle to remember about negotiation is that one of the parties wishes to alter the present relationship with the other (Smeltzer, 1991). If both parties desire a change in the relationship, there is a greater probability of cooperative negotiation. If the dissatisfaction with the relationship is one-sided, the negotiation has a greater chance of being competitive.

Although negotiation implies winning and losing for both parties, as a negotiator, it is important to:

1. win as much as necessary to achieve your goals,
2. lose as little as possible, as losing would keep you from meeting your goals, and
3. make the other party feel satisfied with the outcome of the negotiation.

Many small compromises occur every day in a spontaneous fashion and are successful without any advance preparation. However, if managers wish to be successful in important negotiations such as those involving financial or unit resources, they must be:

1. adequately prepared,
2. able to use appropriate negotiation strategies, and
3. apply appropriate closure and follow-up to the negotiation.

◆ Prior to Negotiation

Three criteria must be met before a manager agrees to begin the negotiation process: the issue must be negotiable, the negotiators must be interested in both giving and taking during the process, and they must trust each other, as well as the negotiating process (Smeltzer, 1991). If these criteria are met, the manager can begin systematically to prepare for the negotiation.

The manager begins by gathering as much information as possible regarding the issue to be negotiated. Because knowledge is power, the more informed the negotiator is, the greater the degree of bargaining power. The other party in the negotiation often attempts to catch the negotiator off-guard, but managers who have done their homework will not be caught in this trap.

It is also important for managers to decide where they want to start in the negotiation. Because they must be willing to compromise, they should choose a goal that is high, but not ridiculous. This selected starting point should be at the upper limits of their expectations, realizing that they may need to come down to a more realistic goal. The minimum that an individual will settle for is often referred to as the *bottom line.*

The wise manager will also have other options in mind when negotiating important resources. An *alternative option* is another set of negotiating preferences that can be utilized so that the manager need not employ the bottom line, but still meet the overall goal. The negotiator also needs to consider other *trade-offs* that are possible. Trade-offs often represent future gains in a conflict situation.

For example, during nursing school individuals may feel intrapersonal conflict because they are unable to spend as much time as they desire with their children. They are able to compromise by considering the trade-off. Eventually everyone's life will be better because of this present sacrifice.

The negotiator must also look for and acknowledge *hidden agendas.* The hidden agenda is the covert intention of the negotiator. There is usually an overt and covert intention behind every negotiation. For example, a new manager may convene a meeting with his or her superior with the established agenda being a discussion of the lack of supplies on the unit. However, the hidden agenda may be that the manager feels insecure and really is seeking performance feedback during their conversation. Having a hidden agenda is not uncommon or wrong by any means. Everyone has them and it is not necessary or wise to always share these hidden agendas. However, managers must be introspective enough to recognize their own hidden agendas so that they are not paralyzed by their acknowledgment and used against them by other parties during the negotiation.

If the manager's hidden agenda is discovered, the manager should admit that it is a consideration but not the "basis" of the negotiation.

For example, your hidden agenda for increasing the number of employees on your unit might be to build your own self-esteem in the eyes of your staff, but there is a legitimate need. If, during your negotiations, the fiscal manager recognizes your hidden agenda and accuses you of wanting to increase your staff just to gain power, you might respond by saying, "It is always important for a successful manager to be able to gain resources for their unit, but the real issue here is an inadequate staff." Managers who protest too strongly that they do not have a hidden agenda make themselves vulnerable.

◆ During the Negotiation

Negotiation is psychological as well as verbal. Because power can be perceived as well as imagined, the effective negotiator always appears calm and self-assured. At least part of this self-assurance comes from having adequately prepared for the negotiation. This preparation includes learning about the type of negotiators they will be working with and determining the strengths and weaknesses of their negotiating personality.

Ridicule, helplessness, guilt, seduction, and flattery are tactics that have been used successfully by some individuals to gain an upper hand in negotiation. These tactics might be conscious or unconscious, but they are used repeatedly because they have proved to be successful for that particular individual. Successful managers do *not* use negotiation tactics that are destructive or manipulative, but because others with whom they may negotiate do so, they must be prepared to counter such tactics.

In addition to developing sensitivity to negotiation tactics and assertiveness skills, there are several things managers can do during negotiation to increase their persuasiveness and foster open communication:

1. Use only factual statements that have been gathered through research. Have accurate information.
2. Listen carefully and watch nonverbal cues.
3. Keep an open mind as negotiations always provide the potential for learning. Do not prejudge. Establish a cooperative rather than a competitive climate.
4. Attempt to understand the viewpoint of the other party. It is likely that what one individual perceives differs from the perception of another. Concentrate on understanding and not only on agreement.
5. Always discuss the conflict. Do not personalize the situation by discussing the parties involved in the negotiation.
6. Try not to belabor how the conflict occurred or try to lay specific blame. Focus on preventing its reoccurrence.
7. Be honest.
8. Be initially demanding so that concessions are possible. It is far harder to escalate demands in the negotiation than to make concessions.
9. When faced with an unexpected development in negotiations, do not attempt to deal with it at that time. Respond that you are not prepared to discuss the particular issue at the moment, or that it was not on the agenda, suggesting that another appointment can be arranged for further discussion. If asked a question to which you do not know the answer, simply state that you do not have the information in question at the present time.
10. Never tell the other party fully what you are willing to negotiate. You may be showing your hand too early.
11. Know your bottom line, but try to *never* resort to it. If you play your bottom line, you must be ready to back it up or lose all credibility. If

you reach your bottom line, tell the other party that you have reached an impasse and cannot negotiate further. Then encourage the other party to think about it and reconsider. Always leave the door open for further negotiation. Be sure to allow the other party and yourself to save face.

12. If either party becomes angry or tired during the negotiation, take a time out. Go to the bathroom or make a telephone call. Remember that neither party can effectively negotiate if enraged.

13. Listen attentively and ask the other parties in the negotiation to further explain any ideas you may not have understood.

14. Be patient: The majority of concessions and settlements occur after original deadlines. Whenever possible, know the competitor's negotiating deadline without revealing your own (Smeltzer, 1991).

◆ Closure and Follow-up to Negotiation

Just as it is important to begin the formal negotiation with some pleasantries, it is also good to conclude on a friendly note. Once a compromise has been reached, restate it so that it is clear to everyone just what has been agreed on. If managers win more in negotiation than expected, they should try to hide their astonishment. At the end of any negotiation, be it a short 2-minute conflict situation in the hallway with another RN, or an hour-long formal salary negotiation, the result should be satisfying to all parties in that each has won something. It is a good idea to follow up formal negotiation in writing by sending a letter or a memo listing what was agreed on.

◆ Summary

When conflict occurs in the unit, managers must be able to discern constructive from destructive conflict. Conflict that is constructive will result in creativity, innovation, and growth for the unit. When conflict is deemed to be destructive, managers must deal appropriately with that conflict or risk an aftermath that may, in fact, be more destructive than the original conflict. Consistently using conflict resolution strategies with a win–lose or lose–lose outcome will create disharmony within the unit. Managers who use optimal conflict resolution strategies with a win–win outcome promote increased employee satisfaction and organizational productivity.

Negotiation, in its most creative form, is similar to collaboration. In its most poorly managed form, it resembles a competing approach. Most often, it represents a compromise of needs, wants, and expectations. This compromise may result in a *lose–lose* situation if either or both parties perceive they have given up more than the other. It is possible for negotiation not to result in a lose–lose situation, but this can only be achieved if both parties cooperate and are willing to give up something of value.

Negotiation is a high-level management skill. Well-prepared managers know who they will be negotiating with and act accordingly. They are prepared with tradeoffs, multiple alternatives, and a clear bottom-line to ensure that their unit acquires needed resources. The manager also recognizes the need for appropriate closure and follow-up to the negotiation.

Although negotiation implies winning and losing for both parties, some degree of satisfaction for both parties is more probable if assertive communications and active listening skills are employed in the negotiation rather than negotiation tactics.

◆ References

Barton A (1991). Conflict resolution by nurse managers. Nurs Manage 22(5):83–86

Bernhard LA and Walsh M (1990). Leadership—The Key to the Professionalization of Nursing, 2nd ed. St. Louis: CV Mosby

Bowditch JL and Buono AF (1994). A Primer on Organizational Behavior. New York: Wiley

Brett JM, Goldberg SB, and Ury WL (1990). Designing systems for resolving disputes in organizations. Am Psychol 45(Feb):162–170

Erwin K (1992). Managing conflict. Nurs Manage 23(3):67

Greenhalgh L (1986). Managing conflict. Sloan Manage Rev 27(4):45–51

Huber D (1996). Leadership and Nursing Care Management. Philadelphia: WB Saunders

Littlefield VM (1995). Conflict resolution: critical to productive schools of nursing. J Prof Nurs 11(1):7–15

Marquis B and Huston C (1996). Leadership Roles and Management Functions: Theory and Application, 2nd ed. Philadelphia: JB Lippincott

Neubauer J (1993). Redesign: managing role changes and building new teams. Sem Nurse Manage 1(1):26–32

Simpson RL (1991). What you need to know about negotiating contracts. Nurs Manage 22(9):22–23

Smeltzer C (1991). The art of negotiation: an everyday experience. J Nurs Admin 21(7/8):26–30

SAMPLE CASE ANALYSIS

THE CASE ◆

You have been working on the oncology unit since your graduation from State College 1 year ago. You have been complimented by your supervisor on your progress and lately she has allowed you to be relief charge nurse on the 3:00–11:00 P.M. shift when the regular charge nurse is not there. Occasionally you have been asked to work other medical-surgical units when your department has a low census. You dislike leaving your own unit, but have cooperated because you felt you could handle the other clinical assignments and wanted to demonstrate your flexibility.

SAMPLE CASE ANALYSIS (CONTINUED)

It is Saturday evening and you have just arrived at work when the nursing office calls requesting that you go to the delivery room to assist as they are very busy. You protest that you do not "know anything about obstetrics" and that it is impossible for you to take the assignment. The supervisor insists that you are the most qualified person and advises to "just go and do the best you can." Your own supervisor is not on duty and the charge nurse says she does not feel comfortable advising you in this conflict. You feel torn between professional, personal, and organizational responsibilities. What should you do?

• •

Assignment

Select the most appropriate conflict resolution strategy for resolving this conflict. Give a rationale for your choice as well as for rejection of the strategies not selected.

• •

Analysis

To begin conflict resolution, the nurse needs to examine his or her own goal, the supervisor's goal, and a possible goal that both could agree upon. The nurse's goal might be the desire to protect his or her license and also not to do anything that would bring harm to a patient. The supervisor's goal might be to provide assistance to an understaffed unit. A possible common goal would be for neither the nurse nor the supervisor to take any action that would invite risk or bring harm to the organization.

In selecting the most appropriate conflict resolution strategy for this situation, the nurse may want to consider and analyze all of the conflict resolution strategies presented in Display 18-1.

Accommodating is the most obvious wrong choice. If the nurse really believes that he or she is unqualified to work in the delivery room, then this is an unsuitable method for handling this conflict. Such a decision would not satisfy the nurse's or the supraordinate goal.

Since the nurse has little power and no one available to intervene on his or her behalf, smoothing or avoiding are inappropriate. The problem can neither be avoided nor smoothed away.

In some situations like this, the nurse might be able to negotiate a compromise, for instance, by saying, "I cannot go to the delivery room, but I will float to another medical-surgical area if there is someone on another medical-surgical unit who has OB experience." Or a compromise could be reached by stating, "I feel comfortable with postpartum and will work in that area, if you have a qualified nurse from postpartum who can be sent to the delivery room."

It is possible that either solution could end the conflict depending on the availability of other personnel and how comfortable the nurse felt in the postpartum area. Often, someone attempting to problem solve, such as the supervisor in this case, becomes so overburdened and stressed that he or she is unable to recognize other available alternatives.

If time allows and the other party is willing to adopt a common goal, collaboration is the preferred method of dealing with conflict. But the power holder must relinquish the status to problem solve if this method of conflict manage-

SAMPLE CASE ANALYSIS (CONTINUED)

ment is to be successful. Perhaps the nurse could convince the supervisor that the hospital and the supervisor could be at risk if an unqualified RN was assigned to an area requiring special skills. Once the supraordinate goal is adopted, the nurse and supervisor would be able to find alternative solutions to the problem. There are always many more ways to solve a problem than any one problem solver can generate.

Normally, competing is not an attractive alternative for conflict resolution, but sometimes it is the only recourse. Before using competition as a method to manage this conflict, the nurse needs to examine his or her motives. Is the nurse truly unqualified for work in the delivery room? Or is the nurse using a lack of experience as an excuse not to float to an unfamiliar area that would produce anxiety? If the nurse is truly convinced that he or she is unqualified, then the nurse possesses information that the supervisor does not have (a criterion necessary for the use of competing as a method of conflict resolution). Therefore, if other methods for solving the conflict, that is, compromising or collaboration, are not effective, the nurse must employ competition to resolve the conflict. The nurse must win at the expense of the supervisor's losing. There is much personal risk for the nurse in using this type of conflict resolution. The nurse may be fired for insubordination, or at best, the supervisor may view the nurse as uncooperative.

The most appropriate method for using competition in this situation is an assertive approach. An example would be repeating firmly, but nonaggressively, "I cannot go to the delivery room to work because I would be putting patients at risk. I am unqualified to work in that area." This approach is usually effective. The nurse must not work in a unit where patient safety would be at risk, as it would be morally, ethically, and legally wrong to do so.

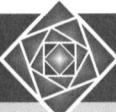 CASES FOR PROBLEM SOLVING

CASE 1

You have been working at an outpatient emergency clinic for 3 months and have begun to feel fairly confident in your new role. However, one of the older diploma nurses working with you constantly belittles baccalaureate nursing education. Anytime you request assistance in problem solving or in learning a new skill she says, "Didn't they teach you anything in nursing school?" The clinic supervisor has given you a satisfactory 3-month evaluation but you are becoming increasingly defensive regarding the comments of the other nurse.

Assignment

Explain how you plan to evaluate the accuracy of the diploma nurse's comments. Discuss how you will cope with this situation and what efforts you can make to improve this relationship. Is the end result worth the time and energy it will take to resolve this conflict?

CASE 2 ◆

Assignment

Read the following two conflict scenarios and select the most appropriate conflict resolution strategy. Give the rationale for your selection, as well as for rejection of those not selected.

Scenario 1

You are a circulating nurse in the OR. Usually you are assigned to Room 3, for general surgery, but today you have been assigned to Room 4, which is for orthopedics. You are unfamiliar with the routines of the orthopedists and have attempted to brush up on them quickly before each case today by reading their preference cards in advance. Thus far you have managed to complete two cases without incident. The next case comes in the room and you realize everyone is especially tense as this patient is the wife of a local physician and is undergoing a bone biopsy for a possible malignancy. You prep the area to be biopsied and the surgeon (who has a reputation for a quick temper) enters the room. You suddenly realize that you have prepped the area with betadine and this surgeon prefers another prep solution. He sees what you have done and yells at you. "You are stupid, you are a stupid, stupid nurse."

What will you do?

Scenario 2

You are the head nurse of an ICU and have just finished a particularly exhausting 8 hours on duty. Working with you today have been two nurses who work 12-hour shifts. You have been assigned two patients each and they have all had high acuity levels. You welcome the opportunity to go out of town tonight to attend an important seminar as you are certainly tired. You are also pleased that you scheduled yourself an 8-hour shift today and that your relief is coming through the door. You will just have time to give your report and catch your plane.

It is customary for 12-hour nurses to continue with their previous patients and that assignments not be changed when 8- and 12-hour staff are working together. Therefore, you proceed to give your report on your patients to the 8-hour nurse coming on duty. One of your patients is an acutely ill FUO (fever of unknown origin) who is in the isolation room. It is suspected that he has meningitis. Your other patient is a multiple trauma victim.

In the middle of your report the oncoming nurse interrupts you and says she has just come from the doctor's office, where she has learned that she is pregnant. She states, "I can't take care of a possible meningitis patient. I'll have to trade with one of the 12-hour nurses."

You approach the 12-hour nurses and they respond angrily, "We took care of all kinds of patients when we were pregnant and we are not changing patients with just 4 hours left in our shift." When you relate this message to the oncoming nurse she says, "Either we trade or I go home!" You quickly telephone the nursing office and they state that because of a flu epidemic among the staff there is absolutely no personnel to call in and all other units are already short staffed. What will you do?

CASE 3 (Marquis and Huston, 1996)

One type of conflict resolution strategy is competing. In this method, one party involved in the conflict pursues goals at the expense of the other party. It is a win–lose conflict resolution strategy and is generally identified as appropriate only when a quick or unpopular decision must be made, or when one party has more information or knowledge about a situation than the other.

You are a middle-level manager of an ICU/CCU. Your responsibilities include strategic planning, budgeting, hiring, discipline, and staffing. Staffing presents challenges even to experienced nursing managers and competing is frequently employed as a conflict resolution strategy.

Your unit has clearly defined policies regarding holidays off, with a choice of two of the following five: Thanksgiving, Christmas Eve, Christmas Day, New Year's Eve, and New Year's Day. Although you have always tried hard to meet individual staff requests, this year, almost all of your staff have requested first and second choices of Christmas Eve and Christmas Day. It is impossible to grant everyone's request without leaving the unit dangerously understaffed. You call a meeting and pose the problem to the staff. None of them is willing to withdraw the request. Some staff feel that their request should be honored because they have the greatest seniority, whereas others feel that their request should be granted because they had to work those holidays last year. Still some maintain that this is not fair, as they had taken the Christmas holidays off last year only to equalize the holiday distribution of days off, and that this is the year they are requesting a preference. Yet others say they are already scheduled to work Thanksgiving, and would not have agreed to do so had they known that they might not have their request for Christmas holidays approved. Some staff have purchased nonrefundable airplane tickets and many have made extensive plans.

* * *

Assignment

It is obvious that some sort of competing approach will be required to resolve this conflict. Identify what criteria you will use to solve this dilemma. Have you considered common good over the needs of the individual? How did your values impact on your problem solving?

CASE 4

You are the supervisor of a medical unit. Two of your youngest nursing assistants come to your office today to report that a young male quadriplegic patient has been making lewd sexual comments and gestures at them when they provide basic care. When you question them about their response to the actions of the patient, they maintain that they normally simply look away and try to ignore him, although they are offended by his actions. They are very reluctant to confront the patient directly.

Because it is anticipated that this patient may remain on your unit for at least several weeks, the nursing assistants have asked you to intervene in this conflict by either talking to the patient or by assigning other nurses responsibility for his care.

CASE 4 (CONTINUED)

. . . .

Assignment

How will you handle this staff–patient conflict? Is avoidance (assigning different staff to care for the patient) an appropriate conflict resolution strategy in this situation? Will you encourage the nursing assistants to confront the patient directly? What coaching or role playing might you use with them if you choose this approach? Will you confront the patient yourself? What might you say?

CASE 5 (Marquis and Huston, 1996)

You are a female, top-level nursing administrator, with a master's degree in health administration, and are about to present your proposed budget to the CEO. You have thoroughly researched your budget and have adequate rationale to support your requests for increased funding. You are aware, though, that the CEO is often moody, and that it will be difficult to predict in advance how he will respond to your proposal.

You also recognize that he has some very traditional views about where women should be, and this generally does not include executive-level positions. Because he is fairly paternalistic, he is charmed and flattered when asked to assist "his nurses with their jobs." The last top-level nursing administrator was recently fired as she was perceived as brash, bossy, and disrespectful by the CEO. In fact, the previous top-level nursing administrator was one of a series of nursing administrators who had been replaced in the last several years for these characteristics. From what you have been told, these perceptions were not shared by the nursing staff.

You sit down and begin to plan your strategy for this meeting. You are conscious that you have greater probability for success in having your budgetary needs met if you dress conservatively, solemnly beseech your need for his assistance and support throughout the presentation, and remain fairly passive in your approach. In other words, you will be required to assume a traditionally effeminate, helpless role. If you appear capable and articulate, you may not achieve your budgetary goals and may not even keep your job. It would likely not be necessary for you to perpetuate this role, except in your interactions with the CEO.

. . . .

Assignment

Are the use of such behavioral tactics ethical if the outcome is desirable? Are the use of such tactics simply "smart negotiation" or are they inappropriate? How would you respond in this situation? Is conflict inevitable?

◆ Bibliography

The following is a list of references to help you solve these cases:

Arnold E and Boggs K (1990). Survival skills in the workplace: what every nurse should know. Learn to manage workplace conflicts. Am Nurses Assoc 148:48–52

Barton A (1991). Conflict resolution by nurse managers. Nurs Manage 22(5):83–84, 86

Booth RZ (1993). The dynamics of conflict and conflict management. In Mason DJ, Talbot SW, and Leavitt JK (eds): Policy and Politics for Nurses, 2nd ed. Philadelphia: WB Saunders

Broom C (1991). Conflict resolution strategies: when ethical dilemmas evolve into conflict. DCCN: Dimen Crit Care Nurs 10(Nov/Dec):354–363

Cavanagh S (1991). The conflict management style of staff nurses and nurse managers. J Adv Nurs 16(8):1254–1260

Christopher P (1991). Difficult co-worker: Dr. Bingham couldn't care less what nurses thought. Nursing 91,21(9):105–107

Deutsch M (1994). Constructive conflict resolution: principles, training, and research. J Soc Iss 50(1):13–32

Dirschel KM (1993). Principled negotiation. In Mason DJ, Talbot SW, and Leavitt JK (eds): Policy and Politics for Nurses, 2nd ed. Philadelphia: WB Saunders

Dixon CV (1991). Conflict resolution. Can Nurse 87(6):8, 10

Evans SA (1991). Conflict resolution: a strategy for growth. Heart Lung 20(2) (Mar):20A, 22A, 24A

Fisher ML (1991). Negotiating a severance agreement. Nurs Econ 9(1):36–39

Gardner D (1992). Conflict and retention of new graduate nurses. W J Nurs Res 14(1):76–85

Huston CJ (1987). A conflict born of insecurity. Imprint 34(3)

Johnson M (1994). Conflict and nursing professionalization. In McCloskey J and Grace H (eds): Curr Issues in Nursing, 4th ed. St. Louis: CV Mosby, 643–649

Kahn RL (1993). Role conflict and ambiguity in organizations. In Management and Organizational Behavior, 5th ed. Matteson M and Ivancevich JM (eds): Illinois: Irwin, 187–198

Larson BA and Martinson DJ (1990). Words can hurt: dealing with verbal abuse in the operating room. Amer Op Room J 52(6):1238–1241

Manion J (1990). Change from within: nurse intrapreneurs as health care innovators. The skills for successful intrapreneurship. Am Nurses Assoc Publ G-178:33–64

Morrill C (1991). Conflict management, honor, and organizational change. Am J Soc 97(3):585–621

Rubin JZ (1994). Models of conflict management. J Soc Iss 50(1):33–45

Tjosvold D, Dann V, and Wong C (1992). Managing conflicts between departments to serve customers. Hum Rel 45(10):1035–1051

Wall Jr. JA and Callister RR (1995). Conflict and its management. J Manage 21:515–558

Ward RP (1990). Negotiators, mediators, and arbitrators. Mic Nurse 63(3):12

Zubek JM, Pruitt DG, McGillicuddy RS, Neil B, and Syna H (1992). Dispute and mediator behaviors affecting short-term success in mediation. J Confl Resol 36(3):546–572

PERSONAL NOTEBOOK

1. It is important for managers to be self-aware regarding how they view and deal with conflict. In your personal life, how do you resolve conflict? Is it important for you to win?

2. When was the last time you were able to settle a dispute by reaching a supraordinate goal with another person?

3. In conflicts with family and friends, are you least likely to compromise values, scarce resources, or role expectations?

4. Does conflict affect you to a greater degree cognitively, emotionally, or physically?

5. Currently, do you feel that you have too little or too much conflict in your life? Do you have any control over the issues that are causing any conflict in your life?

6. What do you perceive as your greatest skills as a negotiator?

Unions in the Health Care Industry

A *labor union* is an organization of wage earners, usually with a strong economic motivation, who join together to gain bargaining power with their employer regarding the terms and conditions of work. *Collective bargaining* may be defined as those negotiations occurring between organized labor and management that affect employee relations. This usually includes the negotiation of formal labor agreements and the day-to-day interactions between the union and management. First- and middle-level managers normally have little to do with the negotiation of the labor contract, but they have a great deal to do with its day-to-day implementation. It is the middle-level manager who has the greatest impact upon the quality of the relationship that develops between labor and management. Other terminology associated with unions and collective bargaining is shown in Display 19-1.

Because collective bargaining can have a major impact on the directing phase of management, managers must develop an understanding of the issues underlying the growth of unionization and recognize that collective bargaining can often be a positive force, as well as a constraint for organizations.

It is necessary to see collective bargaining from four perspectives:

1. the viewpoint of the organization,
2. the viewpoint of the worker,
3. a general historical and societal viewpoint, and
4. a personal viewpoint.

Managers able to gain this broad perspective will have a better understanding of how management and employees can work together within the constraints imposed by unionization. This is an accomplishment of many other industrial-

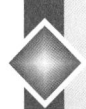

DISPLAY 19-1
Collective Bargaining Terminology

National Labor Relations Board: A labor board formed to implement the Wagner Act. Its two major functions are to 1) determine who should be the official bargaining unit when a new unit is formed and who should be included in that unit, and 2) adjudicating charges of unfair labor practices.

Supervisors: Historically defined as someone who has the authority to hire, fire, transfer, and promote another employee. More recently, court decisions have expanded the definition to include anyone who directs less-skilled employees as part of his or her duties.

Free Speech: The law states that "the expressing of any views, argument, or dissemination thereof, whether in written, printed, graphic, or visual form, shall not constitute or be evidence of an unfair labor practice under any provisions of this Act, if such expression contains no threat of reprisal or force or promise of benefit" (U.S. Congress, Public Law 101, Sec. 8).

Union Shop: Also called a closed shop. All employees are required to join the union and pay dues.

Agency Shop: Also called an open shop; employees are not required to join the union.

Strike: A concerted withholding of labor in an effort to bring economic pressure on the employer to grant employee demands.

Lockout: A closing of a place of business by management in the course of a labor dispute for the purpose of forcing employees to accept management terms.

Grievance: A perception on the part of a union member that management has failed in some way to meet the terms of the labor agreement.

Arbitration: The terminal step in the grievance procedure; always indicates the involvement of a third party. Arbitration may be voluntary on the part of management and labor, or imposed by the government in a compulsory arbitration.

Conciliation and Mediation: Synonymous terms that refer to the activity of a third party to help disputants reach accord. However, unlike an arbitrator, this individual has no final power over decision making.

Fact Finding: Rarely used in the private sector, but frequently used in labor–management disputes that involve government-owned companies. In the private sector fact finding is usually performed by a Board of Inquiry.

ized nations, but an achievement less often realized in the United States. Kearney and Hayes (1994) suggest that, despite our long history of adversarial labor relations in union environments and authoritarian or paternalistic management approaches in nonunion settings, a mutuality of interests is not only possible but desirable between management and labor.

◆ The National Labor Relations Board

The *National Labor Relations Board* (NLRB), a federal agency created in 1935, is charged with administering the nation's laws relating to labor relations in the private and nonprofit sectors. (Some public sector organizations are also under its jurisdiction, but these are less common.) The NLRB is given the power to safeguard employees' rights to organize, to determine through elections whether workers want unions as their bargaining representatives, and to prevent and remedy unfair labor practices (Shafritz, 1988).

Traditionally, all nurses below the level of supervisor or middle-level management were eligible for protection under the National Labor Relations Act (NLRA), with a supervisor being defined as someone who hired, fired, disciplined, transferred, or promoted. However, a Supreme Court ruling in 1994 argued that the definition of a nursing supervisor should be expanded to include any nurse who directs less-skilled employees as part of his or her duties. In essence, this ruling disenfranchised most registered nurses from protection under the NLRA and clouded the issue of whether nurses were eligible for union membership.

In 1996, the NLRB, in a reinterpretation of the NLRA, issued a decision containing a detailed analysis of nursing duties that define true supervisory work according to labor law. In the NLRB decision (in contrast to the Supreme Court decision), nonsupervisory employees continue to have the right to organize for collective bargaining purposes and to engage in other concerted activity (Nursing, 1996). As such, nurses who speak out as a group regarding job conditions or management conditions that they believe may compromise the safety or quality of patient care, should be protected from firing.

The question of when a professional nurse becomes a supervisor will continue to be analyzed and argued for several years. It is clear that with the increased used of unlicensed assistive personnel (UAP) in healthcare, and the current widespread cycle of economically motivated redesign that threatens job security for many nurses, the issue of NLRB protection has great implications for the profession of nursing. One of the most critical lessons to be learned from the debate is that labor law is not static; it is constantly re-evaluated and changed in response to a variety of contemporary forces. Managers then, must be cognizant of current labor law legislation that may affect both them and their subordinates. A second lesson may be that nurses must be more proactively involved in policy decisions that have such a significant impact on their profession.

◆ Historical Perspective of Unionization in America

Unions have been present in America since the 1790s. Early unions were composed of skilled craftsmen, who banded together to protect themselves from wage cuts during the highly competitive industrial era in the United States. An examination of the history of the union movement reveals that membership increases during high employment and prosperity, and decreases correspondingly sharply during economic recessions and layoffs.

For many reasons, collective bargaining was slow in coming to the health care industry. As of 1996, only about 20% of nurses in hospitals were represented by unions. Until labor laws were amended, it was not legally possible for unionization to occur. The long history of nursing as a service industry also contributed to the delay in labor organization of health care organizations.

Collective bargaining in the nursing profession began in government or public health care organizations. This was made possible by Executive Order 10988, authored in 1962, which lifted restrictions preventing public employees from organizing. Therefore, in the 1960s, city, county, and district hospitals and health care agencies began to unionize.

In 1974, the U.S. Congress passed amendments to the Wagner Act, called the Taft–Hartley Act, which extended national labor laws to private, nonprofit hospitals, nursing homes, health clinics, health maintenance organizations, and other health care institutions. These amendments opened the doors to increased union activity for professionals as well as the public employee sector. Indeed, if union membership figures are reviewed, it becomes apparent that since 1960, most collective bargaining activity in the United States has taken place in the public and/or professional sector of industry (Willis, 1988). There has been little growth of unionization in the private and/or blue-collar sector, since membership peaked in the 1950s and 1960s. A Bureau of Labor Statistics survey suggests that between 1961 and 1984, union membership among production employees in metropolitan areas, declined from 73% to 51% (Mosca and Pressman, 1995). See Table 19-1 for a summary of legislation affecting the union movement.

From 1962 through 1983 there were slow but steady increases in the numbers of nurses represented by collective bargaining agents. This increase in union membership was also seen in other professions, most notably, among

◆ TABLE 19-1
Labor Legislation

Year	Legislation	Effect
1935	The National Labor Act—The Wagner Act	Gave unions many rights in organizing; resulted in rapid union growth.
1947	The Taft–Hartley Act	Returned some power to management; resulted in a more equal balance of power between unions and management.
1962	Kennedy Executive Order 10988	Amended the 1935 Wagner Act to allow public employees to join unions.
1974	Amendment to the Wagner Act	Allowed nonprofit organizations to join unions.

faculty at institutions of higher education, teachers at primary and secondary levels, and physicians (Willis, 1988). However, since the air traffic controller's strike and resultant breakup in the early 1980s, labor union influence in nursing decreased, in a manner similar to production workers.

Triggered by work redesign, downsizing, and threats to job security, there has been a resurgence of interest by nurses in labor unions in the 1990s. In an effort to allow nurses to focus on issues specific to their own profession (as opposed to clerical or maintenance workers), the U.S. Supreme Court in 1991 ruled that eight separate bargaining units per hospital could be formed (Supreme Court, 1991; Catalano, 1996). The eight units were:

1. nurses,
2. physicians,
3. all professionals except nurses and physicians,
4. all technical employees,
5. all skilled maintenance employees,
6. all business office clerical employees,
7. all guards, and
8. all other nonprofessional employees.

This move to separate bargaining units in acute care hospitals was opposed by the American Hospital Association, which argued that the cost for a single hospital to contract with eight separate unions could exceed $360,000 for just one round of negotiations (Stearley, 1995). Some advocates of the eight unit ruling argue, however, that because there is an economic incentive to negotiate in a more timely manner, that collaboration between union and management will increase as a result of the ruling.

◆ Collective Bargaining Agents for Nurses

The following are the major organizations acting as collective bargaining agents for nurses:

1. *Service Employees International Union:* the largest, representing almost 400,000 nurses and health care providers nationwide (Strickland and Fishman, 1994);
2. *the State Nurses' Associations of the American Nurses Association:* the second largest, representing 140,000 registered nurses in 840 bargaining units across the United States (Catalano, 1996); and the
3. *National Union of Hospital and Health Care Employees of the Retail, Wholesale, and Department Store Union.*

◆ American Nurses Association and Collective Bargaining

One difficult issue faced by nursing managers, not typically encountered in other disciplines, occurs because of the dual role of their professional organization, the American Nurses Association. This organization, at most state levels, is recognized by the National Labor Relations Board (NLRB) as a collective bargaining agent.

The use of State Nurses' Associations as bargaining agents has been a divisive issue among nurses in the United States. Because management is excluded from union membership, many nurse managers feel they have been disenfranchised by their professional organization. For other nurse managers, this issue presents no conflict.

Regardless of individual values, there does appear to be some conflict in loyalty. There are no easy solutions to the dilemma created by the dual role held by the American Nurses Association. Clarifying these issues begins with the manager examining the motivation of nurses to participate in collective bargaining activities. The manager must make an effort to at least hear and understand the employee's point of view.

◆ Motivation to Join or Reject Unions

Knowing that human behavior is goal directed, it is important to examine what motivates union membership. Nursing managers often tell one another that health care organizations are different than other types of industrial organizations. This is actually a myth, for in reality, most nurses work in large and impersonal organizations that frequently leave the nurse feeling powerless, vulnerable, and alone in a complex institution. Therefore, one of the primary motivations for joining a union is to 1) *increase the power of the individual.* Polls regarding nurses' perceptions of management reveal that, in overwhelming numbers, nurses believe management does not listen to them or care about their needs (California Nursing Review, 1987). This provides a fertile ground for union organizers. Employees know that they are essentially dispensable. Because a large group of employees is much less dispensable, nurses may increase their bargaining power and reduce their vulnerability by joining a union.

Another motivator driving a nurse toward unionization might be 2) *the need most individuals have to communicate their aims, feelings, complaints, and ideas to others.* Since unions emphasize equality and fairness, nurses often join unions because they are 3) *driven by a need to eliminate discrimination and favoritism.* This might be an especially strong motivator in groups that have had past experience with discrimination, for example, women and minorities.

There are a variety of social factors that also motivate nurses regarding union activity. Peer pressure often culminates in 4) *a social need to be accepted.* Sometimes this social need occurs as a result of family pressure. Many working-class families have a long history of strong union ties, and individuals are frequently raised in a cultural milieu that promotes unionization.

Last, nurses join unions because 5) *it is a part of the union contract that all nurses belong to the union.* This formidable force has been an effective motivator among blue-collar workers. However, the *closed shop,* or requirement that all employees belong to the union, has never become prevalent in the health

◆ Labor–Management Relations Laws

The manager needs to be aware of the portions of the Wagner Act (1935) and the Taft–Hartley Act (1947) that address unfair labor practices by employers and unions. The five initial prohibited labor practices were:

1. To interfere with, restrain, or coerce employees in a manner that interfered with their rights as outlined under the Act. Examples of these activities include conducting surveillance at union gatherings and threatening employees with job loss or closure of a company if union organization occurs.
2. To interfere with the formation of any labor organization as well as to give financial assistance to a labor organization. This financial aid provision was included to prevent "employee representation plans" that were primarily controlled by management.
3. To discriminate in regard to such areas as hiring, tenure, and advancement, in order to discourage membership in the union.
4. To discharge because of, or discriminate over, charges filed or testimony before the NLRB.
5. To refuse to bargain in good faith.

The original Wagner Act gave considerable power to the unions of the day. It was necessary in 1947 to enact additional federal legislation to restore a balance of power between labor and management. The Taft–Hartley Act retained the provisions under the Wagner Act that guaranteed employees the right to collective bargaining. But the Taft–Hartley Act added the provision that employees also had the right to *refrain* from taking part in unions. In addition to that provision, the Taft–Hartley Act prohibited the following six unfair labor practices of unions:

1. Requiring a self-employed individual or employer to join a union.
2. Forcing an employer to terminate business affairs with another person. This placed a ban on secondary boycotts, then prevalent in unions.
3. Forcing an employer to bargain with one union when another has already been certified as the bargaining agent.
4. Forcing the employer to assign certain work to members of one union rather than those of another.
5. Charging excessive or discriminatory initiation fees.
6. Causing or attempting to cause an employer to pay for unnecessary services. This prohibited *featherbedding,* a term used to describe union practices that prevented the elimination of positions owing to advances in technology.

◆ Effective Labor–Management Relations

Prior to the 1950s labor–management relations had a turbulent history. History books are filled with accounts of various battles, strikes, mass picketing scenes, and brutal treatment by both management and employees alike. In the last 30 years, employers and unions have substantially improved their relationships. Although there is growing evidence that management has come to accept the reality that unions are here to stay, businesses in the United States are still less comfortable with unions than are their counterparts in many other countries. Likewise, unions have come to accept the fact that there are times when organizations are not healthy enough to survive aggressive union demands.

It is the attitudes and the philosophies of management and the union that determine what type of relationship develops between the two parties in any given organization. In working with unions, managers must be flexible. It is critical that they not try to overwhelm others with power or ignore issues. The rational approach to problem solving must be used.

Once management is faced with dealing with a bargaining agent they have a choice of either accepting or opposing the union. They may actively oppose the union with "union busting" techniques, or they may choose a more subtle form of opposition such as exploiting any attempt to discredit the union. Acceptance may also run along a continuum, as the company may accept the union with reluctance and suspicion. The managers know that the union has legitimate rights, but believe they must be perpetually on guard against further encroachment by the union into traditional management territory.

Lastly, there is an increasingly common type of union acceptance, characterized by approval of the union by management, with both union and management showing mutual respect for each other. When these conditions exist labor and management can establish mutual goals, especially in the areas of safety, cost reduction, efficiency, eliminating waste, and improving working conditions. Porter-O'Grady (1992) feels that this type of relationship has begun to be evidenced between unionized professional registered nurses and health care organizations and refers to this more cooperative interaction as a new model of collective relationship. Admittedly, such cooperation represents the most mature and advanced type of labor–management relations. Mosca and Pressman (1995) suggest that the key to success of unions in the 21st century may lie in the creation of a cooperative atmosphere between labor and management.

◆ Summary

Managers must learn to work collaboratively with unions to assist the organization in meeting organizational goals. The process will seem less burdensome to managers if they remember that unions serve the primary purpose of protecting the rights of employees. If managers perform their jobs well, and work for organizations that desire "to do the right thing" by accepting their social responsibility, unionization can be viewed with less trepidation.

If the organization is nonunionized, the manager must use good communication, fairness, and shared decision making to ensure that employees do not feel unionization is necessary to meet their needs. The manager who is a role model for equity makes a point of knowing unit employees well, and sincerely seeks to meet their needs. This decreases the chances of union activity. In making decisions, the effective manager should always seek to do what is just. Additionally, he or she should seek appropriate assistance before finalizing decisions that involve sensitive contract issues.

◆ References

Catalano JT (1996). Contemporary Professional Nursing. Philadelphia: FA Davis

(1987). Job satisfaction: what nurses have to say. California Nursing Review 9(4)

Kearney RC and Hayes SW (1994). Labor–management relations and participative decision making: toward a new paradigm. Publ Admin Rev 54(1):44–51

Mosca JB and Pressman S (1995). Unions in the 21st century. Publ Pers Manage 24(2):159–166

Porter-O'Grady T (1992). Or rabbits and turtles: a time for change for unions. Nurs Econ 10(3):177–182

Shafritz J (1988). The Dorsey Dictionary of American Government and Politics. Chicago: The Dorsey Press, 367

Stearley H (1995). The rise and fall of nursing unions. J Nurse Empower 5(2):56–59

Strickland OL and Fishman DJ (1994). Nursing Issues in the 1990s. Albany: Delmar

(1991). Supreme Court Okays All-RN unit. Am Nurse 20:1

(1996). Twin triumphs—NLRB findings favor nurses. Nursing 96(April):10

U.S. Congress, Public Law 101 (Taft-Hartley Amendment). 80th Congr. 1st sess., June 23, 1947

U.S. Congress, Wagner Act. 298 U.S. 238, 1935

Willis R (1988). Can American unions transform themselves? Manage Rev 77(2):14–21

SAMPLE CASE ANALYSIS

THE CASE ◆

One of your best performing staff nurses has just returned to work following the death of her father. She had cared for her father in her home the last 6 months of his life; because of the heavy burden this placed on her, she gradually used up all her accrued vacation time. The health department where you are a county health supervisor is under union contract to the county employee association, and the contract allows 3 bereavement days leave for a death in the immediate family.

The nurse, Alice Dole, has used her 3 days but still appears exhausted and weepy. She was out making her home visits yesterday and today she has been in the office all day doing paperwork. She emerges from her office and asks to speak with you. She requests the use of some of her accumulated sick time to recover from her father's illness and subsequent death. You ask if she is ill and she says, "Not really physically ill, but I just can't seem to concentrate and I am so tired." You suggest an unpaid leave of absence but she says she cannot afford to be without an income as she is the sole means of support for her three children (she is a widow).

SAMPLE CASE ANALYSIS (CONTINUED)

You consult the union contract and it states that the employee will accrue one sick day every four weeks to be used in times of legitimate illness. You are unsure if fatigue and emotional stress apply. You would really like to give Mrs. Dole her accrued sick time, but believe you should consult with the health department personnel director. However, your past dealings with him have not gone well. He has been rigid and unwilling to bend whatsoever on any employee issue. Also, he always interprets the union contract in favor of the county and not the employee, which has resulted in several employee grievances, most of which have been won by the employee and the union.

You are tempted to not go to the personnel director and to just give Mrs. Dole her paid time off, but you are concerned that you would be setting an unwanted precedent for other employees. Would or could the union use it against you someday?

•••

Assignment

If you were the manager in this case, what would you do? Outline your plan as well as your rationale. If your approach results in negative consequences for you or Alice Dole, what could you do?

•••

Analysis

Although this manager was severely tempted, she did not act without consulting her superior and the personnel director. The manager included her boss in this situation because she had the same authority as the personnel director and she had always been open to listening to her first-level manager's requests.

Prior to consulting with either her supervisor or the personnel director, the manager outlined her managerial goal for the conflict, which was to provide Mrs. Dole with some needed paid time off.

Initially, the personnel director insisted upon denying the request. He reasoned that all employees would take off and want paid time off, "when they just had an argument with their boyfriend." He maintained that it was precedent setting and that the union would then want to include such a provision in the next contract, that is, the employees would not need to be physically ill to use accrued sick time.

But the manager had done her homework and was prepared to justify her request. She had called numerous health care agencies in the state and been informed that many of them already had a policy stating that employees could use such time for emotional or mental stress. The manager put forth the following argument:

1. Employees only receive one paid sick day every 4 weeks and once the sick time has been used, they must use unpaid time.
2. Therefore, letting Mrs. Dole apply her sick time to emotional stress means that in the event she was physically ill, she would be on unpaid sick leave.
3. The goodwill that the organization creates by allowing Mrs. Dole to use her paid sick leave at this time greatly overrides any potential for strengthening the union contract at a future date.

SAMPLE CASE ANALYSIS (CONTINUED)

4. Mrs. Dole is an excellent and loyal employee and this is a way to reward such employees even though they are unionized. This increases the power of the organization.
5. Last, the manager appealed to both the personnel director and the superior that this was ethically the right thing to do.

The outcome of the manager's presentation was that she convinced the superior to join with her in persuading the personnel director to allow Alice Dole to use her paid sick leave for the emotional stress caused by the death of her father. Eventually, the union did manage to include a clause in the union–management contract that allowed employees to use sick time for emotional or mental stress. It seems ironic that in the *health* professions it has been largely owing to union activity that this provision is now an option for nearly all nurses in any organization, but 15 years ago, it was rarely an option for any nurse.

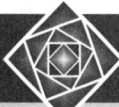 # CASES FOR PROBLEM SOLVING

CASE 1

You are a staff nurse in the intensive care unit at one of the two hospitals in the city where you live. You have worked at this same hospital for 5 years, transferring to the intensive care unit 2 years ago. You enjoy nursing, but are sometimes frustrated in your job due to a short supply of nurses, excessive overtime demands, and the stress of working with critical patients.

The hospital has a closed shop, so union dues are deducted from your pay even though you are not actively involved in the union. The present union contract is up for renegotiation and union and management have not been able to agree on many issues. Management has made their last offer and the new contract was put to a vote by all the nurses and rejected. The old contract has expired, leaving the nurses free to strike if they vote to do so.

You had voted for accepting the management offer, because you have two children to support and it would be devastating to be without income for an extended period. Last night the nurses voted on whether to return to the bargaining table to try and negotiate again with management, or to go out on strike.

Again, you voted against a strike. You have just heard from your friend that the strike vote won. Now you must decide if you are going to support your striking colleagues or if you are going to cross the picket line and return to work tomorrow. Your friends are exerting a great deal of pressure on you to support their cause. You are aware that the union will provide some financial compensation during the strike, but feel it will not be adequate to support yourself and children.

You agree with union demands that the organization has overworked and underpaid you, and that they have generally been unresponsive to nursing needs. On the other hand, you believe your first obligation is to your children.

CASE 1 (CONTINUED)

• •

Assignment

List all the reasons for and against striking. Make a decision about what you will do. Use appropriate rationale from outside literature to support your final decision. Share your decision with the class. Take a vote in class to determine how many would strike and how many would cross the picket line.

CASE 2

Betty Smith, a unit clerk, has come to see you, the manager of the medical unit, to complain of flagrant discriminatory practices against women employees at University General Hospital. She alleges that females at University General Hospital are denied advancement and training opportunities comparable to those available to their male counterparts.

She shows you a petition with 35 signatures supporting her allegations. Ms. Smith has threatened to forward this petition to the Administrator of the hospital, the press, and to the Department of Labor unless corrective action is taken at once.

Being a woman yourself, you have some sympathy for Ms. Smith's complaint. However, you feel, overall, that employees at University General are treated fairly regardless of their gender.

Ms. Smith has been a fairly good employee and has worked on your unit for 4 years. However, she has been creating problems of late, including being reprimanded for taking too much time off for coffee breaks. Personnel evaluations which make recommendations for pay raises and promotions are due next week.

• •

Assignment

How should you handle this problem? Outline your plan and give your rationale for selecting your approach. Should you address the petition at Ms. Smith's personnel evaluation?

CASE 3

Mrs. Stanton, an LVN-LPN on your unit, has been a long-time employee with an extended history of treating patients in a rough manner. After many informal conferences and counseling sessions 1 year ago it became necessary for you to give her a written warning to be placed in her personnel file. You have now received another signed complaint from a patient who says that Mrs. Stanton, "turned him in a rough manner on the night of his surgery." The union contract states that employees must have a series of formal warnings with escalating penalties before they can be dismissed. The first offense results in a written warning notice of the behavior. The second mandates suspension for 5 days without pay and the third time that the *same offense is repeated,* the employee may be discharged.

CASE 3 (CONTINUED)

••

Assignment

What should you do about Mrs. Stanton's latest offense? What action should you take? If you decide to take some formal action, what should you do in order to justify it if this case were to proceed to formal arbitration?

◆ Bibliography

The following is a list of references to assist you in solving these cases:

Chipman D (1993). Strike! J Nurse Empow 3(4):22–25, 81–83

Flarey D, Yoder S, and Barabas M (1992). Collaboration in labor relations. J Nurs Admin 22(9):15–21

Foley ME (1993). The politics of collective bargaining. In Mason DJ, Talbot SW, and Leavitt JK (eds). Policy and Politics for Nursing, 2nd ed. Philadelphia: WB Saunders

Giovinco G (1993). When nurses strike: ethical conflicts. Nurs Manage 24(5):86–90

Grelli AR (1994). Nurses who direct aides are supervisors. High court decides. The Philadelphia Inquirer, May 24

Havens DS and Mills ME (1994). Are nurses getting what they are worth? In McCloskey J and Grace HK (eds). Current Issues in Nursing, 4th ed. St. Louis: CV Mosby

Hoerr J (1991). What should unions do? Harvard Business Review. May/June, 30–45

Hudacek SS (1990). Collective bargaining—not a dinosaur of the past. Advanc Clin Care 5(1):27–28

Kingsbury S (1990). SNA bargaining brings big win for staff RNs. Am Nurse 22(3):19, 21

MacLachlan LD (1990). Meeting the challenges of collective bargaining. Calif Nurse 86(3):1,4–5

Marquis B and Huston C (1994). Motivation to join or reject unions. J Nurs Admin 24(2):4

McDonald DM (1995). Labor relations issues. In Vestal KW (ed). Nursing Management, 2nd ed. Philadelphia: JB Lippincott

O'Connor KS (1994). Why are we seeing more unionization? In McCloskey J and Grace HK (eds). Current Issues in Nursing, 4th ed. St. Louis: CV Mosby

Staff: California Nurses Association (1994). Top ten myths about hospital restructuring and health care reform. J Nurse Empow 4(3):24–25

Stickler KB (1990). Union organization will be divisive and costly. Hospitals 64(13):68–70

PERSONAL NOTEBOOK

1. How do you feel about the states of the American Nurses Association being certified as collective bargaining agents? Do you presently belong to your state student nurses' association? Do you plan to join your state ANA? Why or why not?

2. Examine the following questions. Would you feel differently about unions if you were a supervisor? What influences you the most in your desire to join or reject unions? What experience have members of your group had with discrimination or with feelings of powerlessness in the workplace?

3. Do you agree or disagree with the 1994 Supreme Court ruling that any nurse who directs less skilled employees should be classified as a supervisor? Should the definition of "supervisor" in nursing be different than that used by other professions?

CONTROLLING

Any profession which doesn't monitor itself becomes a technology.

—*Maria Phaneuf*

This unit introduces controlling as the fifth and final step in the management process. Koontz and Weihrich (1988) define controlling as "the measurement and correction of performance in order to make sure that objectives and the plans devised to attain them are accomplished." Marriner-Tomey (1996) views controlling as the function of management that involves setting and measuring performance against standards, reporting the results, and taking corrective action. In both these definitions, it becomes apparent that controlling requires evaluation and subsequent action. It also provides opportunities for growth and learning.

Tappen (1995) suggests that controlling provides a means of clarifying performance expectations, reinforcing constructive behavior, correcting unsatisfactory behavior, providing recognition, increasing self-awareness, and promoting growth and change. Whether control mechanisms are formal or informal depends on the situation and the individuals involved. Regardless, all people and all organizations need to know how they are doing. Employees who know and understand the expectations of their employer have greater control over their destinies, which, in turn, increases their job satisfaction and job performance. Organizations also need to have some control over productivity, quality outcomes, and innovation.

Because the management process, like the nursing process, is cyclic, controlling should never be considered an end in itself; instead, it should be implemented throughout all phases of the management process. Examples of management controlling functions include the ongoing evaluation of unit and agency performance through quality control mechanisms, the measurement of individual and group performance against pre-established standards, and the modification/redirection of organizational member behavior as necessary to achieve organizational goals.

◆ References

Koontz H and Weihrich H (1988). Management. New York: McGraw-Hill

Marriner-Tomey A (1996). Guide to Nursing Management, 5th ed. St. Louis: CV Mosby

Tappen RM (1995). Nursing Leadership and Management: Concepts and Practice, 3rd ed. Philadelphia: FA Davis

Quality Assurance

CHAPTER 20

Quality assurance, a specific type of controlling, refers to activities that evaluate, monitor, or regulate services rendered to consumers. In nursing, the goal of quality assurance is to ensure a quality product while meeting intended purposes. Quality assurance, when viewed simplistically, can be broken down into three basic steps.

1. The criteria or standards must be determined.
2. Information is collected to determine if standards have been met.
3. Educational or corrective action is taken if the criteria were not met.

◆ Quality Assurance as a Process

It is fairly simple to measure quantitative data. However, qualitative data is more elusive and attempts to measure it are more difficult. Accurate assessment of qualitative data requires managers to consistently use a specific and systematic process. The use of a process, such as that shown in Display 20-1, reduces subjectivity and increases the validity and reliability of the measurements.

The first step in Display 20-1 is the establishment of control criteria or standards. It is impossible to measure performance if clearcut standards have not been established. Not only must standards exist, but the manager must see that all subordinates know and understand them. Because they vary among institutions, employees must know the standard expected of them at their particular institution and that their performance will be evaluated in terms of their ability to meet that standard. For example, hospital nurses should provide postoperative patient care that meets criteria specific to their institution. The nurse's performance can only be measured when it can be compared to a preset standard.

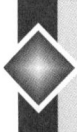

DISPLAY 20-1
Steps in the Auditing of Quality Control

Generate control criteria → Identify the information relevant to the criteria → Determine ways to collect the information → Collect and analyze the information → Compare collected information with the established criteria → Make a judgment about the quality → Provide information and, if necessary, corrective action regarding the findings to appropriate sources → Determine when there is a need for re-evaluation

The second step in the quality assurance process includes identifying information relevant to the criteria. What information is needed for its measurement? In the postoperative patient care example, the data might include the frequency of vital signs, dressing checks, neurological or sensory checks, and so on.

The next step is the identification of information sources. As in all data gathering, the manager must be sure to utilize all appropriate sources. In assessing quality control of the postoperative patient, the manager could find much of the information within the patient chart. Postoperative flow sheets, physician's orders, and nursing notes would probably be most helpful. Speaking to the patient or nurse could also yield information.

The next step in auditing quality assurance is to collect and analyze information. For example, if the standards specified that postoperative vital signs were to be checked every 30 minutes for 2 hours, and every hour thereafter for 8 hours, it would be necessary to examine how often vital signs were taken the first 10 hours after surgery. The frequency of vital signs listed on the postoperative flow sheet would then be compared with the standard set by the unit. The resulting discrepancy or congruency gives managers information for use when making a judgment about the quality or appropriateness of the nursing care. If vital signs were not taken frequently enough to satisfy the standard, the manager would need to obtain further information regarding why the standard was not met, and counsel employees as needed.

The last step in Display 20-1 is re-evaluation. If quality assurance is measured on 20 postoperative charts and a high rate of compliance with established standards is found, the need for short-term re-evaluation is low. If standards are consistently not met or only partially met, frequent re-evaluation is indicated. It is important to remember that quality assurance should not be implemented solely as a reaction to a problem. Effective managers ensure that quality assurance is proactive: identifying areas where care can be improved to maximum standards as well as addressing and eliminating existing problems in early stages, before productivity or quality are compromised.

In order for any quality assurance program to be effective, certain components need to be in place. First, the program needs to be supported by top-level administration, and not merely be an exercise to satisfy various standards set forth by federal or state regulatory agencies. A sincere pledge by the agency, as evidenced by the commitment of time and money, will be a deciding factor in determining and improving the quality of services rendered. In addition, although the organization must be realistic about the economics of the services rendered, if nursing is to strive toward excellence, then criteria in development should be pushed to optimum standards rather than be set at minimum acceptable levels (Marquis and Huston, 1996).

◆ The Development of Standards

A standard is a model of expectation; that is, it is the expected behavior or conduct. It is not an evaluation instrument in itself, but does provide a yardstick for measuring the quality of service provided. Because there is no one set of common standards, each organization and profession must set its own standards to guide individual practitioners in providing safe and effective care. Standards for nursing practice define the scope and dimensions of professional nursing. The American Nurses Association (ANA), as well as specialty groups within the nursing profession, has played a key role in developing standards for the profession since the 1930s. These standards generally exemplify optimal performance expectations and have provided a basis for the development of organizational and unit standards nationwide.

Organizational standards outline levels of acceptable practice within the institution itself. For example, each organization develops a policies and procedures manual that outlines the standards established for that organization. These standards may be minimizing or maximizing in terms of the quality of service expected and allow the organization to more objectively measure unit and individual performance.

◆ Audits as a Quality Assurance Tool

Whereas standards provide the yardstick for the measurement of quality care, audits are the tool. An audit is a systematic and official examination of a record, process, or account to evaluate performance. Auditing in health care organizations provides managers with a means to determine the quality of services rendered. The audits most frequently used in quality control include the following.

PROCESS AUDIT

These audits are used to measure the process of care or how the care was carried out. Process audits are task-oriented and focus on whether or not standards of nursing practice are being met. These audits assume there is a relationship between the quality of the care and the process used to provide care. Process *standards* may be documented in patient care plans, procedure manuals, or nursing protocol statements.

For example, a process audit might be used to establish whether fetal heart tones or blood pressures were checked according to the established policy in a hospital. In a community health agency, a process audit could be used to determine if newborn teaching had been carried out during the first postpartum visit.

STRUCTURE AUDIT

This audit monitors the structure or setting in which patient care occurs (i.e., the finances, nursing service structure, medical records, and environmental structure). These audits assume there is a relationship between setting, quality care, and appropriate structure. Structural *standards,* which are often set by licensing and accrediting bodies, ensure a safe and effective environment but do not address the actual care provided.

Examples of structural audits might include checking to see if patient call lights are in place or if patients can reach their water pitchers. It might also examine staffing patterns to ensure that adequate resources are available to meet changing patient needs.

OUTCOME AUDITS

Naylor and colleagues (1991; 210) define outcomes as the "end results of care; the changes in the patient's health status that can be attributed to the delivery of health care services." Outcome audits determine what results (if any) occurred as a result of specific intervention by nurses for clients. These audits assume the outcome accurately demonstrates the quality of care that was provided. Many experts consider outcome measures to be the most valid indicators of quality care, but until the last decade, evaluations of hospital care have tended to focus on structure and process.

Examples of outcomes traditionally used to measure quality of hospital care include mortality, morbidity, and length of hospital stay. Naylor (1991) suggests that outcome measures more clearly influenced by nursing could include functional status, mental status, stress levels, satisfaction with care, burden of care on families, and cost of care.

◆ Total Quality Management and Benchmarking: Two Strategies for Quality Assurance

Total quality management (TQM), a philosophy developed by Deming and others, and considered the hallmark of highly successful Japanese management systems, has been applied to American health care settings in an effort to provide a practical solution to the "best for less" dilemma (Arikian, 1991). TQM is based on the premise that the individual is the focus of production and service; that is, the environment must be customer responsive. Quality is built into the service or product, rather than assuming that inspection of and removal of errors leads to quality (Kirk, 1992). Thus, it is identifying and doing the right things, the right way, the first time, and the prevention of problems—not inspection and reactive problem solving—that lead to quality outcomes. In TQM, this philosophy is incorporated into the organizational culture and reflected in all attitudes regarding hierarchies, cost containment, and human relations (Arikian, 1991).

Because TQM is a never-ending process, everything and everyone in the organization is subject to continuous improvement efforts. No matter how good the product or service is perceived to be, the TQM philosophy states that there is always room for improvement (Kirk, 1992). Customer needs and experiences with the end product are constantly evaluated. This data collection is done by workers, not by a central quality assurance department, thus providing a feedback loop between administration, workers, and consumers. Any problems encountered are approached in a preventive or proactive mode so that crisis management becomes unnecessary.

Another critical component of TQM is the empowerment of employees by providing positive feedback and reinforcing attitudes and behaviors that support quality and productivity. Based on the premise that employees have an in-depth understanding of their jobs, believe they are valued, and feel encouraged to improve product or service quality through risk taking and creativity, TQM trusts the employee to be knowledgeable, accountable, and responsible and provides education and training for employees at all levels.

Although the philosophy of TQM emphasizes that quality is placed before profit, the resultant increase in quality owing to a well-implemented TQM program attracts more customers, resulting in increased profit margins and a financially healthier organization. Because the health care industry is so vulnerable to the forces of competition, changing technology, reimbursement, and dwindling resources, some experts propose that TQM may be one of the factors guaranteeing the survival of the fittest in the future (Arikian, 1991).

Another tool that has been used to promote quality in health care organizations is benchmarking. Benchmarking or best practices research (BPR) occurs when an organization identifies a weakness and then goes about identifying other organizations (the ideal) who excel in that area. Following communication and role play with the model organization, the deficient organization then goes about trying to emulate the best practices of the excellent organization and even to improve on those practices.

Drachman (1996) suggests that benchmarking provides a means of improved communication between organizations, particularly when those organizations do not have to compete in the market. It is, however, labor intensive and requires constant monitoring and support. In addition, confidentiality agreements should be in place to guard against inappropriate use of the findings such as comparative advertising or promotions (Drachman, 1996).

◆ External Impacts on Quality Assurance

Although few organizations would argue the tremendous benefits of well-developed and accurately implemented quality assurance programs, in health care organizations they evolved primarily as a result of external intervention, and not as a voluntary effort to monitor the quality of services provided. As discussed in Chapter 7, when Medicare and Medicaid (U.S. Government health care reimbursement for the elderly, disabled, and financially indigent) were implemented in the early 1960s, health care organizations had little need to justify costs or to prove that the services provided met clients needs. Reimbursement was based on costs incurred in providing the service and no actual ceilings were placed on the price that could be charged for services. As the cost of these programs skyrocketed, the U.S. Government established regulations requiring organizations to substantiate the need, as well as to monitor the quality of services provided.

The new big brother surveillance and the existence of external controls had a tremendous impact on the health care industry. Health care organizations began to question basic values and were forced to establish new methods for collecting data, keeping records, providing services, and general accounting. Because government programs such as Medicare and Medicaid represented such a large group of clients receiving health care, organizations who were unwilling or unable to meet these changing needs did not survive financially.

In the 1970s, the Joint Commission on the Accreditation of Healthcare Organizations (JCAHO) became involved in quality assurance at the organizational level and mandated each hospital to have a program in place by January 1, 1981. Again, in 1982, JCAHO established standards for nursing care as measured against written criteria. These standards placed an emphasis on quality and the need for continuous review and evaluation of care provided by professional workers. Current JCAHO guidelines state that a quality assurance program should be an integrated, systematic, institution-wide, quality review plan for all care-related services, support services, medical staff, and governing boards (Bushy, 1991). The advent of diagnostic related groupings (DRGs) in the early 1980s added to the ever-increasing need for organizations to monitor cost containment while providing a minimum level of quality. Fiesta (1992) argues that changing health care economics has resulted in a shift from clinical to financial control of medical decisions and that, arguably, the standard of care should be divided into two elements, a clinical standard and a resource utilization standard.

It is clear that DRGs have contributed to increased acuity levels of hospitalized patients and a decrease in the length of patient stay. Although some health care providers have argued that DRGs have resulted in the premature discharge of patients from the hospital, others have countered that quality of care has not been impacted, as these patients' needs are being met through increased out-patient follow-up and through home care, which are more cost effective. The key point, however, is that changing external regulations regarding quality control continue to strongly influence management decisions.

◆ Contemporary Efforts to Promote Quality Assurance

Organizations have become increasingly accountable regarding the internal monitoring of cost containment and quality over the last 30 years. "Numerous efforts to control escalating health care costs continue to be introduced although the bottom line for insurers, administrators, and providers remains unchanged: providing health care at a reasonable cost while maintaining or enhancing the quality of that care" (Naylor, Munro, and Brooten, 1991; 210).

One contemporary effort to promote quality assurance is the use of "critical pathways." Critical pathways, as described by Hurley (1994), are predetermined courses of progress that patients should be making following admission for a specific diagnosis or following a specific surgery. For example, a critical pathway for a specific diagnosis might suggest an average length of stay (ALOS) of 4 days, and that the patient should have certain interventions completed by certain points on the pathway (much like a PERT diagram). Any patient's progress found to not be in compliance with the critical pathway prompts a review of the medical care and a report regarding why the critical pathway has been violated.

The advantage of critical pathways is that they do provide some means of standardizing medical care for clients with similar diagnoses. Their weakness, however, is the difficulties they pose in accounting for and accepting what are often justifiable differentiations between unique clients that have deviated from their pathway. Critical pathway documentation also poses one more paperwork and utilization review function in a system that is already overburdened with administrative costs.

Another contemporary quality performance tool being developed is HEDIS (Health Plan Employer Data and Information Set). HEDIS, which was developed by the National Committee for Quality Assurance, suggests performance indicators that can be used to assess the quality of managed care organizations. Version 2.0 of HEDIS, which was implemented as a "report card" of 21 managed care organizations in 1995, contained 36 performance indicator measures (Grimaldi, 1996). Rather than compare the managed care organizations against each other directly, HEDIS assigns them a grand mean score in the indicators and also provides an analysis of each managed care organization's progress in meeting goals from the U.S. Public Health Service's Healthy People 2000.

Version 2.5 of HEDIS contains approximately 60 performance indicators and was used to create "report cards" of more than 200 managed care organizations in 1996 (Grimaldi, 1996). Version 3.0. will have an even greater number of performance indicators, as an attempt is being made to include performance indicators specific to the growing Medicaid and Medicare segment of the population enrolled in managed care.

The greatest strength of the HEDIS program is that it offers the best promise of an impartial evaluation of managed care programs to date. As performance indicators are developed further and more managed care organizations choose to participate, HEDIS holds great potential to provide meaningful information to assist consumers in selecting an appropriate managed care program.

Another advantage of HEDIS is that it has prompted an offshoot of interest in developing "report cards" for all hospitals. Harris (1994) predicts that hospital report cards, patterned after the HEDIS model, will be used broadly before the turn of the century.

The greatest limitation of the HEDIS program is its infancy. Much more research is needed to determine what are appropriate performance indicators and the best way to measure them. Another limitation is that the data presented in report cards by HEDIS have not yet been prepared in a manner that makes them readily accessible to and understandable by the general public. Report cards issued by HEDIS and other agencies often pose conflicting views, contrary findings, and use language not easily understood by the general public. Such concerns must be addressed. Also, there is an effort underway by the JCAHO to develop a performance indicator report card that may be used as part of the hospital accreditation review process (Harris, 1994).

Another tool that holds promise for improving quality assurance efforts in the future is the Nursing Minimum Data Set (NMDS). The NMDS was developed by Werley and Lang (1988), and represents a decade-long effort to standardize the collection of nursing data. With the NMDS, a minimum set of items of information with uniform definitions and categories are collected to meet the needs of multiple data users. Although in various stages of use across the country, Leske and Werley (1992), suggest that both the use and implementation of the NMDS are in the "stage of infancy."

There are other efforts to measure quality that are continuously done at the organization level. Most acute-care and long-term care agencies continuously collect and analyze quality indicator data as part of meeting accreditation requirements through JCAHO or other accrediting bodies. This data, although important and assistive to the agency in identifying their own quality deficiencies, are unfortunately, often hidden away in a quality assurance department and considered to be "bad laundry," not to be released to the public or other agencies. This severely limits the ability of health care agencies to learn from one another.

Another problem in organizational level data collection is that there are not yet any widely accepted or mandated national quality indicators; thus, each organization is collecting data on what it believes to be a quality indicator and each in whatever way it sees fit. The work of HEDIS and the JCAHO should be instrumental in suggesting national quality indicators that will allow for greater standardization of data collection at the organization level.

◆ Quality Control in the Future

Little is known about how the future will define quality care. It is clear, however, that over time, quality control tools will become more refined and additional objective standards will be developed. Naylor and associates (1991) suggest the need for an increased emphasis on outcome measurement in the future and the linking of outcomes to nursing practices. Waltz and Sylvia (1991) state that both the quantity and quality of the measurement efforts directed toward outcome assessment, especially outcome related to the effectiveness of nursing care, have increased markedly during the past decade and will increase in the future as nurses attempt to document the worth of nursing programs and services.

Omachonou and Nanda (1989) suggest a need for *output* measures in addition to outcome measures, which, in conjunction with DRGs, clarify health care costs and provide a consistent measure across all health care organizations. Outcome measures examine productivity in terms of efficacy, or the potential ability to restore health through nursing or medical intervention. Output measures focus on the dollar value of the services rendered and resources expended. Thus, output measures lend themselves to more objective quantification of results and eliminate the need for the assumption that there is a direct relationship between outcome and quality of care. Output measures are also more suitable to fiscal control than outcome measures.

One quality measurement issue that has not been fully resolved is whether quality assurance in health care in the coming century should be gauged more by consumer satisfaction or by more objective outcome indicators of quality of care. Most industries create product lines based on consumer expectations and satisfaction, whereas nursing has been driven by quality standards set by the profession. These standards measure the quality of nursing care reflected in terms of morbidity rate, incidence of nosocomial infection, length of hospital stay, behavioral changes of the client as a result of new knowledge, and rehabilitative potential. The question is whether consumer expectations and professional standards are complementary.

In a study of 139,830 former patients from 225 hospitals, not one of the top 15 factors determining patient satisfaction had anything to do with whether the patient's health improved during the stay (Modern Health Care, 1992). Patients were more concerned about staff attention to privacy, sensitivity to the inconvenience of hospitalization, overall cheerfulness of the hospital, and the skill level and courtesy of technicians drawing blood.

These findings pose many questions for managers. Should quality assurance measures be designed to gauge consumer satisfaction or standards set by the profession? Should they reflect an integration of both criteria?

In what will perhaps be defined as the seminal work in defining quality indicators thus far, the ANA (1996), based on structured interviews with a nationwide sample of 10 institutions that included at least one academic medical center, public hospital, private hospital, urban hospital, rural hospital, and hospital system, integrate both criteria, in their identification of 10 quality indicators. They include:

1. nosocomial infection,
2. patient injury rate,
3. patient satisfaction with nursing care,
4. patient satisfaction with pain management,
5. patient satisfaction with educational information,
6. patient satisfaction with care,
7. maintenance of skin integrity,
8. nurse staff satisfaction,
9. mix of RNs, LPNs, and unlicensed staff caring for patients in acute care settings, and
10. total nursing care hours provided per patient day.

◆ Who Should Be Involved in Quality Assurance?

Ideally, everyone in the organization should participate in quality assurance because each individual benefits from it. Quality control gives employees feedback about their current quality of care as well as how it can be improved. As direct caregivers, staff nurses are in an excellent position to monitor the impact of nursing practice on patient care. Naylor and associates (1991) maintain that nurses as major providers of health care must assume a leadership role in measuring the quality of their services, as well as documenting their costs. Although it is impractical to expect full staff involvement throughout the quality assurance process, as many staff as possible should be involved in the determination and review of criteria or standards, data collection, or reporting. Patient or client participation and input should also be strong encouraged.

Quality assurance also requires a coordination of other involved health care professionals. Physicians, respiratory therapists, dietitians, physical therapists, and others contribute to client care and outcomes and therefore must be considered in the audit process. However, it is possible to separate the contribution of nursing to the client outcome, and recognition of this accountability is an important step in nurturing the professionalism of nursing.

◆ Summary

Accurately appraising quality allows managers to change problem solving from an unsystematic, unscientific process to an accurate, analytical one. Managers must determine what standards will be used to measure quality care on their unit and then develop and implement a quality assurance program that measures end results against those standards. All managers have a responsibility to monitor the quality of the product that their unit produces—in health care organizations, that product is client care. Managers also have a duty to assess and promote consumer satisfaction whenever possible.

However, the manager cannot operate in a vacuum in determining what quality is and how it should be measured. Demands for hard data on quality have increased as regulatory bodies, consumers, payers, and hospital managers have required substantiation of services provided. Most health care organizations today have complete quality assurance programs and are actively involved in cost containment. Managers must be cognizant of rapidly changing quality assurance regulations and proactively adjust unit standards to meet these changing needs.

◆ References

American Nurses Association (ANA) (1996). Nursing Quality Indicators: Definitions and Implications. Washington, DC: American Nurses Publishing

Arikian VL (1991). Total quality management: applications to nursing service. J Nurs Admin 21(6):46–50

Bushy A (1991). Quality assurance in rural hospitals. J Nurs Admin 21(10):34–39

Drachman DA (1996). Benchmarking patient satisfaction at academic health centers. J Qual Improve 22(5):359–367

Fiesta J (1992). Cost standards, quality and technology. Nurs Manage 23(2):16–17

Grimaldi PL (1996). Monitoring managed care's quality. Managed Care Primer—Supplement to Nursing Management. Oct. 1996, pp. 18–20

Harris N (1994). How hospitals measure up. Business and Health August, 20–24

Hurley ML (ed). (1994) Focusing on outcomes. RN 57(5):57–60

Kirk R (1992). The big picture—total quality management and continuous quality improvement. J Nurs Admin 22(4):24–31

Leske JS and Werley HH (1992). Use of the nursing minimum data set. Comput Nurs 10(6):259–263

Marquis B and Huston C (1996). Leadership Roles and Management Functions: Theory and Application. Philadelphia: JB Lippincott

Modern Health Care (1992). Outliers—what the patients think. June 1, 44

Naylor MD, Munro BH, and Brooten DA (1991). Measuring the effectiveness of nursing practice. Clin Nurse Spec 5(4):210–215

Omachonu VK and Nanda R (1989). Measuring productivity: outcome vs. output. Nurs Manage 20(4):35–38, 40

Waltz CF and Sylvia BM (1991). Accountability and outcome measurement: where do we go from here? Clin Nurse Spec 5(4):202–203

Werley HH and Lang NM (1988). The nursing minimum data set: benefits and implications. In Perspectives in Nursing, 1987–1989. New York: Springer

SAMPLE CASE ANALYSIS

THE CASE ◆

Irene Martin is a public health nurse employed in a small, nonprofit community visiting nurses group. The nursing director has requested that she chair the newly established quality assurance committee because she has had some experience in her past positions with developing audit criteria.

A review of the patient population indicates that maternal–child clients make up the greatest percentage of the visiting nurse's home visits, so the committee decides to examine this area first. They have chosen to develop a tool for a retrospective process audit that would be appropriate for monitoring the quality of an initial home visit of a postpartum client, discharged with infant, after less than 12 hours in a birth center or obstetrical unit, following uneventful delivery. The home visit would occur no longer than 72 hours after the delivery.

SAMPLE CASE ANALYSIS (CONTINUED)

Assignment

Assume you are Ms. Martin. Design an audit tool that would be appropriate and convenient to use for this diagnosis. Specific percentages of compliance, the sources of information, and the number of clients to be audited should be included. Limit your process criteria to 20 items.

Analysis

Rationale for form: In writing audit criteria it is best to define the client population as clearly as possible first, so that your retrieval of information can be expedited. See Display 20-2 for a sample audit form. In this case, abnormal newborns, complicated or cesarean section births, and home births have been eliminated. This was done because those clients would require more in-depth assessment and teaching.

The performance expected was set at 100% compliance, but an allowance was given for those reasons that an exception could be made. This compliance percentage was chosen because it was felt that if any of these criteria were not recorded, there should be some remedial action taken. The client's record was selected as the source of information, as it is an objective source and it is assumed that if the criteria were not recorded, they were not met. Thirty charts were audited because this number can give the agency sufficient data to make adequate assumptions, but is not such a large number that it becomes a burden to review the records.

After the audit committee has concluded their review, they should write a summary of their findings. A typical summary might appear as follows.

Summary of Audit Findings

Nursing diagnosis: Initial home visit, within 72 hours, following uncomplicated delivery, with normal newborn, occurring in a birth center or obstetrical facility.

Number of records audited: 30.

Date of audit: 7/6/97.

Summary of findings: 100% compliance in all areas except mother's temperature (50% compliance) and newborn assessment (70% compliance).

Suggestions for improving compliance: Post results of audit: Remind public health nurses to record temperature of mother in record, even if normal. Time might be a factor in newborn assessment as they are frequently recorded on subsequent visits. Committee agrees that they should be done on first home visit and suggests an inservice for staff regarding this area of noncompliance.

Signed,

Chairman of the Committee

The summaries should be forwarded to the individual responsible for the quality assurance—in this case, the director of the agency. At no time should individual public health nurses be identified as not having met the criteria. Quality assurance must always be separate from performance appraisal.

DISPLAY 20-2
Nursing Audit Form for Visiting Nurses

Diagnosis: Initial home visit within 72 hours, following uncomplicated vaginal delivery, with normal newborn, occurring in a birth center or obstetrical facility.

Source of information: Record of client.

Expected compliance: 100%, unless specified by exceptions.

Number of records to be audited: 30.

	YES	NO
1. Home visit made within 72 hours following delivery	___	___
2. Mother's lochia examined for amount, color, and odor	___	___
3. Mother's episiotomy assessed for tenderness, redness, and edema	___	___
4. Mother instructed on perinatal care	___	___
5. Temperature of mother and infant taken	___	___
6. Mother assisted with breast feeding (Note: exception is not breast feeding)	___	___
7. Mother instructed on dealing with breast engorgement (Note: exception is no breast engorgement)	___	___
8. Mother instructed on feeding infant water	___	___
9. Mother instructed on preparation and feeding of formula (Note: exception is breast feeding)	___	___
10. Mother questioned regarding general systems and condition (voiding, ambulation, discomfort, nutrition, intake, and rest)	___	___
11. Infant bath demonstration given	___	___
12. Newborn physical assessment completed	___	___
13. Assessment made of mother's support system	___	___
14. Assessment made of mother's knowledge of infant care	___	___
15. Assessment of mother–infant bonding	___	___
16. Follow-up plan made	___	___

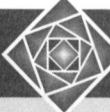 **CASES FOR PROBLEM SOLVING**

CASE 1 (Marquis and Huston, 1996)

Some clients who are ill get well despite nursing care, not as a result of nursing care. Does the quality of the nursing care have an impact on client outcome? Do you feel that quality nursing care can make a difference in clients' lives? Identify five criteria you would use to define "quality nursing care." These criteria should reflect what you believe nurses do that makes the difference.

CASE 2 (Marquis and Huston, 1996)

You have been the nursing coordinator of cardiac services at a medium-sized urban hospital for 6 months. Among the cardiac services provided by the hospital are open heart surgery, invasive and noninvasive diagnostic testing, and a comprehensive rehabilitation program. The open heart surgery program is relatively new, having been implemented just over 1 year ago. Over the last 3 months, you have begun to feel uneasy about the mortality rate of postoperative cardiac patients at your facility. An audit of medical records shows a unit mortality rate approximately 30% above national norms.

You approach the unit medical director with your findings. She becomes very defensive and states that there have been a few "freakish situations to skew the results, but that the open heart program is one of the best in the state." When you propose the statistics be examined further, the director becomes very angry, turns to leave the room, stops and says, "Remember, these patients are leaving the operating room alive. They are dying on your unit. If you stir up trouble, you are going to be sorry."

•••

Assignment

Outline what you will do, identifying areas in your data gathering that may have been misleading or that may have invalidated your findings. If you believe action is still warranted, what are the personal and professional risks involved? How well developed is your power base to undertake these risks? To whom do you have the greatest responsibility?

CASE 3 (Marquis and Huston, 1996)

You are the director of a baccalaureate nursing program. In the early 1980s, your school averaged approximately 200 applicants per 50 student openings each semester. This resulted in great selectivity on the part of the school about which students would be chosen to enter the program. Because entering students traditionally had high cumulative grade point averages (GPAs), and had completed almost all non-nursing requirements, the attrition and drop-out rate was fairly low, and academic failure was rare.

In conjunction with a severe national nursing shortage and a marked decrease in the number of students pursuing nursing as a career, there are barely sufficient numbers of applicants to fill each entering class. As a result, students meeting minimal GPA requirements and having many general studies

CASE 3 (CONTINUED)

course requirements outstanding are accepted into the program. You have seen the attrition and dropout rate quadruple over the last 3 years and believe that much of this attrition is attributable to academic failure.

Recently, the faculty have begun discussing changing the academic failure policy in an effort to increase student retention. The current policy results in automatic dismissal from the program if students fail two courses in the nursing major.

Faculty have recently begun voicing concerns that teaching positions will be cut as a result of the decreased enrollment and high attrition. You are aware that university administration feels that nursing is a costly major, that this situation is not going to improve in the near future, and that budget cuts may indeed be mandated in the near future to reflect the decrease in full-time students.

However, you have grave concerns about eliminating or altering this policy as you believe that in effect, you are lowering program standards and thus, the quality of the end product. You do not believe that students failing two courses in the major would make safe practitioners. You also believe that students having academic difficulties are taking a disproportionate amount of faculty time and energy at the expense of those students who are succeeding.

Assignment

What options are available to you? What obligations do you have to your faculty? To the students? To the public as consumers of health care? To university administration? How do you determine an appropriate course of action when these duties are in conflict?

CASE 4 ◆

Develop three nursing criteria for an outcome audit and three nursing criteria for a process audit for the following nursing diagnoses. In each criteria show a percentage of expected compliance and/or the exceptions to 100% compliance.

Alterations in comfort, acute pain.

Alteration in tissue perfusion, anemia.

◆ Bibliography

The following is a list of references to assist you in solving these cases:

Berkey T (1994). Benchmarking in health care: turning challenges into success. J Qual Improve 20(5):277–284

Betta PA (1992). Developing a successful ambulatory QA program. Nurs Manage 23(4):31–33

Brocka B and Brocka MS (1992). Quality Management: Implementing the Best Ideas of the Masters. Homewood, IL: Richard D. Irwin

Buerhaus PI (1992). Nursing, competition, and quality. Nurs Econom 10(1):21–28

Curtin L (1992). Of commissions, omissions, and just plain missions. Nurs Manage 23(5):7–8

Epstein A (1995). Performance reports on quality: prototypes, problems, and prospects. Sounding board. JAMA 333:57–61

Grimaldi PL (1996). A glossary of managed care terms. Managed Care Primer—a Supplement to Nursing Management. October, 5–7

Hibbard JH and Jewett JJ (1996). What type of quality information do consumers want in a health care report card? Med Care Res Rev 53(1):28–47

Hoesing H and Kirk R (1990). Common sense quality management. J Nurs Admin 20(10):10–15

Kerfoot KM (1992). Achieving excellence: the nurse manager's challenge. Nurs Econom 10(2):140–143

Mahrenholz DM (1991). Outcomes research and nurses. Nurs Connect 4(1):58–61

Masters F and Schmele JA (1991). Total quality management: an idea whose time has come. J Nurs Quality Assur 5(4)July:7–16

Mitchell PH (1993). Perspectives on outcome-oriented care systems. Nurs Admin Quart 17(3):1–7

Neame R (1993). Making the case for healthcare smart cards. Healthcare Inform 10(6):16–20

O'Leary DS (1993). The measurement mandate: report card day is coming. J Qual Improve 19(11):487–491

Porter JE (1995). The benchmarking effort for networking children's hospitals (BENCHmark). J Qual Improve 21:395–406

Roberts GA (1994). Quality outcomes for case managed practices. Aspen's Adv Nurse Exec 9(9):4–6

Schroeder P (1991). From the editor . . . cost and quality are being integrated into clinical settings. J Nurs Qual Assur 5(4)July:viii

Simpson RL (1991). Adopting a nursing minimum data set. Nurs Manage 22(2):20–21

Sorgen LM (1991). Process and outcome measurement in Alberta's coordinated home care program. Home Health Care Serv Quart 12(1):103–113

Wylie DM (1991). Continuous quality improvement. Can J Nurs Admin 4(2)June:5

PERSONAL NOTEBOOK

1. Is the quality of your patient care always as high as you would like it to be? What factors affect its quality? Which ones can you control? In your clinical experiences, have DRGs impacted on the quality of care provided? In what ways?

2. Building in evaluation checkpoints often allows us to make midcourse corrections so that we are able to meet our goals. During the semester, what controls do you use in order to stay on schedule with your course work?

3. Have you ever worked in an organization with a TQM philosophy? Some organizations attempt to implement only select components of such a philosophy. Do you see any inherent difficulties in this approach?

Performance Appraisal

An additional managerial controlling responsibility is determining how well employees carry out the duties of their assigned jobs. No activity of the manager is as personalized as appraising the work performance of others. Because work is an important part of one's identity, individuals are very sensitive to the opinions of others about how they perform. For this reason, performance appraisal becomes one of the greatest tools an organization has to develop and motivate staff. When used correctly, performance appraisal can increase retention and productivity. However, in the hands of an inept or inexperienced manager, the appraisal process may discourage and demotivate staff.

Because a manager's opinions and judgments are used in making far-reaching decisions regarding the employee's life, it is necessary that they be reached in an objective, systematic, and formalized manner. The use of a formal system of performance review reduces the subjectivity of the appraisal.

◆ Using the Performance Appraisal to Motivate Employees

Although systematic employee appraisals have been used in management since the 1920s, it was not until the 1950s that interest was directed toward the use of the appraisal as a method to promote employee growth. Performance appraisal becomes a useless waste of management time if it is merely an exercise to satisfy regulations and does not result in employee growth.

The following factors influence whether an appraisal ultimately results in increased motivation and productivity.

1. The employee must feel that the appraisal is based on a standard to which all other employees are held accountable. This standard must be commu-

nicated clearly to the employee at the time of hire, and may consist of a job description or personal goals set by employees, as in management by objectives (MBO). MBO will be discussed later in this chapter.

2. The employee should have some input into the development of the standards or goals upon which his or her performance is judged. This is *imperative* for the professional employee.

3. The employee must be aware, in advance, what occurs if he or she does not meet expected standards of performance.

4. The employee needs to know how information used to determine his or her performance will be obtained. The appraisal tends to be more accurate if various sources and types of information are solicited. Sources could include peers, coworkers, nursing care plans, patients, and personal observation. The employee should be informed which sources will be used and how such information will be weighted.

5. The appraiser should be someone who directly supervises the employee. For example, the charge nurse who works directly with staff nurses should be involved in their appraisal process and interview. It is appropriate and advisable in most instances for the head nurse and/or supervisor also to be involved. However, employees must believe that the person conducting the major portion of the appraisal is someone who has actually observed the work.

6. The result of the performance appraisal is more likely to be positive if the appraiser is viewed with trust and professional respect. This increases the probability that employees will perceive the appraisal as a fair and accurate assessment of their work performance.

◆ Strategies to Ensure Accuracy and Fairness

If the appraisal is viewed as valuable and valid by the employee, then the outcome of the appraisal can have many positive results. Information obtained during the performance appraisal can be used to develop the employee's potential, to assist employees in overcoming difficulties they have in fulfilling their roles, to point out strengths the employee may not be aware of, and to aid employees in setting future goals. Since the result of an inaccurate or unfair appraisal is negative and demotivating, it is critical that the manager employ strategies that increase the likelihood of an equitable appraisal (Huston and Marquis, 1989). Although there will always be some subjectivity in any performance appraisal, the following steps will assist the manager in arriving at an appropriate assessment.

1. *The appraiser should develop an awareness of personal biases and prejudices.* This helps guard against subjective attitudes and values influencing the appraisal.

2. *Consultation should be sought frequently.* Not only should another manager be consulted when there is a question about personal bias, but in many

other situations as well. For example, it is very important that new managers solicit assistance and consultation when they complete their first performance appraisals. Even experienced managers should seek consultation when an employee is having great difficulty in fulfilling the duties of the job. Consultation must also be used when employees work several shifts; in this way information can be obtained from all the shift supervisors.

3. *Data should be gathered appropriately.* Not only should many different sources be used in gathering data regarding employee performance, but the data gathered needs to reflect the entire time period covered by the appraisal. Frequently, managers will collect data and observe employees just prior to completing their appraisal. This affords an inaccurate picture of job performance, as all employees have periods where they are less productive and less motivated. Thus, data should be gathered systematically and regularly.

4. *Information should be written down and not entrusted to memory.* The manager should make a habit of writing notations regarding observations, comments by others, as well as a periodic review of charts and nursing care plans.

5. *Collected assessments should contain positive examples of growth and achievement as well as examples of areas needing further development.* Nothing delights an employee more than discovering that his or her immediate supervisor is aware of his or her growth and accomplishments and can cite specific instances when good clinical judgment was used. Too frequently, collected data concentrate on the negative aspects of job performance.

6. *The appraiser needs to guard against the three common pitfalls of assessment, namely, the "halo effect," "horns effect," and "central tendency."* The halo effect occurs when the appraiser lets one or two positive aspects or behaviors unduly influence all others in regard to the employee's performance. The horns effect occurs when the appraiser allows some negative aspects of the employee's performance to override the assessment to such an extent that other positive levels of job performance are not accurately recorded. The manager who falls into the central tendency trap is hesitant to risk true assessment, and therefore, rates all employees as average. These errors on the part of the appraiser can lead employees to discount the entire assessment of their work performance.

7. *Some effort must be made to include the self-appraisal of the employee as part of the performance review process.* Self-appraisal may be conducted in several appropriate ways. The employee can be instructed to come to the appraisal interview with some informal thoughts regarding their performance, or he or she can work with the manager in completing a joint assessment. There are both advantages and disadvantages to using self-appraisal as a method of performance review. Introspection and self-appraisal result in growth when the individual is self-aware, but even mature individuals require feedback and validation of their performance.

Some employees may regard their annual performance review as a time to receive positive feedback from their supervisor. This is especially true if they receive infrequent praise on a day-to-day basis. Asking these employees to perform their own performance appraisal would probably be viewed negatively rather than positively (Marquis and Huston, 1996).

In addition, employees often underrate their performance. Thus, it is not wise to allow self-evaluation to be the only form of performance appraisal. When used in conjunction with the manager's assessment, self-appraisal is an effective method of promoting further development of the employee.

Self-evaluation should be done periodically, because if we are truly honest we will find areas in which growth is needed. Ellis and Hartley (1992) suggest outlining areas you wish to evaluate and keeping notes on yourself. An analysis can reveal strengths and weaknesses. Managers should congratulate themselves on identifying strengths as well as planning how to overcome weaknesses.

◆ Performance Appraisal Tools

At various times in the history of personnel management, certain types of tools or review techniques have been popular. Each of the numerous checklists, rating scales, and job dimension scales available for performance appraisal has it own strengths and limitations. Presently, the JCAHO advocates that performance reviews be developed using the employee's job description as the standard. Although the tool selected has some bearing on objectivity, the type of appraisal form used is not as crucial as obtaining information and carrying out the appraisal interview appropriately.

A written narrative or essay is one type of appraisal tool. Most organizations use some sort of narrative, either as an addendum to printed evaluation forms or as the appraisal tool itself. This can be a lengthy essay or a summary of strengths and weaknesses. Often, it includes some type of goal setting for the employee for the coming year.

Other instrument types described by Allen and Sinesi (1996) appropriate for use in performance appraisal are graphic rating scales, forced choice rating, critical incident technique, rank order method, and paired comparison rating. Graphic rating scales are scales in which a range is given, such as satisfactory to unsatisfactory. In forced choice rating, the evaluator reviews groups of statements and determines which best fits or least fits the individual being rated. The critical incident technique requires managers to keep anecdotal notes regarding incidents considered critical to job performance. The rank order method, which has a number of variations, allows the appraiser to rank order employees on a number of job performance standards. And finally, in paired comparison rating, selected criteria are used to evaluate employees against each other.

Management by objectives (MBO) is another appraisal tool that can be used for assessing individual employee progress, as it incorporates the assessments of both the employee and the organization. In MBO, each employee (in consultation with his or her superior) determines their personal goals for the upcoming evaluation period. The employee's next appraisal then focuses on whether these goals were accomplished. Because Drucker's MBO concepts were discussed earlier in this book, the present focus will be on how these concepts are used as an effective performance appraisal method, rather than on their use as a planning technique.

McGregor (1960) probably best outlined how features of MBO can be used effectively in performance appraisal. The following steps guide the employee and supervisor in their roles.

1. The employee and supervisor meet and agree upon the primary duties and responsibilities requisite to the position of the employee. (The job description serves as a guide only, and other information may be included.)
2. The employee sets short-term goals and target dates in cooperation with the manager, who guides the process so that the goals relate to the duties of the position.
3. Both parties agree upon what criteria will be used for measuring and evaluating whether goals have been met.
4. On a regular basis (more than once a year), the employee and supervisor meet to discuss progress. At these meetings some modifications can be made if agreed on by both parties.
5. The role of the manager is supportive, assisting the employee in reaching goals by coaching and counseling.
6. During the appraisal process the manager determines whether goals have been met by the employee.
7. The entire process focuses on results and not personal traits.

Advantages of MBO identified by Marriner-Tomey (1996) are that the standard of evaluation is based on the characteristics of a specific person and job; employees have some input and control over their future; employers are aware of the standard by which they will be judged; there is a better basis for evaluation than personality traits; and it stimulates higher individual performance and morale. In addition, because employees set their own goals, they are more motivated to achieve them, defensive feelings are minimized and a spirit of teamwork prevails. In MBO, the emphasis is on the controllable present and future, rather than the uncontrollable past.

There are disadvantages to MBO as a performance appraisal method as well. Highly directive and authoritarian managers find it difficult to lead employees in this manner. Also, the marginal or demotivated employee may attempt to set easily attainable goals. Perhaps, however, the greatest disadvantage of MBO is that it is not an easy system to implement, requiring ongoing staff and managerial teaching regarding goal setting and evaluation (Marriner-Tomey, 1996).

◆ Peer Review

Another performance appraisal tool or technique is peer review. Peer review is the monitoring and assessment of performance by peers rather than by supervisors. Although the prevailing practice in most organizations is to have managers evaluate employee performance, there is much to be said for peer review.

The opinion the manager formulates of the employee may not be complete unless some type of peer review data are gathered. When implemented properly, peer review provides the employee with valuable feedback that can promote employee growth. Peer ratings are widely used by colleges and universities, as well as by physicians, but have not been as widely accepted by business and industry (Andrusyszyn, 1990).

Health care organizations have been slow to adopt peer review for the following reasons.

1. Poor orientation of staff to the peer review method. Peer review is viewed as very threatening when adequate time is not spent orienting employees to the process and when necessary support is not provided throughout.
2. Peers often feel uncomfortable sharing feedback with coworkers, so they omit necessary suggestions for improving the employee's performance. Thus, the review becomes more advocacy than evaluation.
3. It is viewed by many as more time-consuming than traditional superior–subordinate performance appraisals.
4. Because much socializing takes place in the work place, friendships often result in inflated evaluations, or interpersonal conflict may result in unfair appraisals.
5. Since it shifts the authority away from management, the insecure manager may feel threatened.

Peer review has its shortcomings, as is evidenced by some university teachers receiving unjustified tenure, or the failure of physicians to adequately maintain quality control among members of their profession. Additionally, peer review involves much risk, is time-consuming, and requires a great deal of energy. However, since performance appraisal is part of quality control, it seems reasonable to expect that nurses should have some input into the evaluation of the profession's own members.

Peer review can be carried out in several ways. It may require that reviewers share results exclusively with the individual being reviewed, or with the employee's supervisor as well. The review would never be limited to the employee's supervisor.

The results may or may not be used for personnel decisions. The frequency of observations and the number, qualifications, and classifications of peer reviewers need to be developed for each organization. If peer review is to be successful, the organization must overcome the inherent difficulties by doing the following prior to implementing a peer review program.

1. Peer review appraisal tools must reflect standards to be measured, that is, the job description.
2. Staff must receive a thorough orientation to the process prior to its implementation. The role of the manager should be clearly defined.

3. Ongoing support, resources, and information must be made available to the staff during the process.
4. Applied data needs to be obtained from uniform sources, for example, observations, charts, patient-care plans, and so on.
5. A decision must be made regarding whether anonymous feedback will be allowed. This controversial issue should be addressed in the procedure.
6. It must be decided whether the peer review will affect personnel decisions, and if so, in what manner.

Peer review has the potential to increase the accuracy of performance appraisal. It is hoped that its use in nursing will increase as the profession gains autonomy. However, unless managers fully support and encourage this type of professional, internal control it is unlikely to succeed.

◆ Difficulties with Appraisal Interviews

The most accurate and thorough appraisal will fail to produce growth in employees if the information gathered is *not* used appropriately. Many appraisal interviews have negative outcomes because managers view them only as a time to instruct employees on what they are doing wrong, rather than focusing on employee growth.

Managers often dislike the appraisal interview more than they dislike the actual data gathering for the performance appraisal. One of the reasons managers find this function so distasteful is because of their own past negative experiences with performance appraisals.

Both parties in the appraisal process tend to be anxious prior to the interview, so it is not surprising that the appraisal remains an emotionally charged event. For many employees, it also becomes a traumatizing experience. Since the manager is dealing with adults who are likely to have had previous appraisal interviews, little can be done to completely quell the anxiety created by past experiences, but care should be taken to make the current performance appraisal interview as positive as possible.

Nearly everyone agrees that performance appraisals are necessary and beneficial to both the organization and to individuals. However, *how* the information from the performance appraisal is shared, also has an impact on later performance. The appraisal interviewer must ensure that there is no threat to the individual's self-esteem, because this will circumvent possibilities for a meaningful and constructive relationship between the manager and the employee. For growth to occur in the work place, it is necessary that a constructive relationship exist.

◆ Overcoming Appraisal Interview Difficulties

Feedback is perhaps the greatest tool a manager has for changing behavior, but to be effective the feedback must be delivered in an appropriate manner. There is a greater chance that the performance appraisal will have a positive outcome if the following conditions are present prior, during, and after the interview.

PRIOR TO THE INTERVIEW

1. Ensure that the previously mentioned conditions have been met (i.e., the employee knows the standard by which work will be evaluated and has a copy of the appraisal form).
2. Select an appropriate time for the appraisal conference. Do not choose a period when the employee has just had a traumatic personal experience or when the employee is too busy for a lengthy and meaningful conference.
3. Give the employee advance notice of the scheduled appraisal conference (2 to 3 days) so that he or she can be mentally and emotionally prepared for the interview.
4. Be personally mentally and emotionally prepared for the conference, and if something should happen to interfere with your readiness for the interview, it should be canceled and rescheduled.
5. Schedule time for the interview that will be uninterrupted, and hold it in a private, quiet, and comfortable setting.
6. Plan a seating arrangement that reflects collegiality rather than power. Having the individual seated across a large desk from the appraiser implies a power-status position, but placing the chairs side-by-side infers collaborative status.

DURING THE INTERVIEW

1. Greet the employee warmly and show that you as well as the organization have a sincere interest in his or her future growth.
2. Begin the conference on a pleasant, informal note.
3. Ask the employee to comment on his or her perceived progress since the last performance appraisal.
4. Avoid surprises in the appraisal conference. The effective manager coaches and communicates informally with staff on a continuous basis, so there should be little new information given at an appraisal conference.
5. Coaching techniques should be used throughout the conference.
6. When dealing with employees with several either new or longstanding problems, the employee should not be made to feel overwhelmed at the conference. If there are too many issues to be addressed, select those that are most important.
7. Conduct the conference in a nondirective and participatory manner. Frequent input from the employee should be solicited throughout. The performance of the employee and not his or her personal characteristics must be the theme of the conference.
8. Be prepared with explicit examples of the employee's performance. Be

liberal in the positive examples, and use examples of poor performance sparingly. Use several examples only if the employee has difficulty with self-awareness and requests additional specific examples of problem areas in performance.

9. Never threaten, intimidate, or use status in any manner.

10. Let the employee know that the organization and you are aware of his or her unique qualities, special interests, and valuable contributions to the unit. Remember that all employees make some special contribution to the work place.

11. Use terminology and language that is clearly understood and carries the same meaning for both parties involved. Words that carry a negative connotation should be avoided. Do not talk down to employees or use language that is inappropriate for their level of education.

12. Goal setting for further growth or improvement in performance should be accomplished mutually, including a decision on how goals will be accomplished, how they will be evaluated, and what support is necessary in order for the employee to reach them.

13. Plan on being available for employees who wish to return later to discuss the appraisal review further. There is frequently a need for the employee to return for elaboration if the conference did not go well, or if the employee was given unexpected new information. This is especially true for the new employee.

FOLLOWING THE INTERVIEW

1. Both the manager and the employee need to sign the appraisal form to document that the conference was held and that the employee received the information given. This does not imply agreement on the part of the employee to the information contained in the appraisal. It merely documents that the employee read it. An example of such a form is shown in Display 21-1. There should be a place for comments by you and the employee.

2. End the interview on a pleasant note.

3. Document what mutual goals for further development have been agreed on by both parties. The documentation should include target dates for accomplishment, support needed, and when goals are to be reviewed. This documentation often is part of the appraisal form.

4. If the interview reveals specific long-term coaching requirements, you should develop a method of follow-up to ensure such coaching takes place.

◆ Informal Subordinate Performance Appraisal

As noted previously, the formal evaluation of the employee should not contain many surprises because the effective manager is aware that day-to-day feed-

DISPLAY 21-1
Performance Appraisal Documentation Form

Performance appraisal for:

Name: _____

Unit: _____

Prepared by: _____

Reason: _____
　　　　　　　　(Merit, terminal, end of probation, general reviews)

Date of evaluation or conference: _____

Comments by employee:

　　　　　　　　　　　　　　Employee's signature: _____

(Signature of employee indicates that the evaluation has been read. It *does not* signify acceptance and/or agreement. Space is provided for any comments employee wishes to make.)

Comments by evaluator:

(These comments are to be written at the time of the evaluation conference and in the presence of the employee.)

_____   _____   _____
Employee's signature   Date   Evaluator's signature

_____
(From Huston and Marquis, 1989.)

back regarding performance is one of the best methods for improving work performance and building a team approach. The word *coaching* has become a contemporary term to convey the spirit of the manager's role in informal day-to-day performance appraisals. Coaching techniques should also be used in the formal appraisal interview, but are especially effective for encouraging and/or correcting day-to-day work performance.

When coaching is applied in conjunction with an informal performance appraisal, the outcome is usually a positive modification of behavior. For this to occur, however, the manager must establish a climate where there is a free exchange of ideas. In order for this coaching feedback to be effective and improve the work performance, it should be delivered in the following manner, as suggested by Orth, Wilkinson, and Benfari (1990).

1. Be specific, not general, in describing behavior that needs improvement.
2. Be descriptive, not evaluative, when describing what was wrong with the work performance.
3. Be certain that the feedback is not self-serving; that it also meets the needs of the employee.
4. Direct the feedback toward behavior that can be changed.
5. Use sensitivity in timing the feedback.
6. Make sure the employee has clearly understood the feedback and that the employee's feedback has also been clearly heard.

When employees become aware of their manager's interest in their performance and personal growth, they will experience less anxiety toward the work performance appraisal. When the uneasiness that usually accompanies formal performance appraisals is reduced, the process can be more easily used to set mutual performance goals.

◆ Performance Appraisal of Managers

The manager should use three sources to assess their performance: their superior, their subordinates, and themselves. Everyone generally has someone overseeing their performance. For example, the top-level nursing director may answer to the CEO, the CEO to the board of trustees, and the board of trustees to the community. Normally, the individual who carries out performance appraisals of managers is the one directly above them in the organizational hierarchy.

Subordinates should also be involved in some manner in the performance appraisal of their managers. Unfortunately, this is rarely the case in health care organizations. In academia, however, positive results are frequently achieved as a result of teacher evaluation by students. Likewise, such benefits should be obtained when employees have input into the performance appraisals of their supervisors. It is important, however, to remember that because subordinates rarely possess a full perspective or appreciation for the complete demands of being a supervisor, their ratings should constitute only a portion of the input that comprises a supervisor's performance appraisal. However, such valuable input is totally ignored in most organizations.

◆ Summary

Performance appraisal is a major responsibility in the controlling function of management. Although performance appraisal is never easy, if used appropriately, it produces growth in the employee and increases productivity in the organization.

It is imperative that managers use a formalized system of appraisal and gather data regarding employee performance in a systematic manner, using many sources. The manager should attempt to be as objective as possible, using established standards for the appraisal. The result of the process should provide the manager with the necessary information for meeting training and educational needs of employees. By following up conscientiously on identified performance deficiencies, the manager is able to correct problems before they become habits.

Managers aware of their own biases and prejudices will gravitate toward fairness and honesty in evaluating performance. This, in turn, increases trust in the employees and promotes a team spirit and increased motivation.

Use of day-to-day coaching techniques improves work performance and reduces the anxiety of work performance appraisal. When anxiety is reduced during the appraisal interview the manager establishes a relationship conducive to mutual goal setting, which has a greater potential to result in increased motivation and the correction of deficiencies.

◆ References

Allen RB and Sinesi LA (1996). As found in Decision Making in Nursing. Jones R and Beck S (eds). Albany, NY: Delmar Publishers

Andrusyszyn MA (1990). Faculty evaluation: a closer look at peer review. Nurse Educ Today 10(6):410–414

Ellis JR and Hartley CL (1992). Nursing in Today's World, 4th ed. Philadelphia: JB Lippincott

Huston CJ and Marquis BL (1989). Retention and Productivity Strategies for Nurse Managers. Philadelphia: JB Lippincott

Marquis BL and Huston CJ (1996). Leadership Roles and Management Functions in Nursing. 2nd ed. Philadelphia: JB Lippincott

Marriner-Tomey A (1996). Guide to Nursing Management and Leadership, 5th ed. St. Louis: Mosby

McGregor D (1960). The Human Side of Enterprise. New York: McGraw-Hill

Orth CD, Wilkinson HE, and Benfari RC (1990). The manager's role as coach and mentor. J Nurs Admin 20(9):11–15

SAMPLE CASE ANALYSIS

THE CASE ◆

It is time for Nancy Irwin's annual performance appraisal. She is an RN on a postsurgical unit, dealing with complex trauma patients requiring high-level nursing intensity. You are the evening charge nurse and have worked with Ms. Irwin for the 2 years since she has graduated from nursing school. Last year, in addition to the regular 1–5 rating scale for job expectations, all the charge nurses added an MBO component to the performance appraisal form. Each employee developed five goals, in collaboration with his or her charge nurse, that were supposed to have been carried out over a 1-year period.

In reviewing Ms. Irwin's performance, you use several sources, including your written notes and her charting, and your conclusion is that with her strengths and weaknesses, overall, she is a better-than-average nurse. However, you believe she has not grown much as an employee over the past 6 months. This observation is confirmed by a review of the following:

Objective	Result
1. Conduct a mini inservice or patient-care conference twice monthly for the next 12 months.	Met goal first 2 months. Last 10 months conducted only six conferences.
2. Will attend five educational classes related to work area; at least one of these will be given by an outside agency.	Attended one surgical nursing wound conference in the city and one in-house conference on TPN.
3. Will become an active member of a nursing committee at the hospital.	Has become an active member of the Policies and Procedures Committee and regularly attends meetings.
4. Reduce the number of late arrivals at work by 50% (from 24 per year to 12).	First 3 months: not late. Second 3 months: 3 late arrivals. Third 3 months: 6 late arrivals. Last 3 months: 6 late arrivals.
5. Ensure that all patients discharged have discharge instructions documented in their charts.	Anecdotal notes show that Ms. Irwin still frequently forgets to document these nursing actions.

Assignment

As Ms. Irwin's charge nurse, what can you do to ensure that the current appraisal results in greater growth for her? What went wrong with last year's MBO plan? Devise a plan for the performance appraisal.

Analysis

This case could have several different approaches depending on whether motivation or change theory or another rationale was being implemented to support the decisions. In reality, a manager may employ several different theories in order to increase productivity. However, this case will be solved using only performance appraisal techniques in order to demonstrate that they can also serve as an effective method to control productivity.

SAMPLE CASE ANALYSIS (CONTINUED)

There are several aspects that seem to stand out in the information presented in this case. First, it appears that Ms. Irwin is a person who needs to be reminded. She functions well in objective #3 because she received monthly reminders of the meetings and because she worked with a group of people she was able to make a real contribution to this committee.

The similarities among the other four objectives are that they all required Ms. Irwin to 1) work alone to accomplish them and 2) there were no built-in reminders. Rather than applying this performance appraisal critically, the charge nurse should expend her energy in developing a plan to help Ms. Irwin succeed in the coming months. Nothing is as depressing or demotivating to an employee as failure.

The following plan concentrates only on the MBO portion of Ms. Irwin's performance appraisal and does not center on the rating scale of job performance.

PRIOR TO THE INTERVIEW	RATIONALE
1. Ask Ms. Irwin to review her objectives from last year and to come prepared to discuss them.	1. Gives the employee opportunity for individual problem solving and personal introspection.
2. Set a convenient time for you and Ms. Irwin and allow adequate time and privacy.	2. Shows interest in, and respect for the employee.

AT THE INTERVIEW	RATIONALE
1. Begin by complimenting Nancy on objective #4. Ask her about her work on the committee; what procedures she is working on, and so forth.	1. Shows interest in and support of employee.
2. Review each of the other four objectives and ask for Ms. Irwin's input. Withhold any advice or criticism at this point.	2. Allows the employee to make her own judgments about her performance.
3. Ask Ms. Irwin if she sees a pattern.	3. Guide the employee into problem solving on her own.
4. Tell Ms. Irwin that MBO often works better if objectives are reviewed on a more timely basis and ask how she feels about this.	4. This is an offer to assist the employee in achieving improved performance and is not a punitive measure. It allows the employee to have input.
5. Suggest that she keep her unmet four objectives and add one new one.	5. Employees should be encouraged to meet objectives unless they were stated poorly or were unrealistic.
6. Work with Ms. Irwin in developing a reminder or check point system that will assist her in meeting her objectives.	6. Again this is helping the employee to succeed. Do not simply tell employees that they should do better; help them identify how.
7. Do not sympathize or excuse her for not meeting objectives.	7. The focus should remain on growth and not on the *status quo*.
8. End on a note of encouragement and support. "I know that you are capable of meeting these objectives."	8. Employees often live up to their manager's expectations of them, and if those expectations are for growth, then the chances are greater that it will occur.

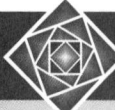 C A S E S   F O R   P R O B L E M   S O L V I N G

CASE 1

Mrs. Merrill is a new LVN-LPN and has been working 3:00–11:00 P.M. on the unit where you are the P.M. charge nurse. It is time for her 3-month performance appraisal. In the facility where you are employed, each employee's job description is used as the standard of measure for job performance appraisal.

Essentially, you feel Mrs. Merrill is performing her job well, but are somewhat concerned because she still relies on the RNs for even minor decisions regarding patient care. Although you are glad that she does not act completely on her own, you would like to see her become more independent. The patients have commented favorably to you on Mrs. Merrill's compassion as well as on her follow through on all their requests and needs.

Mrs. Merrill gets along well with the other LVNs-LPNs and you sometimes believe they take advantage of her hardworking and pleasant nature. On a few occasions you felt they inappropriately delegated some of their work to her.

In preparing for Mrs. Merrill's upcoming evaluation, what can you do to make the appraisal as objective as possible? This will be her first evaluation and you want it to be growth producing.

Assignment

Plan how you will proceed. What positive forces are already present in this scenario? What negative forces will you have to overcome? Support your plan with readings from the bibliography.

CASE 2 (Marquis and Huston, 1996)

You are a middle-level manager in a public health department. One of your closest friends, Janie Forrest, is a registered nurse under your span of control. Today, she called you and told you that she injured her back yesterday during a home visit, after she slipped on a wet front porch. She said that the homeowners were unaware that she fell and there were no witnesses to the accident. She states that she has just returned from her doctor's office and that he is advising 6 weeks of bed rest to allow her back to heal. She requests that you initiate the paperwork for workmen's compensation insurance and disability, as she has no sick days available.

Shortly after your telephone conversation with Ms. Forrest, you decide to take a brief coffee break in the lounge. While there, you overhear a conversation between Jon and Lacey, two additional staff in your department. Jon states that he and Janie were waterskiing last night, when she took a terrible fall, hurting her back. He planned to call her as soon as he finished his break to see how she was feeling.

Your initial response is to feel hurt and betrayed by Ms. Forrest, because she has lied to you. Your second response is to call her and confront her with her dishonesty. You are angry that she has placed you in this position. You are also aware that it may be difficult to prove that the injury is not work-related.

CASE 2 (CONTINUED)

Assignment

1. How should you proceed?
2. In what way (if any) is this case related to performance appraisal?
3. Would it be appropriate to have a conference with Janie? Outline your plan and support your position with your rationale.

CASE 3

Tom Morgan is an LVN-LPN who has been employed on your unit for 10 years. He is a middle-aged man supporting a large family and it is common knowledge that he moonlights at a nursing home on his days off. His work is generally of high quality, but in reviewing his past performance appraisals you notice that in the last 4 years at each evaluation he has been rated unsatisfactory for being on duty promptly, as well as for not attending staff development programs. Since you are the new 3:00–11:00 P.M. charge nurse, you would like to be able to improve Mr. Morgan's performance in these two areas.

You have given him a copy of the evaluation tool and job description and have scheduled his appraisal conference for 10:00 P.M., when the unit will be quiet and you can go into the conference room.

Assignment

How would you conduct this performance appraisal? Outline your plan, including how you would begin. What innovative or creative approach would you employ to provide direction or improvement in the mentioned areas, and how would you terminate the session? Be able to give the rationale for your decisions.

CASE 4

You have been with Mercy Hospital since your graduation from nursing school. Your roommate at school, Dina Post, has also worked at Mercy since her graduation. For the first year you and Ms. Post were assigned to different units, but 6 months ago you both received a transfer to the oncology unit. You both work 3:00–11:00 P.M., and it is the policy for the charge nurse duties to alternate among three RNs assigned to the unit on a full-time basis. Both you and Ms. Post are among those assigned to rotate to the charge position. You have been very much aware lately that when your friend Ms. Post is "in charge" her personality seems to change. She barks orders and seems tense and anxious. She is an excellent clinical nurse, and many of the staff seek her consultation regarding patient care problems. However, you have heard several of the staff grumbling about her behavior when she is in her supervisory mode. As Ms. Post's good friend you do not want to hurt her feelings, but as her professional colleague you feel a need to share your perceptions with her.

CASE 4 (CONTINUED)

....

Assignment

Describe what you would do, how you would set up a meeting, and what you would do and say. Be able to justify your decisions in this matter.

✻ Bibliography

The following bibliography will assist you in solving these cases:

Ackerman N (1991). Effective peer review. Nursing Manage 22(8):48

Basford P (1991). How to . . . use individual performance review. Nurs Times 87(27):59

Beck S (1990). Developing a primary nursing performance appraisal tool. Nurs Manage 21(1):36–38

Bice M (1990). Employee rewards can pay off for hospitals. Hospitals 64(12):56

Buechlein-Telutki MS, Bilak Y, Merrick M, Reich M, and Stein D (1993). Nurse manager performance appraisal: a collaborative approach. Nursing Manage 24(10):48–50

Casebeer L (1990). Personnel decisions: "wheeling" toward better performance. Nurs Manage 21(8):42–44

del Bueno DJ (1990). Evaluation: myths, mystiques, and obsessions. J Nurs Admin 20(10):10–55

Farh J, Cannella A, and Bedeian A (1991). Peer ratings: the impact of purpose in rating quality and user acceptance. Group Organ Stud 16(4):367–386

Gill D and Kendall ER (1994). The abolishment of performance appraisals: Parkview's story. Jt. Comm J Qual Improv 20:669–678

Hoeppner M and Schneller S (1995). Coaching: the staff nurse committee member. Nurs Manage 26(1):53

Kanin-Lovers J and Bevan R (1992). Don't evaluate performance—manage it. J Comp Ben 7(5):51–53

Lukes En (1993). Peformance appraisal: a motivational tool. AAOHN J 41(12):599–600

McConnell TR (1994). Surviving your next performance appraisal. Leadership Health Serv 3(5):42–43

McGee K (1992). Making performance appraisals a positive experience. Nurs Manage 23(8):36–37

McMurray C (1993). Performance appraisal: a measure of effectiveness. Nurs Manage 24(11):94–95

Metgzer NJ (1990). Evaluating supplemental professional nurses. Nurs Manage 21(1):54–55

Pennock D (1992). Effective performance appraisals (really!) Supervision 53(8):14–16

Rosen DI (1992). Appraisals can make or break your court case. Pers J 57(11):81–85

Selvey C (1991). Clinical evaluation day: measuring competency. Nurs Manage 22(4):50–51

Smith ML (1993). Defensible performance appraisals. J Manage Eng 9(2):128–135

Van Slyck A (1991). A systems approach to the management of nursing services: productivity monitoring system, part 4. Nurs Manage 22(6):18–20

PERSONAL NOTEBOOK

1. During your lifetime you have probably had many performance appraisals. These may have been evaluations of your clinical performance during nursing school or as a paid employee. Reflect back on these appraisals; how many of them encompassed the recommendations listed in the text?

2. How did the inclusion or exclusion of these recommendations influence your acceptance of the appraisal?

3. Describe what you perceive as your most constructive performance appraisal.

4. Describe what you perceive as your most destructive performance appraisal.

Discipline and Coaching

The coordination and cooperation necessary to meet organizational goals require that managers control the individual urges of subordinates that are counterproductive to these goals. The manager does this by enforcing established rules, policies, and procedures. Subordinates do this by maintaining self-control.

When employees are unsuccessful in meeting organizational goals, the manager must attempt to identify the reasons for this failure and counsel the employee accordingly. If employees fail because they are unable to follow rules or established policies and procedures, or if they are unable to perform their duties adequately despite assistance and encouragement, the manager has an obligation to discipline the employee.

◆ Constructive versus Destructive Discipline

Scientific management viewed discipline as a necessary means for controlling an "unmotivated and self-centered work force." Because of this philosophy about humans and organizations, managers employed threats and fear as the primary means of controlling behavior. Cautionary written warnings of termination were rampant and the employee was always alert to an impending penalty or termination. This "big stick" approach to management focused on eliminating all behavior that could be considered in conflict with organizational goals, without regard for employee growth. Although this method may succeed on a short-term basis, it is demotivating and reduces productivity over the long term. This occurs because individuals will achieve only at the level they feel is necessary to avoid punishment. This approach is also destructive and demoralizing as discipline is often administered arbitrarily, and is unfair either in the application of rules or in the resulting punishment.

Constructive discipline is used as a means of helping the employee grow, and not as a punitive measure. In fact, the origin of the word "discipline" comes from the Latin term "disciplina," which means teaching, learning (Lewis and Spicer, 1987). Punishment may be applied for improper behavior in constructive discipline, but this is carried out in a supportive, corrective manner. The employee is reassured that the given punishment is a result of their actions, and not because of who they are as a person.

The primary emphasis in constructive discipline is in assisting employees to behave in a manner that allows them to be self-directed in meeting organizational goals. Before employees can focus energy on meeting organizational goals, they must feel secure in the work place. This security develops only when staff know and understand organizational rules and penalties and when rules are applied in a fair and consistent manner. In an environment that promotes constructive discipline, employees are generally self-disciplined to conform with established rules and regulations and the primary role of the manager becomes that of coordinator and helper, rather than enforcer.

◆ Self-Discipline

The highest level and most effective form of discipline is self-discipline. In self-discipline, rules are internalized and become a part of the individual's personality (Curtin, 1996). Ideally, all employees should have adequate self-control and should be self-directed in their pursuit of organizational goals. Unfortunately, this is not always the case.

Although self-discipline is internalized, the manager can play an active role in developing an environment that promotes it. Health Care Education Associates (1987) identified four factors that must be present to foster a climate of self-discipline. The first of these factors is *employee awareness and understanding of rules and regulations that govern behavior.* These must be clearly written and communicated to subordinates. Young and Hayne (1988) stated that the most common reason for unsatisfactory work performance is that employees think they are performing satisfactorily. In other words, the employee does not know there is a problem, frequently because of a lack of feedback. Managers must discuss rules, policies, and procedures with subordinates, explain the rationale for their existence, and encourage questions. It is impossible for an employee to have self-control if he or she does not understand what are acceptable boundaries for his or her behavior. Likewise, an individual cannot be self-directed if they do not understand what is expected.

Another factor that must exist is *an atmosphere of mutual trust.* Managers must believe that employees are capable of, and actively seeking self-discipline. Likewise, employees must perceive the manager as honest and trustworthy. Employees often lack the security for self-discipline if they do not trust their manager's motives.

The third factor is that *formal authority must be used judiciously.* If formal discipline is quickly and widely used, subordinates are not given the opportunity for self-discipline.

Another important factor in self-discipline is that *employees should identify with the goals of the organization.* When the employees accept the goals and objectives of an organization, they are more likely to accept the standards of conduct deemed acceptable by that organization.

◆ Fair and Effective Rules

There are several rules that should be followed if employees are to perceive the manager's purpose for discipline as growth and not retaliation. This does not imply that subordinates enjoy being disciplined, or that discipline should be a regular means of promoting employee growth. However, if implemented correctly it should not result in permanent alienation and demoralization of a subordinate.

McGregor (1967) developed a set of rules for enforcing discipline so as to make it as fair and growth producing as possible. These rules were called "hot stove rules" because they can be compared to someone touching a hot stove. The following rules explain his theory:

1. All individuals must be *forewarned* that if they touch the hot stove (i.e., break a rule), they will be burned (punished or disciplined). They must know the rule beforehand and be aware of the punishment.
2. If the individual touches the stove (i.e., breaks a rule), there will be *immediate* consequences (getting burned). All discipline should be administered immediately after rules are broken.
3. If the individual touches the stove again, he or she will again be burned. Therefore, there is *consistency.* Each time the rule is broken, there are immediate and consistent consequences.
4. If any other individual touches the hot stove, he or she will also get burned. Discipline must be *impartial* and everyone must be treated in the same manner if the rule breaking is the same.

Unfortunately, most rule breaking is not enforced using McGregor's rules. For example, many individuals exceed the speed limit when driving. Generally, individuals are aware of speed limits and signs are posted along the roadway to remind individuals of the regulations. Thus, there is forewarning. However, there is no immediacy, consistency, or impartiality. Many individuals exceed the speed limit for long periods of time before they are stopped and disciplined, or they may never be disciplined at all. Likewise, an individual may be stopped and disciplined one day and not the next, even though the same rule is broken. Finally, the punishment is inconsistent in that some individuals are punished for their rule breaking and others are not. Even the penalty different individuals pay may not be the same.

Continuing with this example, imagine that someday automobiles will be developed that require the driver to place a built-in electronic sensor on the end of his or her finger before the automobile will operate. The purpose of this sensor would be to deliver a low level, but painful, electrical shock to the driver every time his or her car exceeds the posted speed limit. The driver would be forewarned regarding the consequence of breaking the speed limit rule. If each time the rule was broken the driver immediately received an electrical shock, and if all automobiles included this feature, it is the contention of the authors that speeding would be virtually eliminated.

If a rule or regulation is worthwhile, it should be enforced (Marquis and Huston, 1996). When broken rules go unpunished, groups generally adjust to and replicate the behavior of the rule breaker. Likewise, the average worker's natural inclination to obey rules can be dissipated by lax or inept enforcement policies, leading employees to develop contempt for managers who allow rules to be disregarded. The enforcement of rules using McGregor's guide for rule fairness keeps morale from disintegrating and allows for structure within the organization.

However, there should be as few rules or regulations as possible, and all of them should be reviewed on a regular basis to see if they should be deleted or modified in some way. If managers find themselves spending all their time enforcing one particular rule, it would be wise to reexamine it and to consider whether there is something wrong with the rule or how it is communicated.

◆ Discipline as a Progressive Process

Occasionally, employees continue to display undesirable conduct, either by breaking rules, or inadequate job performance. Further action should be taken in these situations. Managers have the authority and the responsibility to take progressively stronger measures when employees continue to fail to meet expected standards of achievement. Most progressive discipline systems utilize the following steps.

1. Generally, the first step of the disciplinary process is the *informal reprimand* or *verbal admonishment.* This reprimand includes an informal meeting between the employee and the manager to discuss the broken rule or performance deficiency. This meeting is always done in private. Suggestions are given to the employee on how his or her behavior might be altered to keep the rule from being broken again. Often, informal reprimand is all that is needed for behavior modification. Because no written record is placed in the employee's file, and the meeting is in private, the manager may want to make a private anecdotal record to prove that a verbal reprimand was given (Marriner-Tomey, 1996). Too formal an approach to handling minor offenses, however, can be counterproductive.

2. The second step is a *formal reprimand* or *written admonishment.* If the undesired behavior recurs after a verbal admonishment, the manager again meets with the employee and issues a formal written warning about the behaviors that must be corrected. This warning is very specific about what rules or policies have been violated, as well as what the

consequences will be if behavior is not altered to meet the expectations of the organization. The written admonishment should include any reference to prior informal reprimands, an employee explanation of the incident(s) in question, a plan of action to achieve the expected change or improvement, and employee feedback regarding that plan (Health Care Education Associates, 1987). Display 22-1 depicts a form that could be used for a written reprimand. Both the employee and the manager should sign the written warning. One copy is then given to the employee and another is retained in the employee's personnel file.

3. The third step in progressive discipline is usually a *suspension from work without pay*. If an employee continues the undesired behavior despite verbal and written warnings, the manager should remove the employee from his or her job for a brief period of time, generally a few days to several weeks.

4. The last step in progressive discipline is *involuntary termination* or *dismissal*. Termination should always be the last resort in dealing with poor performance. However, if the manager has given repeated warnings, and the employee continues to break rules or violate policy, the employee should be terminated. Although this is difficult and traumatic for the employee, the manager, and the unit as well, the costs involved in keeping such an employee in the organization in terms of managerial and employee time and unit morale are enormous.

In using progressive discipline it is important to remember that the steps are followed progressively only for repeated infractions of the same rule. For example, even though an employee has received a prior formal reprimand for an unexcused absence, discipline for a first-time offense of tardiness should begin at the first step of the process. It is also important to remember that although discipline is generally administered progressively, some rule breaking is so serious that the employee may be suspended or dismissed with the first infraction. Table 22-1 presents a guide of progressive discipline for specific offenses for managers.

Another critical aspect of using progressive discipline is that, in all but the most serious infractions, the slate be wiped clean after a predesignated period. There is little justification for perpetually holding infractions against employees if they have since modified their behavior.

◆ Principles of Disciplinary Action

It is vital that managers recognize the power they hold in evaluating and correcting the behavior of the employee. Because an individual's job is very important to him or her (often a factor in self-esteem, as well as livelihood), disciplining or taking away an individual's job is a very serious action and should not be taken lightly. There are several principles the manager should follow to ensure that discipline is fair and produces growth.

DISPLAY 22-1
Sample Written Reprimand Form

Employee name _____

Position _____ Date of hire _____

Person completing report _____

Position _____ Date report completed _____

Date of incident(s) _____ Time _____

Description of incident:

Prior attempts to counsel employee regarding this behavior (cite date and results of disciplinary conferences):

Disciplinary contract (plan for correction) and time frame:

Consequences of future repetition:

Employee comments (additional documentation or rebuttal may be attached):

_____   _____
Signature of individual   Employee signature
making the report

_____   _____
Date   Date

Date and time of follow-up appointment to review disciplinary contract:

TABLE 22-1
Suggested Guide to Disciplinary Actions

Offense	First Infraction	Second Infraction	Third Infraction	Fourth Infraction
Gross mistreatment of a patient.	Dismissal			
Discourtesy to a patient.	Verbal admonishment	Written admonishment	Suspension	Dismissal
Insubordination.	Written admonishment	Suspension	Dismissal	
Use of intoxicants while on duty.	Dismissal			
Neglect of duty.	Verbal admonishment	Written admonishment	Suspension	Dismissal
Theft or willful damage of property.	Written admonishment or dismissal	Dismissal		
Falsehood.	Verbal admonishment	Written admonishment	Dismissal	
Unauthorized absence.	Verbal admonishment	Written admonishment	Dismissal	
Abuse of leave.	Verbal admonishment	Written admonishment	Suspension	Dismissal
Deliberate violation of instruction.	Verbal admonishment	Written admonishment	Suspension	Dismissal
Violation of safety rules.	Verbal admonishment	Written admonishment	Dismissal	
Fighting.	Verbal admonishment	Written admonishment	Suspension	Dismissal
Inability to maintain work standards.	Verbal admonishment	Written admonishment	Suspension	Dismissal
Excessive unexcused tardiness.*	Verbal admonishment	Written admonishment	Dismissal	

* The first, second, and third infractions do not mean the first, second, and third time an employee is late, but the first, second, and third time that unexcused tardiness becomes excessive as determined by the manager.

1. The first principle the manager must follow is to *thoroughly investigate* the situation that has prompted the need for discipline. Has the employee been involved in a situation like this before? Was he or she disciplined for it, and what was the reaction to the corrective action? How serious or potentially serious is the current problem or infraction? Who else was involved in the situation? Does this employee have a history of other types of disciplinary problems? What is the quality of this employee's work performance? Have other employees in the organization also broken this rule? How were they disciplined? Could there be a problem with the rule or policy? Were there any special circumstances that could have contributed to the problem in this situation? What disciplinary action is suggested by organizational policies for this type of offense? Will this type of disciplinary action keep the infraction from recurring? Wise managers will ask themselves all of these questions so that a fair decision can be reached about an appropriate course of action.

2. Another principle of disciplinary action is that *the manager should attempt to recognize unacceptable behaviors early and counsel the employee as soon as a problem is suspected.* "An employee does not usually come to a job performing badly (he or she would not have been hired in the first place), but rather *develops* unacceptable patterns of behavior" (Young and Hayne, 1988). Disciplinary problems, if unrecognized or ignored, generally do not go away; they get worse.

3. The wise manager will also adhere to a policy of *always consulting with a superior or the personnel department prior to dismissing an employee.* Most organizations have very clear policies about which actions constitute grounds for dismissal, as well as how that dismissal should be handled. In an effort to protect oneself from charges of willful or discriminatory termination, managers should carefully document the behavior(s) that occurred, as well as any attempts to counsel the employee.

   It is important to remember that some employees overreact and become aggressive or defensive in response to disciplinary feedback. This often occurs as a result of a basic mistrust of the employer's motives. In return, the manager, who may feel threatened or challenged, may overreact and threaten excessive discipline such as unwarranted suspension or termination (Davidhizar and Vance, 1996). Discussing highly charged disciplinary situations with a superior often helps managers view situations more objectively and less personally so that an appropriate disciplinary decision can be made.

4. A fourth principle of disciplinary action is that *privacy must be maintained.* Because such action may adversely affect the ego of the employee, all discipline, even informal admonishments, should be done in private. Although the manager should administer feedback to the employee as soon as the rule breaking or inappropriate behavior has occurred, it is never acceptable to do this in front of patients or peers. The manager must also be careful not to discuss the reasons for terminating one employee with others, or to make negative comments regarding past employees, which may discourage other employees or reduce their trust. By helping the employee save face, there is less possibility of future resentment and a greater chance for future cooperation.

5. It is recommended that the manager learn to *discipline the employee's actions, not the employee as a person.* When disciplining an employee, the manager should emphasize that it was the act that was unacceptable, not the employee as a person (Marriner-Tomey, 1996).

6. The prudent manager will also follow a policy to *carefully document all*

counseling and disciplinary efforts. Obviously, the more objective, specific, and complete the documentation, the better for all parties involved. This type of documentation does not occur automatically.

◆ Ongoing and Problem-Centered Coaching

Another strategy that can be used by the manager in discipline and limit setting is performance-deficiency coaching. *Coaching* means one person helping the other to reach an optimum level of performance. The emphasis is always on assisting the person in recognizing greater options, in clarifying statements, and in encouraging personal growth.

Coaching may be ongoing or problem centered. In *ongoing coaching,* the manager provides immediate, ongoing feedback to employees. This spontaneous coaching is generally viewed as helpful by the employee and not as a criticism of their ability. Because the role of the coach is less threatening than that of enforcer, the manager has the opportunity to become a supporter, enabler, and helper.

Problem-centered or performance-deficiency coaching is less spontaneous and requires more managerial planning than ongoing coaching. In this type, the manager actively brings areas of unacceptable behavior or performance to the attention of the employee and works with them to establish a short-term plan of correction. Orth, Wilkinson, and Benfari (1990) stated that performance-deficiency coaching should not be viewed as a one-time way of solving problems, but as a way of helping employees, over time, improve (change) their performance (behavior and results) to the highest level of which they are capable. As such, the development, use, and mastery of performance-deficiency coaching should result in improved performance for all. The scenario depicted in Display 22-2 is an example of performance-deficiency coaching.

When coaching is unsuccessful in modifying employee behavior, the manager must take more aggressive steps and use more formal disciplinary measures.

◆ The Disciplinary Conference

After having thoroughly investigated the employee's offense, the manager must confront the employee with his or her findings. This occurs in the form of a disciplinary conference. Health Care Education Associates (1987) have identified the following steps in the disciplinary conference.

1. *State the problem clearly and specifically and refer to previous discussions of the rule violation.* It is important in this situation that the manager not be hesitant or apologetic. Novice nursing managers often feel uncomfortable with the disciplinary process and may provide unclear or mixed messages to the employee regarding the nature or seriousness of a dis-

DISPLAY 22-2
Performance-Deficiency Coaching Scenario

Coach: I am concerned that you have been regularly coming into report late. This interrupts the other employees who are trying to hear report and creates overtime as the night shift must stay and repeat report on the patients you missed. It also makes it difficult for your modular team members to prioritize their plan of care for the day if the entire team is not there and ready to begin at 0700. Why is this problem occurring?

Employee: I've been having problems lately with an unreliable babysitter and my car not starting. It seems like it's always one thing or another and I'm upset about not getting to work on time too. I hate starting my day off behind the eight ball.

Coach: This hospital has a longstanding policy on attendance and it is one of the criteria that is used to judge work performance on your performance appraisal.

Employee: Yes, I know. I'm just not sure what I can do about it right now.

Coach: What approaches have you tried in resolving these problems?

Employee: Well, I'm buying a new car, so that should take care of my transportation problems. I'm not sure about my babysitter though. She's young and not very responsible, so she'll call me at the last minute and tell me she's not coming. I keep her though because she's willing to work the flexible hours and days that this job requires and she doesn't charge as much as a formal day care center would.

Coach: Do you have family in the area or close friends you can count on to help with child care on short notice?

Employee: Yes, my mother lives a few blocks away and is always glad to help, but I couldn't count on her on a regular basis.

Coach: There are employment registry lists at the local college for students interested in providing child care. Have you thought about trying this option? Often, students can work flexible hours and charge less than formal day care centers.

Employee: That's a good idea. In fact, I just heard about a child care referral service that could also give me a few ideas. I'll stop there after work. I realize that my behavior has affected unit functioning and I promise to try to work this out as soon as possible.

Coach: I'm sure these problems can be corrected. Let's have a follow-up visit in 2 weeks to see how things are going.

ciplinary problem. Managers must assume the authority given to them by their role; a major responsibility in this role is evaluating employee performance and suggesting appropriate action for improved or acceptable performance.

2. *Get input from the employee regarding why there has been no improvement.* It is always important to give the employee an opportunity to explain any limiting or extraneous factors that you may not be aware of. Allowing employees to provide feedback in the disciplinary process

assures them recognition as a human being and reassures them that your ultimate goal is to be fair and promote employee growth.

3. *Explain the disciplinary action you are going to take and why.* Although the manager must keep an open mind to new information that may be gathered in step 2, you should have made some preliminary assessments regarding the disciplinary action that is appropriate for the offense. This discipline should be communicated to the employee. The employee who has been previously counseled should not be surprised at the punishment to be given, as the ramifications of future rule breaking should have been discussed at the last conference.

4. *Describe the behavioral change that is expected and list the steps needed to achieve this change. Explain what the consequences of failure to change will be.* Again, it is important that the manager not be apologetic or hesitant. This will create confusion in the employee's mind about the gravity of the rule breaking. Employees who have repeatedly broken rules need firm direction, as they lack self-control. It must be very clear to the employee that follow-up will occur in a timely manner.

5. *Obtain agreement and acceptance of the plan. Let the employee know that you are interested in him or her as a person, and give your support.* Because discipline is aimed toward promoting employee growth, rather than just punishment, the manager must be a humanist. Although the expected standards must be very clear, the manager should impart a sense of genuine concern for and desire to help the employee grow. This approach helps the employee recognize that the discipline is directed at the offensive behavior and not at the individual. The manager must be cautious, however, not to relinquish the management role in an effort to nurture and become a counselor for the employee. The manager's role is to provide a supportive environment and structure so that the employee can make the necessary changes.

In addition to understanding what should be covered in the disciplinary conference, the manager must be sensitive to when the discipline should be administered. If more than an informal admonishment is required, the manager should inform the employee of the unacceptable action and then schedule a formal disciplinary conference for further discussion later.

All formal disciplinary conferences should be scheduled in advance at a time agreeable to both the employee and the manager. The employee will want time to reflect on the situation, as will the manager. Allowing this lag time should reduce the emotional intensity of the situation. It also promotes self-discipline on the part of the employee, as he or she is more apt to have had the chance to construct a plan for keeping the behavior from recurring.

Besides advance scheduling, the length of the disciplinary conference also is important. It should neither be so long that it degenerates into a debate, nor so short that both the employee and manager cannot adequately state their position. The facts of the situation should be examined and each party should provide input. If the employee seems overly emotional, or if there are great discrepancies between the perception of the manager and that of the employee, an additional conference should be scheduled. Employees often need time to absorb what they have been told and to develop a plan that is not defensive in nature.

◆ The Termination Conference

On occasion, the disciplinary conference must also be a termination conference. Although many of the principles are the same, the termination conference differs from a disciplinary conference in that planning for future improvement is eliminated. The following steps should be followed in the termination conference.

1. *Calmly state the facts of the situation, and explain the reasons for termination.* It is important that the manager not appear angry or defensive. Although he or she may express regret that the outcome is termination, the manager must not dwell on this or give the employee reason to think that the decision is not final. The manager should be prepared to give examples of the behavior(s) in question.
2. *Explain the termination process.* State the date of termination, as well as the role of the employee and the organization in the process.
3. *Ask for employee input and respond calmly and openly.* Listen to the employee, but do not allow yourself to be drawn emotionally into his or her anger or sorrow. Always stay focused on the facts of the case.
4. *End the meeting on a positive note if possible.* It is important that the manager express confidence in the employee and wish him or her success in the future. The manager should also inform the employee what, if any, references will be supplied to prospective employers in the future. Finally, it is usually best to allow the employee who has been terminated to leave the organization immediately, since it can be demoralizing for everyone who works there (Health Care Education Associates, 1987).

◆ Disciplining the Unionized Employee

It is hoped that all managers would be fair and consistent in disciplining employees regardless of whether there is a union present. The presence of a union does, however, usually entail more procedural and legal safeguards in administering discipline, as well as a well-defined grievance process for employees who feel they have been disciplined unfairly.

For example, the manager of nonunionized employees has greater latitude in selecting which disciplinary measure is appropriate for a specific infraction. This gives the manager greater flexibility and latitude, but may result in an inconsistency of discipline among employees. On the other hand, unionized employees generally must be disciplined according to specific, preestablished steps and penalties within an established time frame. For example, the union contract may be very clear that an unexcused absence from work initially must be disciplined by a written reprimand, followed by a 3-day suspension from work, and then termination. This type of discipline structure is generally fairer to the employee, but allows little flexibility for the manager in evaluating the extenuating circumstances of each case.

Another aspect of discipline that may differ between unionized and nonunionized employees is the need for management to follow *due process* in disciplining union employees. Due process means that management must provide union employees with a written statement outlining disciplinary charges, the resulting penalty, and reasons for the penalty. The employee then has the right to defend him- or herself against such charges and to settle any disagreement through formal grievance hearings.

Another difference between unionized and nonunionized employee discipline lies in the burden of proof. In disciplinary situations with union employees, the burden of proof for the wrongdoing and the need for subsequent discipline falls on management. This means that managers disciplining union employees must keep detailed records regarding misconduct and attempts to counsel employees. In nonunionized employees, the burden of proof may fall to the employee.

Union contracts generally recognize the right of employees to submit grievances when they feel these actions have been taken unfairly or are discriminatory in some way. Each manager must know all union contract provisions regarding discipline that may affect how discipline is administered on the unit.

◆ Grievances as a Result of Disciplinary Action

Growth from discipline can only occur when employees perceive that the constructive feedback given and disciplinary action taken is fair and just. When the employee's perceptions of equitable discipline differ from the managers, most nonunion and virtually all unionized organizations have an established procedure that must be followed to resolve the discrepancy. This *grievance* procedure, as it is called, is essentially a procedure to follow when one feels that a wrong has been committed (Huston and Marquis, 1989). The grievance procedure is not limited to resolving disciplinary discrepancies, and can be used by an employee on any occasion in which an employee feels that he or she has been treated unfairly by management.

Grievances should, however, meet the following criteria to be considered valid.

1. The grievant must be able to show that he or she was adversely affected by whatever action was taken.
2. The grievant must be able to demonstrate that an official action was taken that was either unreasonable or not generally or specifically authorized in the labor contract.
3. If the action follows a written or implied policy, the grievant must demonstrate that the policy is either unreasonable or not generally or specifically authorized.

4. The grievant must show that the remedy sought will not effectively result in special favoritism for him or her or prejudice against others.

Most grievances or conflicts between employees and management can be resolved informally through communication, negotiation, compromise, and collaboration. Generally, though, even this *informal process* has well-defined steps that should be followed in seeking resolution. If the employee and management are unable to resolve their differences informally, a formal grievance process begins.

The steps of the *formal grievance process* are outlined clearly in all union contracts or administrative policy and procedure manuals. If the differences cannot be settled through a formal grievance process, the matter is finally resolved in a process known as *arbitration.* In arbitration, a neutral third party listens to the arguments of both parties and makes a ruling that is binding to both parties.

◆ Rights and Responsibilities of the Employee and Employer in Resolving Grievances

Although the employee and employer have some separate and distinct rights and responsibilities in grievance situations, it is more common that they overlap. However easy it is to be drawn into the emotional aspects of a grievance that focuses on "one's perceived contractual rights," it is imperative that the employer and employee remember that both parties in a grievance have rights, and that these rights have concomitant responsibilities (Huston and Marquis, 1989). For example, although both parties have the right to be heard, there is an equal responsibility by both parties to listen without interrupting. The employee has the right to a positive work environment, but has the responsibility to communicate needs and discontent to the supervisor. The employer has the right to expect a certain level of productivity from the employee, but has the responsibility to provide a work environment that makes this possible. The employer has the right to expect employees to follow rules, but has the obligation to see that these rules are clearly communicated and fairly enforced.

Smooth labor relations require both the employee and the employer to honor existing labor contracts and to show good will in resolving differences when grievances do arise. This means that both parties must be open to discussion, negotiation, and compromise, and that an attempt should be made to solve the grievance at the earliest point possible. The ultimate goal of the grievance should not be to win, but to seek a resolution that results in maximum worker and unit productivity and satisfaction. In many cases, the manager can eliminate or reduce the risk of being involved in a grievance by fostering a work environment that emphasizes clear communication and fair, constructive discipline.

◆ Constructive Growth as a Result of Grievances

Although grievance procedures extract a great deal of time and energy from both the employee and the manager, they serve several valuable and needed purposes. Perhaps the most important outcome of a grievance is the legitimate opportunity it provides for employees to resolve conflicts with their superiors. Employees who are not given an outlet for resolving work conflicts can become demoralized, angry, and dissatisfied. This impacts on unit functioning and productivity. Even if the outcome of the grievance is not in the favor of the grievant, he or she will know an opportunity was given to present his or her case to an objective third party, and the chances for constructive conflict resolution will be greatly increased. In addition, managers tend to be fairer and more consistent when they know that employees have a method of redress for arbitrary managerial action.

◆ Employees with Special Needs

Progressive discipline is generally appropriate for dealing with employees who elect not to follow established rules or procedures or to meet organizational goals. However, it is inappropriate for employees who are impaired as a result of disease or by degree of ability. Such employees include chemically impaired employees and marginal employees. Chemically impaired employees are employees impaired owing to alcohol or other drug addiction. Marginal employees are those whose quantity or quality of work standards are consistently below that considered acceptable by the unit or organization, although they are working to the highest potential possible. These employees disrupt unit functioning because they are unable to carry their share of the work load. Both chemically impaired and marginal employees have special needs and require active coaching, support, and often professional counseling to be productive. It is essential that managers be able to distinguish between employees needing progressive discipline and employees who are impaired, so that the employee can be managed most appropriately.

◆ Summary

When discipline is constructive, fair, and consistent, it provides the structure needed for high unit morale and productivity. When discipline is destructive, vindictive, and inconsistent, unit morale and productivity plummet. It is the first- and middle-level managers who establish the climate for and administer discipline on the unit level. The ultimate goal for any manager is to mold or encourage employees toward displaying self-discipline. The manager may assume the role of supporter, motivator, enabler, or coach to meet this goal.

When employees lack self-discipline, or when they do not adhere to established rules, policies, and procedures, the manager must quickly intervene before the problem becomes worse. Often, the undesired behavior occurs because the employee does not understand established rules, policies, or procedures, and thus does not realize there is a problem. If this is not the case, managers have the authority and the responsibility to take progressively stronger measures until employees meet expected standards of achievement.

This progressive discipline system may include a verbal or written reprimand, suspension without pay, and finally, termination.

Although good managerial practices greatly reduce the need for discipline, some employees will always require external direction and discipline to meet organizational goals. In these situations, discipline will allow the violating employee, as well as all other employees, to clearly understand the organization's expectations, as well as the penalty for not meeting those expectations. Thus, discipline can be growth-producing for all involved.

◆ **References**

Curtin L (1996). Ethics, discipline, and discharge. Nurs Manage 27(3):51–52

Davidhizar R and Vance A (1996). Overreacting—a manager's dilemma. Nurs Manage 27(3):41–42

Health Care Educ Assoc (1987). Models of Excellence for Nurse Managers. St. Louis: CV Mosby

Huston CJ and Marquis BL (1989). Retention and Productivity Strategies for Nurse Managers. Philadelphia: JB Lippincott

Lewis EM and Spicer JG (1987). Human Resource Management Handbook: Contemporary Strategies for Nurse Managers. Rockville, MD: Aspen

Marquis B and Huston CJ (1996). Leadership Roles and Management Functions: Theory and Application, 2nd ed. Philadelphia: JB Lippincott

Marriner-Tomey A (1996). Guide to Nursing Management, 5th ed. St. Louis: CV Mosby

McGregor D (1967). The Professional Manager. New York: McGraw-Hill

Orth CD, Wilkinson HE, and Benfari RC (1990). The manager's role as coach and mentor. J Nurs Admin 20(9):11–15

Young LC and Hayne AN (1988). Nursing Administration: From Concepts to Practice. Philadelphia: WB Saunders

S A M P L E C A S E A N A L Y S I S

THE CASE ◆

At the facility where you are the night charge nurse, one of your LVN-LPNs repeatedly falls asleep at night, usually during nonbusy times, and must be frequently awakened to answer patients' call lights.

This has been a longstanding problem with this employee. You have personally spoken with her on several occasions and in reading her personnel file, you find this behavior mentioned in several past performance appraisals.

SAMPLE CASE ANALYSIS (CONTINUED)

Former appraisals identify her as an average employee overall. She has worked at the facility for 6 years. Her clinical performance has been satisfactory, but she is fairly dependent on others for direction and lacks initiative. You are aware that she is a single parent with four children; two of them have had some difficulties with minor infractions of the law.

As a new charge nurse you feel it is your responsibility to provide some type of structure to assist this employee in staying within the accepted policy of the facility, that is, "employees are not to sleep on duty."

••

Assignment

Outline your plan(s) for dealing with this problem employee. What would be your first, second, and so on, approach? Who else (if anyone) would be involved?

••

Analysis

Step I: In attempting to solve this case, the first action the charge nurse should take is to define the problem and the overall goal in solving it. Sometimes it is also helpful to be able to state who owns the problem. In this case, a problem analysis might be:

Problem Statement: The LVN-LPN frequently deviates from standard hospital policy. It is important to note that the case already reveals that this is repeated behavior; the action would be very different for a first-time offense. The case also stated that there was a standard or policy; in all performance appraisals there should be an established criterion for measurement.

Identify whether the employee owns the problem: We are unsure at this point if the LVN-LPN accepts this as her problem, but do know the charge nurse views it as a problem. This is a key point, because an employee has to acknowledge that there is a problem before he or she will change his or her behavior. Perhaps the nurse needs to make the LVN-LPN aware that the continued behavior will result in some action that will affect the LVN-LPN.

Determine the overall goal: Consistent improvement in this behavior. Rather than having a goal of elimination of an undesired behavior, also a possibility, the goal selected was consistent improvement, which represents a more realistic goal.

Step II: The second step in solving this case would be fact finding. Here, the nurse wants to find out as much as she can about why the problem is occurring. Is the employee getting enough sleep? Would assigning duties paced throughout the shift keep her awake? Is the employee working at another job in order to support her family? Does the employee see nothing wrong with sleeping on duty? Is it possible for the employee to take a short nap on her employee break in the lounge? What steps have been taken to correct this problem? Has there been fair and consistent supervision? Is it possible that the employee is bored?

Step III: Once the data have been gathered, a plan of action needs to be formulated. At this point, the charge nurse may wish to discuss the plan with his or her immediate supervisor. In arranging a counseling session with the employee,

SAMPLE CASE ANALYSIS (CONTINUED)

provisions for privacy and sufficient time for a full discussion of the problem are required. The charge nurse should be specific about what the employee must do, and if possible, work with the employee in writing a contract for behavior. The charge nurse must let the employee know that he or she believes improvement is possible, being specific about what will result if there is not consistent improvement in behavior. Relief charge nurses should also be made aware of this action so they can follow through on the regular charge nurse's nights off.

Step IV: There should be consistent follow-up by the charge nurse. The employee should be supported in her effort to improve and should receive recognition for any improvement. However, any deviation from this improvement should be dealt with immediately. If there is not noticeable and consistent improvement, further action needs to be taken, such as a formal written notice placed in the employee's file.

Note: The information regarding the possible personal problems of the employee was purposely included to see how individuals solving this case would use that information. This material has no real bearing on the case. The charge nurse may discover some additional personal information in Step II that would cause her to refer the LVN-LPN to a referral source for assistance, for example, a family counselor, or a physician for a medical checkup. However, the charge nurse should not assume the role of personal counselor for the employee. The manager can be supportive to the employee or even be empathetic to an employee's personal problems, but the charge nurse should not become confused about the purpose of the counseling session, which is to correct poor work behavior. Any other counseling is inappropriate for the managerial role.

•••

Conclusion

There is no one right or wrong way to solve this case, and similar cases would be handled differently depending on the individual circumstances present. Step III or Step IV might be somewhat different depending on what the charge nurse discovered in Step II.

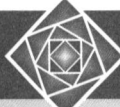 **CASES FOR PROBLEM SOLVING**

CASE 1

You are the supervisor of a neurological care unit. One morning you arrive at work and receive a report from the RNs from the night shift. Neither of the nurses report anything out of the ordinary except that the young head injury patient has been particularly belligerent and offensive in his language. This particular young man seemed especially annoying because he appeared rational at

CASE 1 (CONTINUED)

times, and then would suddenly become abusive. His language was particularly vulgar. You recognize that this is fairly normal behavior in a head injury, but yesterday morning his behavior became so offensive to his neurosurgeons that one of them threatened to "wash his mouth out with soap."

After both nurses leave the unit, you receive a phone call from the night house supervisor, who relates the following information. When the supervisor made her usual rounds to the neuro unit, nurse Caldwell was on a coffee break. Nurse Daly reported that Ms. Caldwell became very upset with the head injury patient because of his abusive and vulgar language and had taped his mouth shut with a 4-inch piece of adhesive tape. Ms. Daly had observed the behavior and had gone to the patient's bedside, removed the piece of tape, and suggested that Ms. Caldwell go get a cup of coffee. The supervisor observed the unit several times following this and nothing else appeared to be amiss. She stated that Ms. Daly said "no harm had come to the patient and that she was reluctant to report the incident, but felt perhaps one of the supervisors should counsel Ms. Caldwell."

After you thank the night supervisor, you ponder the facts in this case.

1. Ms. Caldwell has been an excellent nurse, but has occasionally been judgmental.
2. Ms. Caldwell is a very religious young woman who has led a sheltered life.
3. Taping a patient's mouth with a 4-inch piece of adhesive tape is very dangerous, especially for someone with questionable chest and abdominal injuries, as well as neurological injuries.
4. Ms. Caldwell has never been reprimanded before.

You call the physician and explain what happened. He says that he feels there was no harm done. He agrees with you that it is up to you whether to discipline the employee and to what degree. However, he feels most of the medical staff would want the nurse fired.

You phone the nurse and arrange for a conference with her. She tearfully admits what she did. She states that she "lost control." She asks you not to fire her, although she agrees this is a dischargeable offense. You consult with the administration and everyone agrees that you should be the one to decide the disciplinary action in this case.

....

Assignment

Decide what you would do, remembering your duty to patients, the hospital, and your staff. List at least four possible courses of action. Select from among these choices and justify your decision.

CASE 2

You are the coordinator of a small respiratory rehabilitation unit working with two other nurses in a small hospital. Because of the all-professional staff, you have applied a democratic approach to management and leadership. This approach has worked well and productivity has always been high. The other two nurses design their own schedules so that there are always two nurses on

CASE 2 (CONTINUED)

duty (including yourself) during the week and they take turns covering the weekends, at which time there is only one RN on duty. With this arrangement, it is therefore possible for three nurses to be on duty one day during the week, if there is no holiday or other time off scheduled by either of the other two RNs.

Several months ago you told the other RNs that the State Licensing Board was arriving on Wednesday, October 16 to review the unit, and that it would be necessary for both of them to be on duty as you would be with the inspectors all day. You have reminded them on several occasions since that time. Today is Tuesday, October 15, and you are staying late preparing files for tomorrow's inspection. Suddenly, you notice that one of the RNs has taken his name off tomorrow's schedule. Alarmed, you phone Mr. Stevens, the RN who is scheduled to be off. You remind him of the inspection and state that it will be necessary for him to come to work tomorrow. He says that although he is sorry that he forgot about the inspection, he has dental surgery scheduled and that considering how long it had taken to get the appointment, he feels he cannot cancel his surgery. After a considerable length of time it becomes obvious to you that Mr. Stevens really is not coming to work tomorrow. You say to him, "Mike, I feel this borders on insubordination. I really need you tomorrow and I am requesting that you come in. If you do not come to work I will need to take appropriate disciplinary action." Mr. Stevens replies, "I'm sorry to let you down, do what you have to do. I just cannot cancel my appointment."

• •

Assignment

What action could you take? What action should you take? Outline some alternatives. Decide what you should do, giving the rationale for your decision.

CASE 3 ◆

You are the professional staff coordinator of a small, emergency care clinic. Historically, the clinic is busiest on weekend evenings. This is when the majority of drunk driving injuries, stabbings, and gunshot wounds occur. In addition, many individuals use the clinic on weekends to take care of non-emergency medical needs that were not addressed during physician office hours during the week. Mr. Ketchum, an RN, has worked at the clinic since it opened 2 years ago. He is well-liked by all the employees and provides a sense of humor and lightheartedness in what is usually a highly stressful environment.

Mr. Ketchum has a reputation for being a "party animal." He is known to begin drinking after work on Friday night, and close down the bars Saturday morning. During the last 3 months, he has called in sick five of the seven Saturday evenings he was scheduled to work. This has resulted in the other employees working understaffed on what is generally the busiest night of the week, and they are becoming angry. They have asked you to talk to Mr. Ketchum or to schedule an additional employee on the Saturday evenings that he is assigned to work.

CASE 3 (CONTINUED)

• •

Assignment

You have decided to begin performance-deficiency coaching with Mr. Ketchum. Write a possible coaching scenario that includes the following:

1. The problem stated in behavioral terms,
2. An explanation to the employee of how the problem is related to organizational functioning,
3. A clear statement of the possible consequences of the unwanted behavior,
4. A request for input from the employee,
5. Employee participation in solving the problem, and
6. A plan for follow-up.

CASE 4 (Marquis and Huston, 1996)

You are the supervisor of a pediatric acute care unit. One of your patients, Joey, is a 5-year-old who sustained 30% third-degree burns, which have been grafted and are now healing. He has been a patient in the unit for approximately 2 months now. His mother stays with him nearly all waking hours and is generally supportive of both him and the staff.

In the last few weeks, Joey has begun expressing increasing frustration with basic nursing tasks, has frequently been uncooperative, and has, in the opinion of your staff, become very manipulative. His mother is frustrated with his behavior but feels that it is understandable, given the trauma he has experienced in the last 2 months. She has begun working with the staff on a mutually acceptable behavior modification program.

Although you have attempted to assign the same nurses to care for Joey, today it is not possible. This lack of continuity is especially frustrating today as the night shift reported frequent tantrums and uncooperative behavior. The nurse you have assigned to Joey is Ms. Steele.

Although a good nurse, Ms. Steele has demonstrated a lack of patience in the past working with uncooperative patients. During the morning, you are aware that Joey is continuing to "act out," and although Ms. Steele begins to look more and more harried, she states that things are under control.

When you return from lunch, Joey's mother is waiting at your office. She furiously reports that her son told her that the nurse hit him and told him he was a "very bad boy" after his mother had gone to lunch. She states that she feels physical punishment was totally inappropriate, and that she wants this nurse to be fired. She also states that she has contacted Joey's physician and that he is on his way over.

You call Ms. Steele into your office, where she emphatically denies all allegations. She states that during the lunch hour, Joey refused to allow her to check his dressings, and that she followed the behavior modification plan and discontinued his TV privileges. She believes his accusations are a further reflection of his manipulative behavior. You then approach Joey, who tearfully and emphatically repeats the story he told to his mother. He is consistent regarding the details and swears to his mother that he is telling the truth. All of your staff state that they were not within earshot of Joey's room at the time of the alleged incident. When Joey's doctor arrives, he demands that Ms. Steele be fired.

CASE 4 (CONTINUED)

. . . .

Assignment

Determine what you will do. You do not have proof to substantiate either party's story. You feel that Ms. Steele is capable of the accusations that have been leveled against her, but remain reluctant to implement any type of discipline without proper proof. What factors weigh the most in your decision?

CASE 5

Situation A

Grading students is a difficult task that represents a tremendous responsibility for faculty, as grades assigned to students can have both immediate and long-term effects on their lives. Despite efforts to assign representative and impartial grades, the pressure to do well makes the whole process of assigning and receiving grades an emotional one.

It is not surprising then that a discrepancy over perceptions of performance can occur between the instructor and the student, particularly in the clinical setting. In the majority of these situations, the instructor and the student can resolve this disagreement informally through discussion. Should an informal resolution fail, most academic institutions have formal grievance procedures that are then implemented.

. . . .

Assignment

Outline the formal and informal student grievance procedure at your educational institution. What responsibilities do the students and instructors have in trying to resolve the discrepancy? What rights do the student and instructor have, respectively? How can student grievances be avoided?

. . . .

Situation B

Assignment

Likewise, management and supervision of employees is very difficult and always contains an element of subjectivity. If you are presently employed in any capacity, determine what the grievance procedures of the organization are, and outline the steps that you would need to go through in order to file. What types of offenses would possibly cause you to take this type of action? What rationale could you use to justify your actions?

✳ Bibliography

The following is a list of references to help you solve these cases:

Anthony CE and del Bueno D (1993). A performance-based development system. Nurs Manage 24(6):32–34

Brooke PS (1990). Firing for cause. J Nurs Admin 20(9):45–50

Calfee BE (1995). Was it really wrongful termination? Nursing 25(4):65

Davidhizar D (1990). The manager as coach. Advanc Clin Care 5(3)May/June:42–44

Harmon S (1991). Giving constructive criticism with aplomb. Medic Lab Obs 23(3):24–27

Klann S (1990). Procedures for disciplining employees. OR Manager 6(4):14,16

Lammer M (1992). The investigation and discipline process. ConceRN 21(1):22–23

Manthey M (1993). Discipline without punishment. Nurse Educ 18(2):8–9

Maratea JM (1991). If performance palls, look below the surface. Medic Lab Obs 23(5):19

Martin BJ (1990). A successful approach to absenteeism. Nurs Manage 21(8):45–49

Medical Economics (1995). How to discipline your staff without getting sued. Med Econ Jan. 23,72(2):63

Raper JL and Myaya SN (1993). Employee discipline: a changing paradigm. Health Care Super 12(2):67–77

Tammelleo AD (1995). "Stern tone" or verbal abuse? Disciplinary action. Regan Rep Nurs Law 35(11):2

Vestal K (1990). Fired! Managing the process. J Nurs Admin 20(6):14–16

Wieczorek B (1990). An alternative approach to discipline. Ped Nurs 16(6):587–588

PERSONAL NOTEBOOK

1. Try to recall when an authority figure (i.e., a parent, teacher, boss) set limits or enforced rules in such a way that you became a "better" child, student, or employee. What made this disciplinary experience produce growth as opposed to being destructive?

2. Do you put off taking action such as being assertive until your anger builds up and you are forced to act?

3. Some rules need to be changed. Can you think of a rule or policy that needs to be updated? What could you do to update this rule?

RELATED ISSUES IN MANAGEMENT DECISION MAKING

Several related issues affect all phases of the management process and determine in part both long-term outcomes and management effectiveness. Because nursing is a profession, the nursing manager must remain cognizant of professional issues and laws and legislation directly related to nursing practice. In addition, the ethical ramifications of management are especially important for nursing managers because they direct their management skills toward an end that concerns consumers in need of health care. Ethics, legal constraints, and professional practice boundaries all provide additional controls for management and nursing practice.

The first chapter in this unit is devoted to professional issues in nursing. Nurse managers remain professional nurses and what affects the profession should be of major concern to them. It behooves them to keep abreast of professional issues, to become involved in professional organizations, and to advance the cause of nursing. Since nurse managers have a large sphere of influence they need to examine their role in the greater society of humankind and when possible use their collective power to improve health care for all. For example, the changing demographics of the national citizenry requires an examination of how well the needs of a culturally diverse patient population are being met.

Managers must promote the growth of their employees, encourage advanced education, and become role models of lifelong learning to subordinates. There is also the responsibility to promote a climate of mutual respect, caring, and collegiality.

The second chapter in this unit addresses the many legal and legislative issues of the nursing profession and health care management. All managers have a responsibility to be aware of changing legislation that impacts on their sphere of management, but because of the rapid changes occurring in the health care field this is an area of great importance for nursing managers.

Ethical issues, the final chapter in this section, provide the reader with a background of ethical terminology and a brief overview of ethical frameworks for decision making. Because ethical considerations are inherent in every phase of the management process and in many decisions the manager makes, this chapter provides the foundation for ethical management.

Managers have a responsibility to promote ethical behavior both within and above their sphere of influence. It often takes only one individual in a organization to speak out about an unethical decision to affect changes in the work place.

Whereas previous units have given the reader a sound foundation in management, this unit is devoted to issues that assist the manager in developing leadership skills that are so vital to effective management.

Professional Issues for Managers

As professional nurses, managers have a responsibility beyond the organization and its employees and consumers. They are also responsible to their colleagues and the profession of nursing. Often nurse managers develop a loyalty to the organization that supersedes their commitment to nursing. Therefore, managers should periodically examine their behavior critically to determine if it demonstrates support for the profession as well.

Quinn and Smith (1987) maintain that when individuals choose to enter a profession they voluntarily bite off a chunk of the human condition. This means that they are choosing to become involved (with expertise and commitment) in an area of human life in which important elements of human welfare are at stake and in which people must depend on experts. Thus, entry into a profession involves a personal and public promise to serve others with the special expertise that the profession can provide and that society legitimately expects.

At times the individual manager may feel that the problems of nursing are too big for them to make a difference but this is not true. A single manager can set the climate for increased professionalism among subordinates and promote professional career development.

This chapter focuses on three aspects of professionalism and the role of the manager in each of these areas. The first is the fundamental element of creating an environment that supports professional relationships and professional commitment. The second is the role of the manager as advocate. The third is the responsibility for promoting an organizational educational climate by developing personal career goals and assisting staff with career planning.

◆ Creating a Caring Environment

One of the characteristics of a profession is that its members have some shared values. One of the important values of nursing is that of caring (Duffield and Pelletier, 1995). Within professional relationships a caring focus may take many forms. Some forms, such as mentoring and preceptoring, have been discussed in previous chapters and are related to the manager's role. Other professional relationships that should be encouraged by the manager are caring, collegiality, and networking. In addition, the manager should be a role model of a compassionate individual who is deeply committed to the nursing profession.

We should not deny the significance of caring in our professional relationships. The manager must be a role model to ensure that staff care for one another as well as their clients. Caring fosters cohesiveness and unity that strengthen the profession. An open, caring work environment forms the basis for positive interaction that occurs among colleagues. This environment is likely to lead to greater job satisfaction for all employees.

To determine the level of caring within a unit a manager should assess how often the following behaviors are observed in the work place.

1. Sharing of tasks and flexibility among employees.
2. Recognition, praise, and mutual respect for others by individual staff members.
3. Courtesy and compromise.
4. The ability to give and take constructive criticism.

Empathy, understanding, and concern for others are fundamental in creating a climate of support (Mills and Pennoni, 1990). Managers who demonstrate caring values have the potential to increase self-esteem and job satisfaction among employees. Stenger (1996) claims there should be mutuality in the work place. She states that mutuality is about giving and taking and developing an interdependent connection and not seeking to control or needing to escape someone else's control.

◆ Encouraging Collegiality

Collegiality, the joining together of colleagues, is a valuable commodity for both individuals and the profession as a whole. It is essential to developing professional strength, peer support, and networking. Only after we have forged stronger intraprofessional relationships will we be able to develop improved relationships with other health professions.

As we learn to respect and support each other we will begin to acknowledge our worth to ourselves and each other. Some intraprofessional differences will always exist but acknowledgment of such differences and informed debate will lead to greater unity. With such unity comes power, credibility, professional maturity, and empowerment.

There are unlimited opportunities to demonstrate professional collegiality. Supporting nurses who have been challenged about a good decision they have made is an effective way for a manager to role model this concept. Adapting unit shared decision making and problem solving are other collegial approaches. Implementing a self-governance organizational structure has perhaps the greatest potential for promoting collegiality.

◆ Networking Possibilities

Networking unlocks sources of information and advice that can expedite work activities. Networking is a deliberate process of developing and using contacts for information, leads, referrals, advice, ideas, and moral support (Umiker, 1989). In this way the benefits of collegiality are extended. The networking process is active and purposeful and encourages development of political and professional power through communication and mutual support. The collegiality involved in networking is a way to create a power base for change. Major sources of networking possibilities for the nurse manager are peers and professional organizations.

Networking establishes channels for disseminating information and generating solutions to common problems. When nurses are linked together for a common purpose, the communication and relationships that are formed promote professional collegiality.

At the unit level preceptorships foster networking. Through this process of sharing information and guidance, bonds are forged. Another forum for networking could be a newsletter where nurses share ideas and creative approaches to patient care.

◆ Professional and Societal Accountability

Managers should demonstrate, to their staff, a personal commitment to the nursing profession and to consumers of health care. It is the manager who establishes the common frame of reference for the way staff approach both nursing practice and patient care (Clifford and Wandel, 1993). The following are ways the manager can role model behaviors of professional commitment.

1. *Demonstrate Lifelong Learning.* When Nightingale defined the role of the nurse manager (then called superintendent), she emphasized the need for personal lifelong learning (Henry, Woods, and Nagelkerk, 1990). Managers should share content from personal learning through classes and/or conferences and with staff at unit meetings. When staff have recently cared for a patient with an unusual diagnosis or assisted with an infrequent procedure, they should be encouraged to share new information and technology with other staff. Promoting a learning atmosphere that permeates the agency or department benefits consumer and staff alike.

2. *Serve the Community and Profession.* Managers should look beyond their organization for ways to foster nursing's image. Becoming active in nursing organizations and serving on boards or committees of community service groups has many positive results. It is good networking, builds collegiality, strengthens nursing's political base, and provides good public relations for the organization. The manager's involvement in these activities can be shared with staff and they should be encouraged to actively become involved in professional and community organizations.
3. *Encourage the Use of Research in Practice.* Participation in research is another way to enhance the profession. Clinical research drives innovations in practice and validates current practice. Managers can encourage the reading of research articles and use new research as the motivating force to update and change procedures.
4. *Become Politically Active.* If nursing is to advance as a profession, practitioners and managers must broaden their sociopolitical knowledge base to have a better understanding of the bureaucracies in which they live. This includes speaking out on consumer issues, continuing and expanding attempts to influence legislation, and increasing membership on governmental health policy-making boards and councils (Nelson, 1988).

Managers are looked on as leaders of the discipline of nursing. It behooves them to keep abreast of health care issues. Nursing's legislative efforts to shape the future of the discipline and healthcare are more necessary now than ever. In recent years nursing has been able to defend nursing practice acts in state legislatures from attempts by those outside of nursing to constrain nursing practice (Strader and Decker, 1995). When managers are politically involved they demonstrate empowerment, a willingness to advocate for nursing and seize control of the future.

◆ Advocacy

Through helping others to grow and self-actualize, advocacy becomes a leadership role. In addition to advocating for the profession, managers, by virtue of their many roles, must be advocates for clients and subordinates. Advocacy differs from ethics or good nursing practice, although it is often defined as one or both (Marquis and Huston, 1996).

Technological advances and the accompanying need to distribute scarce and expensive resources have created new problems and ethical dilemmas. For example, although DRGs may have eased the strain on government fiscal resources, they have created new ethical problems such as patient dumping, premature patient discharge, and inequality of care (Huston and Marquis, 1989). It is the first- and middle-level manager who is in the best position to advocate for patients affected by problems like these.

The future will see an even greater culturally diverse patient population. Managers must ascertain that patients of different cultures, languages, and social orientation have their unique needs met. To do this the manager must periodically examine the patient population to determine its cultural makeup and to ensure that language difficulties and cultural differences are being handled appropriately. Perhaps there is no more important advocacy role for the manager than maintaining the right of patients to view health and illness issues within the context of their own culture.

The manager is also an advocate for subordinates. Subordinate advocacy is a neglected concept in management theory but an essential part of the management role. It requires that managers recognize what subordinates are striving for, as well as the goals and values they consider appropriate (Quinn and Smith, 1987). Managers can then guide subordinates toward actualization while defending their right to autonomy. In this area of advocacy, the organization provides some *direction* in solving ethical dilemmas involved in staffing, duties of personnel, and conflicts between medicine and nursing, but it is the manager who must *resolve* such problems and live with the solutions at the unit level.

Upper-level managers advocate for subordinates in a different way. For example, the health care industry often faces crises of inadequate human resources during nursing shortages. Many organizations make quick, hasty decisions to find short-term solutions to a severe, long-term problem. New workers have been recruited at a phenomenally high cost without the development of solutions to the problems that cause high worker attrition (Huston and Marquis, 1989). The upper-level manager must advocate for subordinates in solving problems and making decisions about how best to use limited resources. These decisions must be made carefully following a thorough examination of the political, social, economic, and ethical costs.

◆ Career Development

Career development is the planning and implementation of career plans (Vogel, 1990). This can be accomplished through assessment, job analysis, education, training, job search and acquisition, and work experience. Before the 1970s, organizations did little to help employees plan and develop their careers. In the last two decades, however, the impact of career development programs has been repeatedly documented as being a positive force in successful organizations (Peters and Waterman, 1982; Kramer and Schmalenberg, 1988).

Since Peters and Waterman's work was published, organizations have taken an interest in assisting employees with career development. Recently organizational theorists have determined that to be competitive, organizations must develop a culture of learning—a philosophy that requires everyone in the organization be committed to the concept of continuous learning (Senge, 1990).

Most successful managers will agree they have succeeded because they consciously set career goals, and worked diligently to meet those goals. Career planning provides individuals with a choice in career outcome rather than leaving it to chance (Madison, 1995).

Much of the career development offered by organizations in the past centered around developing managers within the organization. Presently, however, it is recognized that managers should assist all workers with their career plans, encouraging them to achieve more education and to seek out new learning experiences. In addition, managers should encourage workers to diversify in terms of certifications, skill capabilities, and knowledge areas, so they can remain more employable in the event of reorganization or reduced resources. Many nurses do not understand the importance of career planning and for many reasons allow their careers to be undirected.

Vestal (1987) maintains that career planning is an ongoing conscious and deliberate process that is much more difficult than it sounds. It should be a lifelong event, and not an activity inspired by promotion or termination. Thus, like other types of planning, it should be proactive rather than reactive. Vestal (1987) suggests that career planning is easier when a career planning map is created to assist in developing a long-term master plan. A career planning map is shown in Figure 23-1.

In phase 1 of the career planning map, needs and interests are clearly identified. It is important at this point to not allow others to initially limit an individual's scope or to minimize one's ability. Instead, the individual should be specific about his or her goals, both long- and short-term. Interpersonal resources such as knowledge, experience, talents, and so on, as well as weaknesses should be assessed.

In phase 2, all available opportunities are examined within as well as outside the current work place. It is at this point that the individual must have some self-awareness regarding priorities, wants, and needs.

In phase 3, the career plan is implemented; action is taken. The individual may use networking to establish contacts both within and outside the immediate work environment. Resources and time constraints are identified.

In the last phase, progress is periodically evaluated and if necessary, goals are reassessed. Validation is made as to whether priority goals have been accomplished.

Nursing offers many career options; thus, it is necessary for nurses to consciously examine their needs and wants so that they will select the option that brings them the most satisfaction.

One of the greatest values in career planning is being able to work through the process so that participants can become more aware of what factors are shaping their lives. Some plans may fail because of forces beyond their control, but having plans succeed is not as essential as planning. What is important in career planning, is that individuals take an active role and make decisions about their career rather than trusting it to fate. Planning eventually will lead them forward.

Although individuals should be encouraged to plan their own career goals, the manager can assist through advising and providing employees with information about promotions, transfers, and opportunities within the organization. Sharing knowledge of educational opportunities and encouraging employees is also a manager's role.

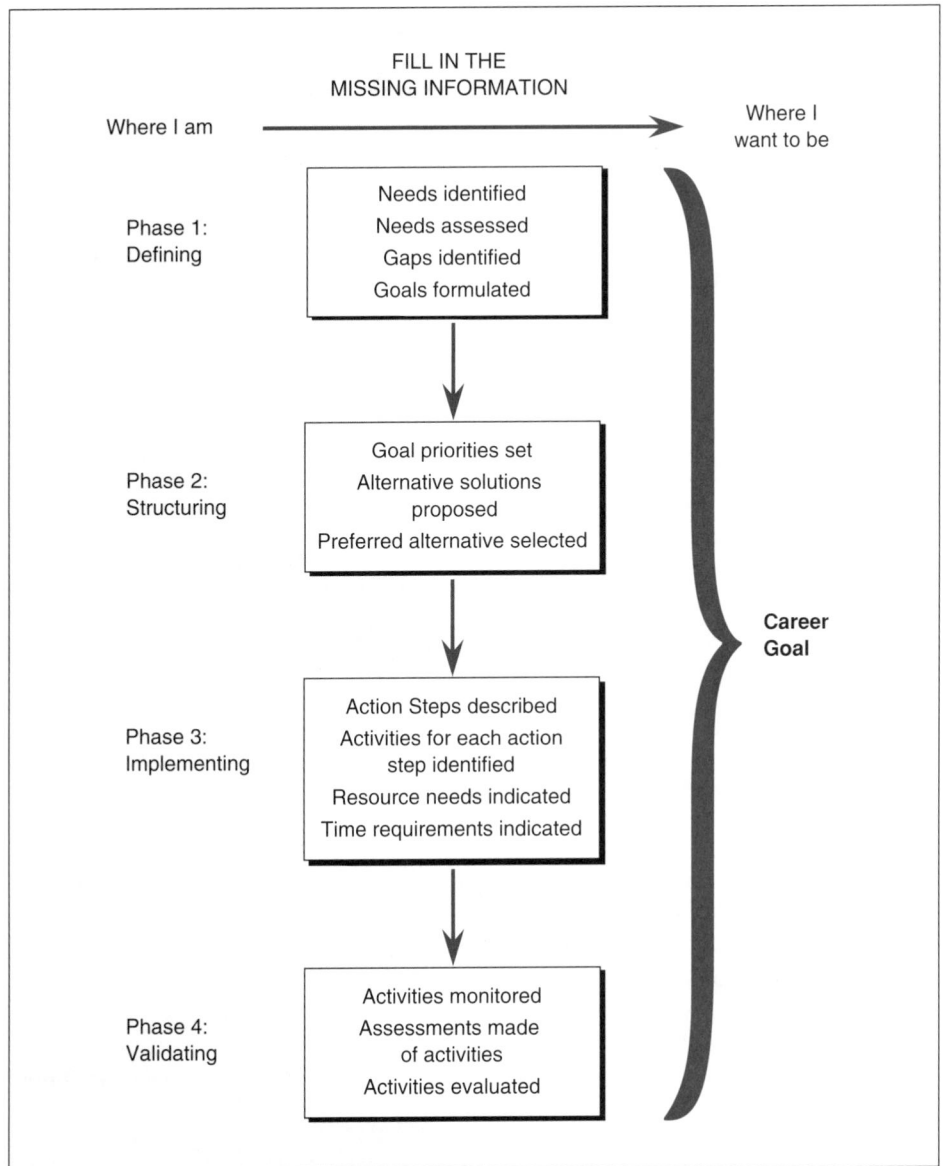

FIGURE 23-1. A Career Planning Guide for a Professional Nurse.

◆ Summary

Because nursing managers are professionals, they have a responsibility to the discipline of nursing. Promoting the profession through networking and political activism is a role of the manager.

Encouraging caring and collegiality among staff members is an excellent method of promoting professional relationships. Managers should also be role models by demonstrating commitment through their involvement with nursing organizations and other forms of networking.

Advocacy is considered one of the most vital roles of the nursing profession. Taking risks, sharing vision, building self-confidence, articulating needs, and being assertive are all behaviors employed in the advocacy role.

Although career development programs benefit all employees and the organization, there is an added bonus for the professional nurse. When nurses have the opportunity to experience a well-planned career development program, a greater vitality for and increased commitment to the profession are often evident.

◆ References

Clifford JC and Wandell JC (1993). Creating a supportive work environment. In Mason DJ, Talbot SW, and Leavitt JK (eds). Policy and Politics for Nurses, 2nd ed. Philadelphia: WB Saunders

Duffield C and Pelletier (1995). Supporting the profession. In Nolan A and Hazelton L (eds). The Practising Nurse. Sydney, Australia: WB Saunders

Henry B, Woods S, and Nagelkerk (1990). Nightingale's perspective of nursing administration. Nurs Health Care 11(4):201–205

Huston CJ and Marquis BL (1989). Retention and Productivity Strategies for Nurse Managers. Philadelphia: JB Lippincott

Kramer M and Schmalenberg C (1988). Magnet hospitals: institutions of excellence, part I. J Nurs Admin (1):18

Madison J (1995). Career development. In Nolan A and Hazelton L (eds). The Practising Nurse. Sydney, Australia: WB Saunders

Marquis B and Huston C (1996). Leadership Roles and Management Functions: Theory and Application, 2nd ed. Philadelphia: JB Lippincott

Mills DS and Pennoni M (1990). A nurturing work environment in philosophy and practice. Cancer Nurs 9(3):117

Nelson ML (1988). Advocacy in nursing. Nurs Outlook 36(3):31–34

Peters TJ and Waterman RH Jr (1982). In Search of Excellence. New York: Harper & Row

Quinn CA and Smith MD (1987). The Professional Commitment: Issues and Ethics in Nursing. Philadelphia: WB Saunders

Senge P (1990). The Fifth Discipline: The Art and Practice of the Learning Organization. New York: Doubleday

Stenger E (1996). Creating New Relationships: A Guide to Mutuality. Cincinnati, OH: Relationship Works

Strader MK and Drecker PJ (1995). Role Transition. Norwalk, CT: Appelton and Lange

Umiker W (1989). Networking: a vital activity for health care professionals. Health Care Super 7(3):65–69

Vestal KW (1995). Management Concepts for the New Nurse. Philadelphia: JB Lippincott

Vogel G (1990). Career development: an integrated process. Holistic Nurs Pract 4(4): 34–38

S A M P L E   C A S E   A N A L Y S I S

THE CASE ◆

You have been the head nurse of a small neurological unit, staffed by an all-licensed staff, for 2 years. You have just completed a management course that emphasized the concepts of mutuality and collegiality. In an effort to promote these concepts and to seek feedback for your own personal growth, you have decided to request some input from subordinates regarding your performance as a supervisor. You realize that there are risks involved, but you believe that the potential benefits from the feedback outweigh the risks. However, because you want to provide some structure for the evaluation, you spend time designing the appraisal tool and developing your plan.

Assignment

What type of tool will you design? What is your overall goal? Will you show the results of the appraisal to your supervisor? How will you use the information obtained? Would the appraisal forms be signed or anonymous? Who would be included in the evaluation group? Be able to support your answers with an appropriate rationale.

Analysis

The first problem to be addressed here is the goal for the involvement of the subordinates in the appraisal of the head nurse. Managers should examine their motives for involving subordinates in their own personnel appraisal. Hidden agendas in this case may include the manager's certainty that he or she is a good supervisor, but because managers receive such infrequent encouragement from their bosses, they feel the need to elicit "strokes" from the staff. If the manager can sincerely examine his or her motives and find that the goal is truly feedback regarding performance as a supervisor, then the appraisal feedback should be anonymous. The form should be designed in such a way that it forces employees to address negative as well as positive aspects of performance. This will indicate that the manager trusts their judgment and is aware that all individuals possess both strengths and areas of needed improvement.

Because this is the first time the manager has used this technique, he or she may wish to wait until the information the appraisal form generates is known before deciding with whom (if anyone) it will be shared. The manager will have gained some political clout with the staff by involving them, but appropriate power communications would support waiting on this decision.

Since this is a small unit with only licensed personnel, the manager decided to include the entire group. However, the distinction is made to have the appraisers state their worker category and length of service as the more recent employees or the LVNs-LPNs may have a less clear picture of the manager's responsibilities and their comments would need to weighed accordingly.

An example of an appropriate performance appraisal tool is shown in Display 23-1. Rather than focusing on whether the staff like or dislike the manager, this form stresses goals, an assessment of management quality, and constructive criticism. Although there is a concluding section for additional comments, the

SAMPLE CASE ANALYSIS (CONTINUED)

form has been designed to enable employees to concentrate on improving the supervision of their unit rather than on individual trivialities. Constructing this type of form greatly reduces the risk to the manager and increases the chances that information gathered will be of value.

DISPLAY 23-1
Sample Supervisor Appraisal Form

All staff on R-West are requested to fill out the following performance appraisal of their head nurse. The appraisal is anonymous, but if you wish, you may make an appointment with me and discuss your appraisal in person.

List my three best strengths as a manager.

1.

2.

3.

List three areas where I could improve as a manager.

1.

2.

3.

What changes instituted on the unit in the past year had positive results?

What changes instituted on the unit in the past year had disappointing or negative outcomes?

What two new goals would you recommend for the unit to pursue in the coming year?

Additional Comments:

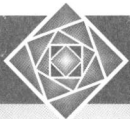

CASES FOR PROBLEM SOLVING

CASE 1

Mr. Carter is a 49-year-old automobile salesman admitted with severe back pain. You are assigned to be his primary care nurse and have established a rapport with him. Mr. Carter has a "type *A* personality" and has been very critical of much of his hospitalization. He has been very upset by the level of his pain following his laminectomy.

You have agreed that you will ambulate him on your shift three times, at 4:00 P.M., 7:00 P.M., and 10:30 P.M., so that he would only need to be ambulated once during the day shift. (He did not care for many of the day staff and felt that you did this better than anyone else.) You noted the ambulating routine on his nursing orders.

Yesterday Joan Martin, a day nurse, was assigned to Mr. Carter and she felt his bowel sounds were somewhat diminished. She urged him to ambulate more on the day shift, but he refused to do so (the doctor had ordered ambulate q.i.d.). When Mr. Carter's physician visited, Ms. Martin told him, "Mr. Carter refused to ambulate more than once on our shift." She did not elaborate further to the doctor. The physician proceeded to talk very sternly with Mr. Carter and told him he was to "get out of bed three times on day shift." Ms. Martin did not mention this incident to you in her report.

By the time you arrived on duty Mr. Carter was very, very angry. He threatened to sign himself out AMA (against medical advice). You spoke with his doctor, had the order changed, and finally managed to calm Mr. Carter down. You then wrote a nursing order that read "Nurse Martin is not to be assigned to Mr. Carter again."

When Ms. Martin came on duty this morning, the night shift pointed out the notation left by you. She was very angry and went to see the head nurse about it.

Assignment

Should you have done anything differently? If so, what? Could the evaluation of clinical performance by both you and Ms. Martin have been done in a manner that would not have resulted in conflict? If you were Ms. Martin, what could you have done to prevent the conflict? Be able to discuss this case in regard to its relationship to professional trust, peer review, and assertive communication.

CASE 2

You are a staff nurse at South Central Hospital. The patient census and acuity at South Central have been very high for the past 6 months. A higher turnover than usual has occurred recently and a coordinated recruitment effort to refill these positions has been largely unsuccessful. The nursing staff is demoralized and frequently call in sick or fail to show up for work. Today, you arrive at work and find that you are again being asked to work shorthanded. You will be the only RN on the floor for 30 patients. Although you have two LVNs and two CNAs assigned to work with you, you are concerned that patient-care safety could be

CASE 2 (CONTINUED)

compromised. A check with the nursing office ascertains that there is no additional help available.

You feel that you have "reached the end of your rope." The administration at South Central Hospital has been receptive to employee feedback about the acute staffing shortage and you believe they have made some efforts to try to alleviate the problem. However, you also maintain that the efforts have not been at a sufficient level, and that the hospital will continue to operate short-handed as long as staff accept the situation as it is. You have considered quitting, but really enjoy your work and feel a moral obligation to your coworkers, the patients, and even your superiors. Today, it occurs to you that you could anonymously phone the State Licensing Bureau and report South Central Hospital for consistent understaffing of nursing personnel leading to unsafe patient care. You believe this could be the impetus needed to improve the quality of care. You are also aware of the political ramification of this approach.

Assignment

Discuss whether or not you would take this action. What is your responsibility to the organization? To yourself? To the patients? How do you make decisions that have conflicting moral obligations?

CASE 3

You are a faculty member of a college of nursing at a major university in the midwest. In addition to your teaching and committee responsibilities in nursing, you are a member of a university-wide committee that selects outstanding faculty from across the campus in recognition of their excellence in teaching as well as their professional accomplishments. You have learned a great deal on this committee and believe that you have been an objective and contributory member.

Recently, the committee met to determine the winner of the Outstanding Educator Award. Several faculty from the school of nursing have been nominated. In reviewing the applicant files, you find that one file from one school of nursing faculty member contains many overstatements and several misrepresentations. You know for a fact that this faculty member did not complete several of the accomplishments listed, as she is a friend and close colleague. She did not, however, know that you were a member of this committee and thus would be aware of this deception.

When the university committee met, several members commented on the impressive file of this faculty member. Although you were able to covertly dissuade them from further considering her nomination, you are left with many uneasy feelings as well as some anger and sadness.

You realize that as she did not receive the nomination for Outstanding Educator, there is minimal actual danger regarding the deceptions in the file being used inappropriately at this time. However, you do recognize that you will not be on the university committee next year and that if she were to submit an erroneous application again, she could, in fact, be widely considered for the award. You also understand that even with the best of intentions and the most therapeutic of communications techniques, confronting your friend with her deception will

CASE 3 (CONTINUED)

cause her to lose face and will probably result in an unsalvageable friendship. In addition, even if you did confront her, there is little that you could do to stop her from repeating her actions, short of formally reporting her conduct to your dean.

Assignment

Determine what you will do. Do the potential costs outweigh the potential benefits? Be realistic about what you would do in this situation.

CASE 4

You are a senior baccalaureate nursing student in your sixth week of an advanced medical-surgical practicum. Your instructor assigns two students to work together caring for a group of four to six patients. The students alternate leader and follower roles, as well as providing total patient care. This is the second full day that you have worked as a team with Dorothy Williams, a fellow student.

Last week, when you were assigned with Ms. Williams, she was the leader and made numerous errors in judgment. She ambulated a patient who was on strict bedrest, gave an IV medication to the wrong patient, and administered morphine too soon as she forgot to record the prior dose in the medication record. Also, she frequently did not seem to know what was wrong with her patients.

Today you have been the leader and you observed her contaminate a dressing and forget to check arm bands twice while giving medications. When you asked her about checking the placement of the nasogastric tube, she did not know how to perform this skill or that she was required to do so. You have overheard some of the other students complain about Ms. Williams.

Assignment

State your obligation to your patients, your fellow students, the clinical agency, and your instructor. Delineate what you would do first, second, and so on. Give the rationale for your decisions.

CASE 5

You are a 25-year-old female in your senior year at a baccalaureate nursing school in the Midwest. One of your assignments for an issues class in nursing is to make a 20-year strategic plan for your career. Be sure you introduce flexibility within your plan.

Assignment

1. What is your overall career goal?
2. What are your strategic plans for reaching that goal? Did you consider financial, geographical, and family constraints?
3. What alternatives did you include in your plan?
4. Is marriage or parenthood part of your plan? Did you plan for aging parents?
5. What are your target dates? Are they feasible and realistic?

◆ Bibliography

This bibliography will assist you in solving these cases:

Ackerman N (1991). Effective peer review. Nurs Manage 22(8):48

Aiken L and Fagin C (1992). Charting Nursing's Future. Philadelphia: JB Lippincott

Deloughery GL (1991). Issues and Trends in Nursing. St. Louis: CV Mosby (1990). From A to Z: Tips and time-savers for career development. Nursing 90:139–149

Gardner D (1992). Career commitment in nursing. J Prof Nurs 8(3):155–160

Haller KB (1991). Diversity, debate and discourse. J Obstetr Gynecol Neonat Nurs 20(4):283

McCloskey J and Grace HK (1994). Current Issues in Nursing, 4th ed. St Louis: Mosby

Moloney M (1992). Professionalization of Nursing: Current Issues and Trends, 2nd ed. Philadelphia: JB Lippincott

Nativio DG (1991). On peer review. J Am Acad Nurse Pract 3(1):134

Parker ME, Gordon SC, and Brannon PT (1992). Involving nursing staff in research: a non-traditional approach. JONA 22(4):58–64

Wuest J (1994). Professionalism and the evolution of nursing as a discipline: a feminist perspective. J Prof Nurs 10(6):357–367

PERSONAL NOTEBOOK

1. Is it easier for you to give constructive feedback to a friend or to someone who is merely an acquaintance?

2. What types of feedback from others have helped you grow and gain insight?

3. Are you presently involved in a nursing organization? If so, describe how you are involved. Is your involvement adequate for you to advocate for the profession?

4. What pending legislation in your state has the greatest possiblility to impact nursing practice? How might you become more involved in advocating for or against this legislation?

CHAPTER 24

Legal Issues in Management

Another professional issue that guides the actions of nurses is legislative constraints. All managers have a degree of responsibility for ensuring that subordinates and their own nursing practice adheres to state nursing practice codes. Other areas of legal concern for the manager are patients' rights, and federal, state, and local laws that affect the organizational environment, employee and management rights, and patient care. Managers must have an awareness of a wide range of legal issues they may encounter in their work including legal considerations of working with a diverse work force. Contracts, fire and safety codes, child abuse, substance abuse, labor and employment law, and malpractice are some of the legal issues that concern managers. Although this chapter is not meant to be a complete legal source, it can serve as a basic guide for managers regarding their responsibility for legal constraints.

◆ The Legal Practice of Nursing

The legal basis for nursing practice comes from statutes (Guido, 1988). The 51 Nurse Practice Acts representing all the states and the District of Columbia are examples of statutes. These Nurse Practice Acts define and limit the practice of nursing (Fiesta, 1990). The State Board of Registered Nursing in each state is responsible for administration of its Nursing Practice Act.

It is important for all nurses to understand what legal controls for nursing practice exist in their state. Managers are responsible for applying those controls in their own professional practice, for monitoring the practice of employees under their charge, and for ensuring that all subordinate personnel maintain current and valid state licensure.

Because the Nurse Practice Act in most states is nonspecific, the individual employer often has established, clearcut guidelines for practice within their organization. These guidelines cannot exceed the scope of practice delineated in the state Nurse Practice Acts. Managers need to be cognizant of the specific interpretations of nursing practice in their organization and ensure that subordinates follow established practice.

◆ Professional Negligence

Historically, physicians were held liable for all care given to a patient, including care performed by nurses and other health care members. Nurses were rarely held accountable for their own acts and hospitals were usually exempted because of *charitable immunity*. However, following precedent-setting cases in the 1960s, employers became liable for nurses' acts under a concept known as *vicarious liability*. One form of vicarious liability is *respondent superior*, from a Latin term meaning that the master is responsible for the acts of his servants. The difficulty in interpreting respondent superior is that it is often unclear if the nurse is acting on behalf of the employer or the physician. In recent years the concept of *joint liability*, where the nurse, physician, and employing organization are all held liable, has become more common, and probably more accurately reflects the higher level of accountability now present in the nursing profession.

One concept that all nurses must understand is that of *personal liability*, which says that every person is liable for his or her own conduct (Goldstein, Perdew, and Pruitt, 1989). Others might share liability, but no one can relieve another of his or her own liability. Occasionally, in nursing and medicine, someone will make a statement that he or she will assume another's liability should something go wrong. Nurses should never act on this statement, since the law does not allow one individual to assume personal liability for another.

Because of the authority, autonomy, and accountability nurses have gained in the last 20 years, nurses are now routinely performing functions that were traditionally reserved for medical practice. This has resulted in an increase in the number of malpractice cases that seek damages from nurses as individuals.

Malpractice is the failure of a person with professional training to act in a *reasonable and prudent manner*. Reasonable and prudent generally imply the average judgment, foresight, intelligence, and skill that would be expected of a person with similar training and experience. Malpractice is also called *professional negligence*.

◆ Elements of Liability

There are five elements that must be present in order for a nurse to be held liable for malpractice. These factors represent the minimum requirements that define acceptable practice (Guido, 1988) (see Table 24-1).

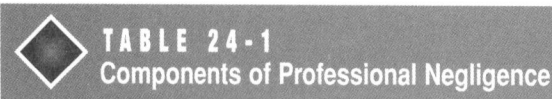

TABLE 24-1
Components of Professional Negligence

Elements of Liability	Explanation	Example: Giving Medications
1. Duty to use due care (defined by the standard of care).	The care that should be given under the circumstances (what the reasonably prudent nurse would have done).	A nurse should give medications accurately, completely, and on time.
2. Failure to meet standard of care (breach of duty).	Not giving the care that should be given under the circumstances.	A nurse fails to give medications accurately, completely, or on time.
3. Foreseeability of harm.	The nurse must have reasonable access to information about whether the possibility of harm exists.	The drug handbook specifies that the wrong dosage or route may cause injury.
4. A direct relationship between failure to meet the standard of care (breach) and injury can be proven.	Patient is harmed because proper care is not given.	Incorrect dosage causes patient to have a convulsion.
5. Injury.	Actual harm results to patient.	A serious or permanent complication occurs.

First, a *standard of care* must have been established, outlining the care that should have been given and was expected. Examples of standards of care include policy and procedure statements in a health care facility, job descriptions, and student guidelines.

Second, there must have been a failure to meet that standard of care—there must have been a *breach of duty.* This breach of duty is defined by other nurses called to testify as expert witnesses.

Third, the nurse must have had prior knowledge or information available that failure to meet the standard of care could result in harm. This is called *foreseeability of harm.* Being uninformed is not a justifiable excuse if the average prudent person could have anticipated that the consequences of an action could result in harm. For example, not reading a medication insert is not a sufficient excuse in regard to forseeability of harm. A different example might be a charge nurse who has assigned another RN to care for a critically ill patient. The assigned RN commits a medication error that injures the patient in some way. If the charge nurse had reason to believe that the RN was incapable of adequately caring for the patient (foreseeability of harm), or failed to provide adequate supervision, both nurses could be held liable. However, if the charge nurse had sufficient evidence that the RN should have been fully capable and was available as needed for supervision, then the charge nurse should not be held liable.

The fourth element of liability is that the failure to meet the standard of care must have the *potential to cause injury* to the patient. There must be a provable correlation between improper care and resultant injury to the patient (Marquis and Huston, 1996).

The fifth and final element is that actual patient *injury* must occur. This injury must be more than transitory. The plaintiff must show that the action of the defendant directly caused the injury and that the injury would not have occurred but for the actions of the defendant.

◆ Additional Legal Issues for the Manager

Many legal regulations involving managers have been discussed in units on hiring and dealing with unions. There are several other regulations and legal issues that influence management action.

1. *The Occupational Safety and Health Act* (OSHA). This broadly written piece of legislation addresses the requirements of the employer to provide a place of employment that is free from recognized hazards that may cause physical harm. It is impossible for the Department of Labor to physically inspect all facilities; therefore, most of their inspections are initiated because of an employee complaint or at the request of an employer for an inspection. The act does allow for fines to be levied if employers continue with unsafe conditions.

   Since the risk of detection, and the subsequent fine if discovered, are both low, some employers may choose to ignore unsafe working conditions. Managers are in a unique position to call attention to hazardous conditions in the work place, and should communicate such concerns to higher authority. Evra (1992) believes that nurses are exposed to four types of hazards: biological, chemical, physical, and psychological.

   Most states also have occupational and safety regulations. The more stringent of the two regulations are those with which the employer must comply. Many of the state licensing boards have additional health regulations that may differ in some manner from the federal regulations.

2. *State Health Facilities Licensing Boards.* In addition to health and safety requirements, many state boards regulate staffing requirements. It is the ultimate responsibility of top-level management to maintain the state license that permits them to operate. However, each manager is responsible for knowledge of and compliance to the regulations that apply to his or her unit or department.

   For example, if the manager of an ICU has a state regulation that mandates 12 hours of nursing care per patient, and also requires that the ratio of RNs to other staff be 2:1, the supervisor is obligated to staff at that level or above. If, during times of short staffing, supervisors are unable to meet this level, they must apprise upper-level management so there can be joint decision making to resolve the situation.

3. *Patient Rights.* Until the 1960s, the primary sources of patient rights were the legislative controls of nursing practice. Patients had very few rights; in fact, many times they were denied basic human rights. Since that time, the National League for Nursing, the American Hospital Association, and many states have passed a Bill of Rights for patients (see sample shown in Display 24-1). A Bill of Rights that has become law or a state regulation has the most legal authority as it provides the patient with legal recourse. A Bill of Rights issued by health care organizations and professional associations is not legally binding, but may influence funding and certainly should be considered professionally binding.

Today, patients are more assertive and involved in their health care. They have more information to examine when deciding on treatment options and are demanding to be participants in decisions about their health care. The right to information and to participate in decisions regarding medical care has led to conflicts in the areas of informed consent and access to medical records. Although the manager has a responsibility to ensure that all patient rights are met in the unit, the areas that are particularly sensitive involve the right to privacy and personal liberty, both guaranteed by the U.S. Constitution.

4. *Informed Consent.* An *informed consent* is one given by the person who is having a procedure or surgery performed and is obtained by a physician. The physician must describe the procedure and/or surgery to the patient in terms understood by the patient. The description must include potential benefits to the patient as well as possible risks, and should not imply any guarantee of result. Only a competent adult can legally sign to show informed consent. Spouses or other family members cannot give consent unless there is an approved guardianship or conservatorship.

In emergency cases, the physician can invoke *implied consent.* If the patient is unable to sign, the physician may state this in the medical record. Most organizations require that two physicians document that the patient is unable to sign, and this is usually written in the progress notes. Physicians do not sign the consent form for the patient.

Nurses frequently seek *expressed consent* from patients by witnessing them sign a standard consent form. In expressed consent, the responsibility of the nurse is to be certain that the patient has informed consent and to seek a remedy if he or she does not. Although nurses have an obligation to teach and to clarify information given to patients by their physician, they should be careful not to give new information that may contradict information given by the physician, thus interfering in the physician–patient relationship. At times, this can be a cloudy issue, both legally and ethically.

5. *Medical Records.* One source of information people apply in helping make decisions about their health care is their medical record; nurses have a legal responsibility for accurately recording appropriate information in the client's medical record. Although the patient owns the information in the medical record, the actual record belongs to the facil-

DISPLAY 24-1
List of Patient Rights in California

1. Exercise these rights without regard to sex or cultural, economic, educational, or religious background or the source of payment for care.

2. Expect considerate and respectful care.

3. Have knowledge of the name of the physician who has primary responsibility for coordinating care and the names and professional relationships of other physicians who will care for them.

4. Receive information from the physician about the illness, the course of treatment, and the prospect for recovery in terms that can be understood.

5. Receive as much information about any proposed treatment or procedure needed in order to give informed consent or to refuse this course of treatment. Except in emergencies, this information shall include a description of the procedure or treatment, the medically significant risks involved in this treatment, an alternate course of treatment or nontreatment and the risks involved in each, and knowledge of the name of the person who will carry out the procedure or treatment.

6. Be able to participate actively in decisions regarding medical care. To the extent permitted by law, this includes the right to refuse treatment.

7. Have full consideration of privacy concerning the medical care program. Case discussion, consultation, examination, and treatment are confidential and should be conducted discreetly. The patient has the right to be advised as to the reason for the presence of any individual.

8. Have confidential treatment of all communications and records pertaining to their care and stay in the hospital. Written permission of the patient shall be obtained before medical records can be made available to anyone not directly concerned with care.

9. Expect reasonable responses to any reasonable requests made for service.

10. Be able to leave the hospital even against the advice of the physician.

11. Reasonable continuity of care and knowledge in advance of the time and location of the appointment, as well as the physician providing the care.

12. Be advised if the hospital–personal physician proposes to engage in or perform human experimentation affecting care or treatment. The patient has the right to refuse to participate in such research projects.

13. Be informed by the physician or a delegate of the physician of continuing health care requirements following discharge from the hospital.

14. Be able to examine and receive an explanation of any bill regardless of the source of payment.

15. Know which hospital rules and policies apply to conduct as a patient.

16. Have all patient's rights apply to the person who may have legal responsibility to make decisions regarding medical care on behalf of the patient and improper care and injury to the patient.

ity that originally made it and is storing it. Although patients must have "reasonable access" to their records, the method for retrieving the record varies greatly from one institution to another. Managers should be aware of the procedure for procuring patients' medical records at their facility. Often, a patient's attempts to secure medical records are the result of a lack of trust, or a need for additional teaching and education. Nurses can do a great deal to reduce this confusion and foster an open, trusting, relationship between the patient and his or her health care providers.

6. *Extended Liability.* A situation that is somewhat different from malpractice but for which individuals may be held liable involves *product liability.* When a product is involved, negligence on the part of the health care provider does not have to be proven. This type of liability is often referred to as *strict liability* and is a gray area within the nursing profession. Essentially, strict liability holds that a product may be held to a higher degree of liability. In other words, if it can be proven that the equipment or product had a defect that caused an injury, then it would be debated in court using all the elements essential for negligence (i.e., duty, breach, etc.). Therefore, equipment and other products fall within the scope of nursing responsibility.

◆ Legal Considerations of Managing a Diverse Work Force

It is predicted that within 50 years minorities will comprise one third of the labor force (Peel, 1992), with a significant growth in the number of Hispanic, Asian, and Black employees (Sabatino, 1993). As discussed in the communication chapter, a primary area of diversity is language, including word meanings, accents, or dialects. Problems arising from this could be misunderstanding or reluctance to ask questions. Staff from cultures where assertiveness is not promoted may find it difficult to disagree with or question others. Blouin and Brent (1994) maintain that when employees' cultures differ dramatically the consequences may lead to conflict and unfilled expectations; therefore, how the manager handles these manifestations of cultural diversity is of major importance.

If the manager's response is seen as discriminatory, the employee may file a complaint with one of the state or federal agencies that oversee civil rights or equal opportunity enforcement. Such things as overt or subtle discrimination is protected by Title VII (Civil Rights Act of 1964). Managers have a responsibility to be fair and just. Tullman (1992) states that lack of promotions and unfair assignments may occur with minority employees just because they are different.

According to Carelli (1994), English-only rules in the work place may be viewed as discriminatory under Title VII. Such rules may not violate Title VII if employers require English only during certain periods of time. Even in these circumstances the employees must be notified of the rules and how they are to be enforced (Carelli, 1994).

Blouin and Brent (1994) maintain that managers should be taught how to deal sensitively and appropriately with a rapidly increasing diverse work force. Enhancing self and staff awareness of personal cultural biases, developing a comprehensive cultural diversity program and role modeling cultural sensitivity are some of the ways that managers can effectively avoid many legal issues associated with discriminatory management. However, it is hoped that future goals for the manager would go beyond compliance with Title VII and move toward understanding and respect of other cultures.

◆ Summary

Legislation of nursing practice has been established to both clarify the boundaries of practice and to protect patient's rights. Other legal constraints concern discrimination and supervisory responsibility. Since laws and legal considerations are constantly evolving, managers must continually keep abreast of legislation that may affect the scope of nursing practice and their role as manager. The manager has a legal obligation to uphold the laws, rules, and regulations impacting on the organization, the patient, and their nursing practice.

◆ References

Blouin AS and Brent NJ (1994). Managing a culturally diverse staff: legal considerations. JONA 21(11):13–14

Carelli R (1994). Court seeks advice on english only job rules. Chicago Daily Law Bulletin 140(55)1:16

Evra G (1992). Nurses in the OR. Revolution 2(2):64–66

Fiesta J (1990). The law and liability. Nurs Manage 21(8):20–21

Goldstein AS, Perdew S, and Pruitt S (1989). The Nurses Legal Advisor. Philadelphia: JB Lippincott

Guido GW (1988). Legal Issues in Nursing: A Source Book for Practice. Norwalk, CT: Appleton and Lange

Huston CL and Marquis BL (1989). Retention and Productivity Strategies for Nurse Managers. Philadelphia: JB Lippincott

Marquis BL and Huston CJ (1996). Leadership Roles and Management Functions for Nurses. Philadelphia: JB Lippincott

Peel KC (1992). Learning to value differences. Health Progr 73(7):44

Sabatino F (1993). Cultural shock: are U.S. hospitals ready? Hospitals 67(10):23–24

Tullman DF (1992). Cultural diversity in nursing education: does it affect racism in the nursing profession? J Nurs Educ 31(7):323

SAMPLE CASE ANALYSIS

THE CASE ◆

Mrs. Moore has been diagnosed as having invasive cancer and has been receiving daily radiation treatments. Her spouse is a frequent visitor and seems to be a devoted husband. Because they are both very interested in her progress and prognosis, they have asked many questions. You have given truthful answers, but there is not much that you know because the physician has not shared much information with the staff. Today, you walk into Mrs. Moore's room and find Mr. Moore sitting at his wife's bedside reading her chart. The radiation orderly had inadvertently left it in the room when Mrs. Moore returned from the x-ray department.

Assignment

Discuss what you would do, and why. What is the problem here? What should your follow-up be?

Analysis

The nurse needs to determine what is the most important goal in this situation. Possible goals include (1) getting the chart away from Mr. Moore as soon as possible, (2) protecting Mrs. Moore's privacy, (3) gathering more information, or (4) becoming a patient advocate for Mrs. Moore.

In solving the case, it is apparent that not enough information has been gathered. Mr. Moore now has the chart and it seems pointless to take it away from him. Usually, the danger in patients' families reading their chart lies in the possibilities of a) not understanding the chart and thereby confusing information obtained or b) an invasion of privacy because the patient has not given consent for family access.

Using this as the basis for the rationale, the nurse should use the following approach:

1. Clarify that Mr. Moore has his wife's permission to read the chart by asking her directly.
2. Ask Mr. Moore if there is any information in the chart that he did not understand or anything that he questioned. You may even ask him to summarize what he has read. Clarify those aspects that are appropriate for the nurse to address (hospital terminology, procedures, nursing care, etc.).
3. Refer questions that are inappropriate for the nurse to answer to the physician and let Mr. Moore know that you will assist him in speaking with the physician regarding the medical plan and prognosis.
4. When the nurse finishes speaking with Mr. Moore, he or she should request the chart and place it in the proper location. The incident should then be reported to the nurse's immediate supervisor.
5. The nurse should follow through by discussing the incident and Mr. Moore's concerns with the physician and by assisting the Moores in obtaining the information that they have requested.

SAMPLE CASE ANALYSIS (CONTINUED)

Conclusion

The nurse first gathered more information before becoming the patient advocate. It is possible that the Moores only had simple questions to ask and that the problem was a lack of communication between staff and their clients, rather than a physician–patient communication deficit. Legally, the patient has the right to understand what is happening and that should be the basis for the decisions in this case.

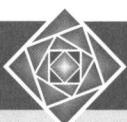 **CASES FOR PROBLEM SOLVING**

CASE 1

You are a surgical nurse working at Mercy Hospital. At 4:00 P.M. you receive a patient from the recovery room who has had a total hip replacement. You note that the hip dressings are saturated with bright red blood, but are aware that total hip replacements frequently have some postoperative oozing from the wound. There is an order on the chart to reinforce the dressing prn and you do so. When you next check the dressing at 6:00 P.M., you find the reinforcements saturated, as well as drainage on the bed linen. You call the physician and tell him that you believe the patient "is bleeding too heavily." The physician reassures you that the amount of bleeding you have described is not excessive, but to continue to monitor the patient closely. You recheck the patient's dressings at 7:00 and 8:00 P.M. You then call the physician again and tell him that "the bleeding still looks too heavy." He reiterates his reassurances and tells you to continue to watch the patient closely. At 10:00 P.M., the patient's blood pressure drops precipitously and she goes into shock. You summon the doctor, who arrives immediately.

Assignment

What are the legal ramifications of this case? Could the nurse be held liable for malpractice? Is the physician guilty of malpractice? Justify your answers.

CASE 2

Mrs. Keller is a 68-year-old cancer patient who has been admitted to the oncology unit at Ridgetop Hospital. Her diagnosis is liver cancer. Her admitting physician has advised chemotherapy, even though he feels there is little chance of its success. The patient asks her doctor, in your presence, if there is an alternative treatment to chemotherapy. He replies, "Nothing else has been proven to be

CASE 2 (CONTINUED)

effective. Everything else is quackery, and you would be wasting your money."
After he leaves, the patient and her family ask if you know anything about alternative treatments. When you indicate that you do have some current literature
available they beg that you share your information with them.

Assignment

What do you do? What is your legal responsibility to your patient, the doctor,
and the hospital? Using your knowledge of the legal process, the Nursing
Practice Act, patient rights, and legal precedents (Tuma versus Board of
Nursing, 1979), explain what you would do and defend your decision.

CASE 3

You are a staff nurse on a surgical unit. Shortly after reporting for duty, you
make rounds on all your patients. Mrs. Newman is a 38-year-old woman scheduled for a bilateral salpingoopherectomy and hysterectomy. In the course of
the conversation, Mrs. Newman comments that she is glad that she will not be
undergoing menopause as a result of this surgery. She elaborates by stating
that one of her friends had surgery that resulted in "surgical menopause" and
it was devastating to her. You return to the chart and check the surgical permit and doctor's progress notes. The OR permit reads "bilateral salpingoopherectomy and hysterectomy" and it is signed by Mrs. Newman. The physician has noted "discussed surgery with patient" in his progress notes.

   You return to Mrs. Newman's room and ask her what type of surgery she is
having and she states, "I'm having my uterus removed." You phone the physician and relate your information to the surgeon. He says, "Mrs. Newman
knows that I will take out her ovaries if necessary; I've discussed it with her.
She signed the permit. Now, please get her ready for surgery—she is the next
case."

Assignment

Discuss what you should do at this point. Why have you chosen this course of
action? What issues are involved here? Be able to discuss the various ramifications of this case. Describe your approach to problem solving.

CASE 4

You have been the evening charge nurse in the Emergency room at Lakeside
Hospital for the past 2 years. In addition to yourself, you have two LPN-LVNs
and four RNs working in your department. Your normal staffing is to have two
RNs and one LPN-LVN on duty Monday–Thursday, and one LPN-LVN and three
RNs on during the weekend.

   It has become apparent that one of the LPN-LVNs, Ms. Kurtz, resents the
recently imposed limitations of LPN-LVN duties as she has had 10 years experience in nursing, including a long tour of duty as a medic in the armed forces.

CASE 4 (CONTINUED)

The emergency room physicians admire her and are always seeking her assistance with any major wound repair. Occasionally, she has exceeded her job description as an LPN-LVN at Lakeside Hospital, although she has done nothing illegal. You have given her satisfactory performance evaluations in the past, despite everyone being aware that she sometimes pretends to be a "junior physician." You also suspect that the physicians sometimes allow her to suture wounds and perform other duties outside her licensure, but you have not investigated or actually seen this yourself.

Tonight you return from supper and find Ms. Kurtz suturing a deep laceration as the physician looks on. They *both* realize that you are upset and the physician takes over the suturing. Later, the doctor comes to you and says, "Don't worry, she does a great job and I'll take the responsibility for her actions." You are unsure what you should do. Ms. Kurtz is a good employee in all other respects, but you are frustrated with the situation.

Assignment

What are the legal ramifications of this case? Discuss what you should do, if anything. What are the responsibilities and liabilities of the physician, Ms. Kurtz, and yourself? Use an appropriate rationale to support your decision.

CASE 5 ◆

At the hospital where you are employed, it is a policy that employees have a current, valid license, in keeping with the state licensing code. It is always difficult to get people to bring their license in to verify that it is, in fact, current. You have just come from a meeting with the director, who reminds you that you must not have people performing duties with an expired license. You decide to issue a memo stating that you will hold the payroll checks of all employees who have not verified their license with you.

Following this, all the LVN-LPNs brought their licenses in for verification. However, one of them has an expired date on her license. When she is questioned, she admits that she did not mail her payment for relicensure until after she had read your memo. She was hoping to delay showing her license, as she is in a financial crisis that caused the delayed payment. You phone the licensing board and they state that it will be 6 weeks before the employee will receive her license. They *will not* verify her active license status over the telephone. You ponder the following facts:

1. It is illegal to perform duties requiring a license without one.
2. The LVN-LPN had prior knowledge of the licensing laws and hospital policy.
3. The LVN-LPN has been a good employee with no record of prior disciplinary action.

Assignment

Decide what you should do. What alternatives do you have? Provide the rationale for your decision.

◆ **Bibliography**

The following is a list of sources to assist in solving these cases:

Betts VT (1993). Nursing and the courts: a strategy for shaping public policy. In Mason DJ, Talbott SW, and Leavitt JK (eds): Policy and Politics for Nurses, 2nd ed. Philadelphia: WB Saunders

Fiesta J (1990). Safeguarding your nursing license. Nurs Manage 21(8):20–21

Fiesta J (1993). Legal aspects—standards of care, Part II. Nurs Manage 24(8):16–17

Fiesta J (1993). Staffing implications: a legal update. Nurs Manage 24(6):34–35

Flarey DL (1992). Legal and ethical issues in HIV testing, Part I. JONA 22(10):14–20

Hall JK (1990). Understanding the fine line between law and ethics. Nursing 90,20(10):37

Kjervik DK (1994). Advance directives: implications for nursing, in McCloskey J, Grace HK (eds): Current Issues in Nursing, 4th ed. St. Louis: CV Mosby

McPherson DC and Jackson MM (1994). The costs fo safety precautions to reduce risks of exposure to bloodborne pathogens, in McCloskey J, Grace HK (eds): Current Issues in Nursing, 4th ed. St. Louis: CV Mosby

Mittelstadt PC and Hart MA (1993). Legislative and regulatory processes, in Mason DJ, Talbott SW and Leavitt JK (eds): Policy and Politics for Nurses, 2nd ed. Philadelphia: WB Saunders

Smejkal CM and Hill FJMcD (1990). Life-sustaining treatment: a legal-ethical dilema. JONA 20(7/8):49–52

PERSONAL NOTEBOOK

1. Do you feel there are unnecessary lawsuits in the health care industry?

2. Have you ever advised a friend or family member to sue for damages you believed he or she suffered as a result of poor quality health care?

3. Do you think you will make future clinical errors in judgment as a nurse? What steps will you take to reduce the likelihood of this happening?

4. Are you willing to risk losing your job in order to ensure patient rights?

Ethical Decision Making for Managers

Legal guidelines for management decision making were examined in Chapter 24. This chapter concerns ethical decision making. Ethics is the study of what our conduct and actions ought to be with regard to ourselves, other human beings, and the environment. It is the justification of what is considered right and good, and the study of what our lives and relationships ought to be—not necessarily what they are (Aroskar, 1987). "Ethics has to do with actions we wish people would take, not actions they must take" (Hall, 1990).

Sometimes, separating legal and ethical issues is difficult. Legislation affecting nursing practice is generally clearer and philosophically impartial. Although legal controls assist the manager in problem solving, many issues or decisions the manager is involved in require some sort of value judgment that may or may not coincide with what is legal.

The conflict between legal and ethical behavior, especially in larger corporations, is under the scrutiny of media, regulators, and public interest groups (Sullivan and Brown, 1991a). Professionals once held in high esteem by society are now being held accountable for abusing their autonomy and enriching their lives at the expense of the clients they represent (Siler et al., 1990).

As in the private sector, the health care industry is facing an era of markedly limited physical, human, and fiscal resources; thus, nearly all decision making by health care managers involves some ethical component. However, the following forces ensure that ethics will become an even greater dimension in health care management decision making in the 1990s: increasing technology, regulatory pressures, competitiveness among health care providers, national nursing shortages, reduced fiscal resources, spiraling costs of supplies and salaries, and the public's increasing distrust of the health care delivery system and its institutions (Marquis and Huston, 1996). Woolery (1990) also suggests that the design and implementation of nursing information systems will create new ethical dilemmas for nursing managers in the coming decade.

In addition, because responsibilites to self, to the organization, to subordinates, and to consumers differ, there is a great potential for managers to experience intrapersonal conflict. Multiple advocacy roles and accountability to the profession further increase the likelihood that managers will be faced with ethical dilemmas in their practice.

Ethical dilemmas can be defined as making a choice between two equally undesirable alternatives. Haddad (1992) defines ethical dilemmas as novel, complex, and ambiguous problems that do not lend themselves to programmed or routine problem solving for which a precedent has been established.

Not all problems have an ethical component or result in an ethical dilemma. Generally a problem is considered to be an ethical dilemma if it cannot be solved using only empirical data, is complex and perplexing to analyze and results in far-reaching consequences (Curtin, 1992).

Curtin also distinguishes ethical dilemmas from moral dilemmas. Morality comprises the degree of congruency between a person's perception of what is right or good and their subsequent behavior. Curtin says that in *ethical* dilemmas, the individual does not know what is the appropriate thing to do. In moral dilemmas, the problem exists because one knows what is right, but does not want to do it.

It is important to remember that the way managers approach and solve ethical dilemmas is influenced by their values and basic beliefs about the rights, duties, and goals of all human beings. Self-awareness, then, is a critical part of ethical decision making, just as it is in so many other aspects of management.

◆ Ethical Problem Solving and Decision-Making Models

Because individual values, beliefs, and personal philosophy play a major role in moral or ethical decision making, how do managers decide between right and wrong in everyday decisions? What if there is no right or wrong answer? What if both answers are wrong?

As in all decision making, these decisions must be made using a professional approach that eliminates trial and error and that centers on proven decision-making models or problem-solving processes. Using a systematic approach to problem solving allows managers to make better decisions and increases the probability that they will be able to accept the ethical decisions they have made.

There are many systematic approaches to ethical problem solving that are appropriate for the nursing manager. These approaches include the use of theoretical problem-solving and decision-making models, ethical frameworks, and ethical principles.

Although not recognized specifically as an "ethical" problem-solving model, the *traditional problem-solving process,* discussed in Chapter 1, can be very effective in solving ethical problems. The following case study provides an example of how the traditional problem-solving process might be applied to a management ethics problem.

S A M P L E   C A S E   A N A L Y S I S

THE CASE: THE MARGINAL EMPLOYEE

You are the oncology supervisor in a 400-bed hospital. There are 35 beds on your unit, which is generally full. It is an extremely busy unit and your staff needs high-level assessment and communication skills in providing patient care. Because the nursing care needs on this floor are unique, and you utilize primary nursing, it has been very difficult in the past to float staff from other units when additional staffing was required. Although you have been able to keep the unit adequately staffed on a day-to-day basis, there are two open positions for RNs on your unit that have been unfilled for almost 3 months.

Historically, your staff have been excellent employees. They enjoy their work and are highly productive. Unit morale has been exceptionally good. However, in the last 3 months, the staff have begun complaining about Ms. Cintron, a full-time employee who has been working on the unit for 4 months. Ms. Cintron has been a registered nurse for 15 years and has worked in oncology units at other facilities. References from former employers identified her work as competent, although little other information was given. At Ms. Cintron's 6-week and 3-month performance appraisals, you coached her regarding her barely adequate work habits, assessment and communications skills, and decision making. She responded that she would attempt to improve her performance in these areas, as working on this unit was one of her highest career goals. Although Ms. Cintron has been receptive to your coaching and has told you of her efforts to improve her performance, there has been little observable difference in her behavior. You have slowly reached the conclusion that she is probably currently working at as high a level as she is capable; she is a marginal employee.

The other staff feel that Ms. Cintron is not carrying her share of the work load and have asked that you remove her from the unit.

••

Analysis (From Marquis and Huston, 1996)

1. *Identify the problem:* The marginal performance of one employee is affecting the morale on the unit.
2. *Gather data to analyze the causes and consequences of the problem:* The following information should be gathered and considered by the manager:
     Ms. Cintron has been an RN for 15 years, and probably has always been a marginal employee.
     She states she is highly motivated to be an oncology nurse.
     She has been coached on several occasions regarding how she might improve her performance and no improvement has been seen.
     It is difficult to recruit and retain staff nurses for this unit.
     The unit is already short two full-time RN positions.
     Ms. Cintron's performance is not unsatisfactory: It is only marginal.
     The other nurses on the floor consider her performance disruptive enough to ask you to remove her from the floor.
3. *Explore alternative solutions:*
     Alternative 1—Terminate Ms. Cintron's employment.
     Alternative 2—Transfer her to another floor.

S A M P L E   C A S E   A N A L Y S I S   (C O N T I N U E D)

Alternative 3—Continue coaching Ms. Cintron and help her identify specific and realistic goals about her performance.

Alternative 4—Do nothing and hope that the problem resolves itself.

Alternative 5—Work with the other staff nurses to create a work environment that will make Ms. Cintron want to be transferred from the floor.

4. *Evaluate the alternatives:*

Alternative 1—Although this option would provide a rapid solution to the problem, there are many negative aspects. Ms. Cintron, although performing at a marginal level, has not done anything that warrants termination. Even though some staff have requested her removal from the unit, this action could be viewed as arbitrary and grossly unfair by a silent minority. Thus, employee security and unit morale could decrease even more. In addition, it would be difficult to fill the position.

Alternative 2—This choice would remove the supervisor's immediate problem and would probably please the staff. This alternative, however, merely transfers the problem to a different unit, which is counterproductive to organizational goals. This might be an appropriate alternative if the supervisor could show that Ms. Cintron could be expected to perform at a higher level on another unit. It is difficult to predict how Ms. Cintron would feel about this alternative. She is probably aware of the staff's frustration with her, and a transfer would provide at least temporary shelter from her colleagues' hostility. In addition, she would appropriately view the transfer as a failure on her part to meet unit expectations. This recognition is demoralizing and the opportunity for her to fulfill a long-term career goal would be denied.

Alternative 3—This requires a long-term and time-consuming commitment on the part of the manager. There is inadequate information given in the case to determine whether the supervisor can make this type of commitment. In addition, there is no guarantee that setting short-term, specific, and realistic goals will improve Ms. Cintron's work performance. It should, however, increase her self-esteem and reinforce her supervisor's interest in her as a person. It also retains an RN who is difficult to replace. This alternative does not address the dissatisfaction of the staff.

Alternative 4—There are few positive aspects to this choice other than that the supervisor would not have to expend energy at the present time. However, the problem will probably snowball and unit morale will get worse.

Alternative 5—Although most individuals would agree that this approach is morally corrupt, there are some advantages. Ms. Cintron would voluntarily leave the unit and the supervisor and staff would not have to deal with the problem. The disadvantages are similar to those cited in Alternative 1.

5. *Select the appropriate solution:* As in most decisions with an ethical component, there is no one right answer and, in fact, all the alternatives have desirable and undesirable facets. Alternative 3 probably presents the least number of undesirable attributes. The cost to the supervisor is in time and effort. The supervisor really has little to lose in attempting this plan to increase employee productivity, as there are no replacements to fill the position anyway. Losing Ms. Cintron by termination or transfer merely increases the workload for other employees because of short staffing. It also cannot help the employee.

6. *Implement the solution:* In implementing Alternative 3, the supervisor should be very clear with Ms. Cintron about her motives. She must also be certain

that the goals they set are specific and realistic. Although the staff may continue to voice their unhappiness with her performance, the supervisor should be careful not to discuss confidential information about Ms. Cintron's coaching plan with them. The supervisor should, however, reassure the staff that she is aware of their concerns and that she will follow the situation closely.

7. *Evaluate the results:* The supervisor elected to review the problem solving 6 months after the plan was implemented. What was found was that although Ms. Cintron was satisfied with her performance and appreciative of her supervisor's efforts, performance had not improved appreciably. She continued to be a marginal employee, meeting minimal competency levels. The supervisor did find, however, that the staff seemed more accepting of her level of ability and rarely expressed their dissatisfaction with her again. In general, unit morale increased.

It is important to recognize that even if the outcome of the selected alternative had yielded negative consequences, the supervisor did make a "good" decision. It was a "good" decision because a structured approach to problem solving was used. This structured approach resulted in the gathering of a great deal of important information about the problem that was then applied in thoroughly analyzing multiple alternatives. Then, regardless of the outcome, the supervisor could feel comfortable that the best possible decision was made at the time with the information and resources available.

Another problem-solving model not specifically designed for ethical analysis, but effective for its use, is the nursing process. The cyclic nature of the nursing process allows for feedback to occur in the decision making at any given step. It also allows the cycle to repeat until adequate information is obtained to make a decision. It does not, however, require clear problem identification. The following case study analysis shows how the nursing process might be used as an ethical decision-making tool.

SAMPLE CASE ANALYSIS

THE CASE: ONE APPLICANT TOO MANY (From Marquis and Huston, 1996)

The reorganization of the public health agency has resulted in the creation of a new position of community health liaison. A job description has been written and notice of the job opening has been posted. As the Chief Nursing Executive of this agency, it will be your responsibility to select the best individual for the position. Because you are aware that all hiring decisions have some subjectivity, you want to eliminate as much personal bias as possible in arriving at your choice. Two individuals have applied for the position, and one of them is a close personal friend.

S A M P L E   C A S E   A N A L Y S I S   (C O N T I N U E D)

Analysis

Assess—As the nursing executive, you have a responsibility to make personnel decisions as objectively as you can. This means that the hiring decision should be based solely on which employee is best qualified for the position. You do recognize, however, that there may be a personal cost in terms of the friendship.

Plan—You must plan how you are going to collect this data. The tools you have selected are applications, resumes, references, and personal interviews.

Implement—Both applicants are contacted and asked to submit personal resumés and three letters of references from recent employers. In addition, both candidates are scheduled for structured format interviews with you and two of the agency board members. Although they will be asked to provide feedback regarding the applicant interviews, you have reserved the right to make the final hiring decision.

Evaluate—As a result of your plan, you have discovered that both candidates meet the minimal requirements posted for the job. One candidate, however, clearly has higher level communications skills while the other candidate (your friend) has more experience in public health and is more knowledgeable regarding the resources in your community. Both employees have complied with the request to submit resumes and letters of reference and these are of similar quality.

Assess—Your assessment of the situation is that you need more information to make the best possible decision. You must measure whether strong communication skills or public health experience and familiarity with the community would be more valuable in this position.

Plan—You need to obtain more information about what the employee will be doing in this newly created position.

Implement—If the job description is inadequate in providing this information, it may be necessary to backtrack and perform further job analysis and design. You may want to gather information from other public health agencies with a similar job classification.

Evaluate—Through job design and analysis, you now feel that excellent communications skills are absolutely essential for the job. The candidate who has these skills also has an acceptable level of public health experience, and seems motivated to learn more about the community and its resources. This means that your friend will not receive the job.

Assess—Now it is necessary for you to examine whether a good decision has been made.

Plan—You intend to evaluate your decision in 6 months using the established job description as a basis for your evaluation criteria.

Implement—You are unable to initiate your plan as this employee resigns unexpectedly 4 months after she takes the position. Your friend is now working in a similar capacity in another state. Although you correspond on an infrequent basis, the relationship has changed as a result of your decision.

SAMPLE CASE ANALYSIS (CONTINUED)

Evaluate—Did you make a wise decision? This decision was based on a carefully thought out process that included adequate data gathering and a weighing of alternatives. Variables beyond your control resulted in the employee's resignation and there was no apparent reason for you to expect that this would happen. The decision to exclude or minimize personal bias was a conscious one and you were aware of the possible ramifications of this choice. The decision making appears to have been appropriate.

Crisham (1985) developed a model for ethical decision making incorporating the nursing process and principles of biomedical ethics. This model is especially useful in clarifying ethical problems that occur as a result of conflicting obligations. Managers frequently have conflicting duties as a result of their differing responsibilities to patients, subordinates, self, and to the organization. This model is represented by the acronym MORAL representing:

M—Massage the dilemma; collect data about the ethical problem and who should be involved in the decision-making process.

O—Outline options; identify alternatives and analyze the causes and consequences.

R—Review criteria and resolve; weigh the options against the values of those involved in the decision. This may be done through a weighting system or grid.

A—Affirm position and act; develop the strategy for implementation.

L—Look back; evaluate the decision making.

A systematic approach to ethical decision making was also developed by Murphy and Murphy (1976). This model is specifically geared for ethical decision making as it helps the individual clarify the basic beliefs and values of those involved. The steps of this model include:

1. Identify the problem.
2. Determine why the problem is an ethical one.
3. Identify the people involved in the ultimate decision.
4. Define the role of the decision maker.
5. Consider the short- and long-term consequences of each alternative.
6. Make the decision.
7. Compare the decision with the philosophy of the decision maker's ethics.
8. Follow up on the results of the decision in order to establish a baseline for future decision making.

This type of systematic decision-making approach differs from problem-solving models already discussed as it does not attempt to solve the underlying problem. It is a decision-making model, however, as it requires the individual to make a decision. The solved case at the end of this chapter shows how Murphy and Murphy's model could be used to make a human resource management decision with ethical ramifications.

Sullivan and Brown (1991b) suggest the use of an *incremental process* in administrative decision making regarding ethical problems. Their common-sense, proactive model includes positive analysis and action as delineated in the following six steps:

1. *Determine the salient facts and ethical norms.*
2. *Look at the facts objectively.* What people are involved directly or indirectly? What are the causes and consequences? How are factors interrelated?
3. *Determine the problem.* Is it economic, psychosocial, legal, or biomedical in nature?
4. *Reflect on the ethical problem.* How does the problem stand up against personal and professional codes? What alternatives for problem solving exist? Who will benefit and lose most, respectively, with each alternative?
5. *Take action.*
6. *Evaluate the outcomes and process.*

◆ Ethical Frameworks for Decision Making

In addition to problem-solving and decision-making models, *ethical frameworks* for decision making have been identified that can assist the manager in problem solving. These frameworks do not solve the ethical problem, but assist the individuals involved in the problem solving in clarifying their values and beliefs. Four of the most commonly used ethical frameworks include (1) utilitarianism, (2) duty-based reasoning, (3) rights-based reasoning, and (4) intuitionism.

Using an ethical framework of *utilitarianism* encourages the manager to make decisions based upon what provides the greatest good for the greatest number of individuals. In doing so, the needs and wants of the individual are diminished. In the case study, "The Marginal Employee," the manager utilizing a utilitarian approach would have dismissed Ms. Cintron in order to provide good for the greatest number (her staff).

Duty-based reasoning is an ethical framework which says that some decisions must be made because there is an obligation to do what is right. There is a duty to either do something, or to refrain from doing something. In the case "One Applicant Too Many," the supervisor felt a duty to hire the best-qualified individual for the job, even if the personal cost was high. In "The Marginal Employee," the supervisor felt a duty to help Ms. Cintron perform at the highest possible level through coaching. In doing so, the supervisor refrained from terminating her as an employee.

Rights-based reasoning is based on the belief that some things are a person's just due; that is, that each individual has basic claims, or entitlements that should not be interfered with. Rights are different from needs, wants, or desires. The supervisor in "One Applicant Too Many" believed that both applicants had the right to fair and impartial consideration of their application.

work to see that pay raises are reflective of performance and not simply length of service.

6. *Truth telling and deception:* These principles are used to explain how the individual feels about the need for truth or the acceptability of deception. A manager who feels that deception is morally acceptable if it is done with the objective of beneficence may tell all applicants rejected for a specific job that they were highly considered, whether they were or not.

◆ Summary

No rules, guidelines, or theories exist that will ever cover all the aspects of the ethical dilemmas managers will face. Ethical issues affect every aspect of management, and managers must make decisions every day that involve complex ethical components. Because these decisions can be so difficult and the cost of a poor decision so high, it is critical that managers learn to make the best possible decisions with the least possible cost, in terms of human and fiscal resources. This requires the manager to become an expert at using systematic approaches to ethical problem solving and decision making, such as theoretical models, ethical frameworks, and ethical principles. The use of a systematic approach reduces personal bias, facilitates better decision making, and lets managers feel more comfortable about decisions they have made. To be good ethical problem solvers and decision makers, managers must also be self-aware regarding their values and basic beliefs about the rights, duties, and goals of human beings.

The quality of ethical problem solving or decision making should always be evaluated in terms of the process used to reach the decision. Many outcomes are beyond the control or foresight of the problem solver, and even the most ethical courses of action can have undesirable and unavoidable consequences. If a structured approach is used, data gathering is adequate, and multiple alternatives are carefully analyzed, then regardless of the outcome, the manager should feel comfortable that the best possible decision was made at the time with the information and resources available.

◆ References

Aroskar MA (1987). The interface of ethics and politics in nursing. Nurs Outlook 25(6)

Crisham P (1985). Moral: how can I do what is right? Nurs Manage 16(3)

Curtin L (1992). On writing a column on ethics. Nurs Manage 23(7):18–20

Etziony MB (ed.) (1973). The Physician's Creed. Springfield, IL: Charles C. Thomas

Haddad AM (1992). Ethical problems in home healthcare. J Nurs Admin 22(3):46–51

Hall JK (1990). Understanding the fine line between law and ethics. Nursing 90 20(10):37

Huston C and Marquis B (1989). Retention and Productivity Strategies for Nurse Managers. Philadelphia: JB Lippincott

Marquis B and Huston C (1996). Leadership Roles and Management Functions: Theory and Application, 2nd ed. Philadelphia: JB Lippincott

Murphy M and Murphy J (1976). Making ethical decisions systematically. Nursing 76 6(5):13–14

Siler JF, Garland SB, Yang C, Foust F (1990). Pressure on professionals. Bus Week 23 July:24–25

Sullivan PA and Brown T (1991a). Common-sense ethics in administrative decision making; part I, preparatory steps. J Nurs Admin 21(10):21–23

Sullivan PA and Brown T (1991b). Common-sense ethics in administrative decision making; part II, proactive steps. J Nurs Admin 21(11):57–61

Woolery LK (1990). Professional standards and ethical dilemmas in nursing information systems. J Nurs Admin 20(10):50–53

S A M P L E   C A S E   A N A L Y S I S

THE CASE: LITTLE WHITE LIES? (Huston and Marquis, 1989)

Mr. Hill is the nursing recruiter for Metro Hospital, which is experiencing an acute nursing shortage. He has been instructed to do or say whatever is necessary to recruit professional nurses so the hospital will not have to close several units. He has also been told that his position will be eliminated if he does not produce a substantial number of applicants as a result of nursing career days that will be held the following week. Mr. Hill loves his job and is the sole provider for his family. Because many other organizations in addition to his are experiencing severe nursing shortages, the competition for employees is keen. After his third career day without a single prospective applicant, he begins to feel desperate. On the fourth and final day, Mr. Hill begins making many promises to potential applicants regarding shift and unit preferences, salary, and advancement that he is not sure he can keep. At the end of the day, he has a lengthy list of interested applicants, but also feels a great deal of free-floating intrapersonal conflict.

••

Assignment

Apply Murphy and Murphy's (1976) ethical problem-solving model in analyzing the conflict felt by Mr. Hill.

••

Analysis

1. *Identify the problem:* In a desperate effort to save his job, Mr. Hill finds he has taken action that has resulted in high intrapersonal conflict regarding his values.
2. *Identify why the problem is an ethical problem:* This is an ethical problem because it involves personal values and beliefs, has far-reaching implications for all those involved, and presents several alternatives for decision making that are equally undesirable.
3. *Identify the people involved in the ultimate decision:* Mr. Hill has the ultimate responsibility for knowing his values and acting in a manner congruent with his values system. The organization is, however, involved in the values conflict in that their values and expectations may be in conflict with Mr. Hill's. The potential applicants are also involved, as there is some responsibility on the part of Mr. Hill and the organization to these applicants, although this responsibility is one of the values in conflict.

SAMPLE CASE ANALYSIS (CONTINUED)

4. *Identify the role of the decision maker:* Because this is Mr. Hill's problem, and it is an intrapersonal conflict, he must decide the appropriate course of action. His primary role is to examine his values and act accordingly.

5. *Consider the short- and long-term consequences of each alternative:* Mr. Hill has several alternatives:

Alternative 1—Quit his job immediately. This would prevent *future* intrapersonal conflict provided that Mr. Hill becomes aware of his values system and behaves in a consistent manner in the future. It does not, however, solve the immediate conflict about the action Mr. Hill has already taken. This solution also takes away his livelihood.

Alternative 2—Do nothing. Mr. Hill could choose not to be accountable for his own actions. This will require that he rationalize that the philosophy of the organization is, in fact, acceptable or that he has no choice regarding his actions. Thus, the responsibility for meeting the needs and wants of the new employees is shifted to the hospital. Although Mr. Hill will have no credibility with the new employees, it will, however, have a negligible impact on his ability to recruit at least on a short-term basis. Mr. Hill will continue in his job and be able to support his family.

Alternative 3—If, after values clarification, Mr. Hill has determined that his values are in conflict with the hospital's directive to do or say whatever is necessary to recruit new employees, he could approach his superior and share these concerns. Mr. Hill should be very clear about what his values are, and to what extent he is willing to compromise them. He also should include in this meeting, what if any action should be taken to meet the needs of the new applicant employees. It is important that Mr. Hill be realistic about the time and effort usually required to change the values and beliefs of an organization. He also must be aware of his bottom line if the organization is not willing to provide a compromise resolution.

Alternative 4—Mr. Hill could contact each of the applicants and tell them that recruitment promises made may not be possible, however, he will do what he can to see that they are fulfilled. This alternative is risky. The applicants will probably be justifiably suspicious of both the recruiter and the organization, and Mr. Hill has little formal power at this point to fulfill their requests. This alternative also requires a time and energy commitment by Mr. Hill and does not prevent the problem from recurring.

6. *Make the decision:* Mr. Hill chose Alternative 3.

7. *Compare the decision with the decision maker's philosophy of ethics:* In values clarification, Mr. Hill discovered that he valued the truth. Alternative 3 allows him to present a recruiting plan to his superior that includes a bottom line that this value will not be violated.

8. *Follow up on the results of the decision in order to establish a baseline for future decision making:* Mr. Hill approached his superior and was told that his beliefs were idealistic and inappropriate in an age of severe worker shortages. He was terminated. Mr. Hill did, however, believe that he made an appropriate decision. He did become self-aware regarding his values and had attempted to communicate them to the organization in an effort to work out a mutually agreeable plan. Although Mr. Hill was terminated, he knew that he could find some type of employment to meet immediate fiscal needs. He also utilized what he had learned in this decision-making process to more carefully evaluate the recruitment philosophy of the organization in relation to his own values system before accepting another job.

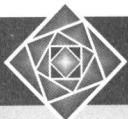

CASES FOR PROBLEM SOLVING

CASE 1

You are a nurse on a pediatric unit. One of your patients is a 15-month-old female with a diagnosis of failure to thrive. The mother has stated that the child appears "emotional" and cries a great deal and does not like to be held. You have been taking care of the infant for the 2 days since admission and she has smiled and laughed and held out her arms to be held by everyone. She has eaten well.

There is something about the child's reaction to the mother's boyfriend that bothers you. She appears to draw away from him when he visits. The mother is very young and seems to be rather immature, but appears to care for the child.

This is the second hospital admission for this child. Although you were not on duty at the time of the first admission 6 weeks ago, you review the records and find that the child was admitted with the same diagnosis.

While you are on duty today, the child's father calls and inquires about the child's condition. He lives several hundred miles away and requests that the child be hospitalized until the weekend (it is Wednesday) so that he can "check things out." He tells you that he feels the child is mistreated. He says he is also concerned about his ex-wife's 4-year-old child from another marriage and is attempting to gain custody of that child, in addition to his own child. From what little the father said, you are aware that the divorce was very bitter and that the mother has full custody.

You speak with the physician at length. He says that after the last hospitalization he requested that child protective services assess the family. Their subsequent report to him was that the 4-year-old appeared happy and well and that the 15-month-old appeared clean, although underweight. There was no evidence to suggest child abuse. However, the agency plans to continue follow-up on the children. He says the mother has been responsible about keeping doctor appointments and has kept the children's immunizations up to date.

The pediatrician proceeds to write an order for discharge. He says that although he also feels somewhat uneasy, there is no justification for continued hospitalization and the state medical aid will not pay for additional days.

You are present when the mother and her boyfriend come to pick up the baby. The baby clings to you and refuses to go to the boyfriend, and is also very reluctant to go to the mother. Throughout the discharge you are extremely uneasy. When you see the car drive away you experience a deep sadness.

Upon returning to the unit you talk with your supervisor. He listens carefully and questions you at length. Finally he states, "It seems as if you have nothing concrete and are only experiencing feelings. I think you would be risking a lot of trouble for yourself and the hospital if you acted rashly at this time. Accusing people with no evidence and making them go through a traumatic experience is something I would hesitate doing."

You leave the supervisor's office still feeling troubled. He did not tell you that you could do nothing, but you feel he would disapprove of further action on your part. The doctor also felt strongly that there was no reason to do more than was already being done. The child will be followed by child protective services. Perhaps the disgruntled ex-husband was just trying to make trouble for his ex-wife and her new boyfriend. You would certainly not want anyone to have reported you or created problems regarding your own children. You remember how often your 5-year-old bruised himself when he was that age. He often looked like an abused child. You go about your duties and try to shake off your feeling. What should you do?

CASE 1 (CONTINUED)

Assignment

Identify the problem and several alternative solutions to solving this ethical dilemma. What should you do and why? What are the risks? How does your value system play a part in your decision? Be able to justify your final solution.

CASE 2

You are the charge nurse of the evening shift in the recovery room. You have just admitted a 32-year-old female who was a passenger thrown from a jeep 2 hours ago. She had been rushed to the ER and subsequently to surgery, where cranial burr holes were completed and an intracranial monitor was placed. No further cranial exploration was attempted, as the patient had received massive neurological damage. She is not expected to survive your shift. The plan is to hold her in recovery room for 1 hour and if she is still alive to transfer her to ICU.

Shortly after receiving the patient in the recovery room you are approached by the evening house supervisor who says that there is a young woman who states she is the patient's sister pleading to be allowed into the recovery room. Normally, visitors are never allowed in the recovery room, but occasionally exceptions have been made. Tonight the recovery room is empty except for the aforementioned head injury case. You decide to bend the rules and allow the young woman's sister into the recovery room.

The visiting sister is near collapse and it is obvious from her words that she had been the driver of the jeep. As the visitor continues to speak to the comatose patient her behavior and words make you begin to wonder if she is indeed the sister.

Within 15 minutes the house supervisor returns and states, "I have made a terrible mistake, the patient's family just arrived and they say that the visitor we just allowed into the recovery room is not a member of the family, but is the patient's lover. They are very angry and demand that this woman not be allowed to see the patient."

You approach the visitor and confront her in a kindly manner regarding the information you have just received. She looks at you with tears streaming down her face and says, "Yes, it is true. June and I have been together for 6 years. Her family disowned her as a result. But we were everything to each other. She has been my life and I have been hers. Please, please let me stay. I will never see her again. I know the family will not allow me to attend her funeral. I need to say my goodbyes. Please let me stay. It is not fair that they have the legal right to be family when I have been the one to love and care for June."

Assignment

You must decide what to do. Recognize that your own values system will play a part in your decision. List several alternatives that are available to you for problem solving. Give your rationale for your decision.

CASE 3 ◆

One of your patients (that you have been following on an outpatient basis as a community health nurse) has been hospitalized. Both Doris Bly and her husband Charles suffer from COPD. Both are cigarette smokers and generally have poor health habits. You have been following this couple for 5 years and have developed a trusting relationship with them, coming to accept their chosen lifestyle and quality of life. They enjoy each other's company and have few friends. They live on a small pension and social security disability. Their days are spent watching television, drinking, and smoking.

You discover, on your arrival at the hospital, that Mrs. Bly has been placed in ICU with a diagnosis of acute pneumonia that is greatly aggravated by her chronic lung condition. Her condition is critical but may be curable with aggressive treatment. The physician is considering placing her on a mechanical ventilator (either using a tracheostomy or endotracheal tube). The physician has been discussing Mrs. Bly's condition with Mr. Bly when you arrive at the hospital. Mr. Bly is adamant that his wife not be placed on a "breathing machine." He clings to you when you arrive and reminds you that Mrs. Bly has always said, "She don't want none of those breathing machines, remember." She used to say, "Don't ever hook me up to a machine to die, Charlie."

You do recall that Mr. and Mrs. Bly were very clear to you regarding their fear of being made to live by artificial means. Mr. Bly looks at you and says, "Help me convince the doc."

··

Assignment

What will you do? What action will you take? How will you be a patient advocate? List your alternatives. Give rationale for your choice.

CASE 4 ◆ (Marquis and Huston, 1996)

Beverly Watson, a 35-year-old full-time nurse on the day shift, has been employed in your facility for 10 years. There have been rumors for some time now that Ms. Watson has been coming to work under the influence of alcohol. Staff have reported the smell of alcohol on her breath, unexcused absences from the unit, and an increase in the number of medication errors she has made. You have not directly observed any of these behaviors. When you arrive at work one day, you observe Ms. Watson covertly drinking from a dark colored flask in her locker. You immediately confront her with your observation and inquire as to whether she is drinking alcohol while on duty. Ms. Watson tearfully admits that she is drinking alcohol, but states that this is an isolated incident and begs you to forget it. She promises not to ever consume alcohol at work again.

In an effort to reduce the emotionalism of the event and to give yourself time to think, you send Ms. Watson home and reschedule a conference with her for later in the day. At this conference, she is defensive and states that she does not have a drinking problem and that you are overreacting. You share the data you have gathered during the day, which support that Beverly is probably chemically impaired. Ms. Watson offers no explanation for these behaviors.

PERSONAL NOTEBOOK

1. Did you agree with the solved case studies in this chapter? What values affected your answer?

2. List your 10 most important values. Attempt to rank order them.

3. Which of the ethical frameworks or principles do you use most often in your ethical problem solving? Which ones do you use least?

Index

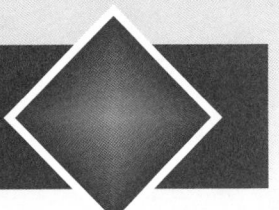

Note: Page numbers in italics *indicate illustrations; those followed by* d *indicate display material; those followed by* t *indicate tables.*

Absenteeism, 227–228
Acceptance Priority Rule, 27–28, 28d
Acceptance Rule, 27, 28d
Accidental change, 79
Accommodation, in conflict resolution, 315
Accountability, 121
Achievement, as motivational factor, 242–243
Acuity–based staffing, 227
Acuity index, 98d, 225d
Ad hoc organizational structure, 122
Administrative decision making, 22d, 22–23
Administrative man, vs. economic man, 22d, 22–23
Admonishments
  verbal, 388
  written, 388–389, 390d
Adult learning, 207–209, 208t
Advocacy, 414–415
Affective conflict, 313, *314*
Affiliation, as motivational factor, 243
Affirming the consequences, 14
Agency shop, 331d
Aggressive communication, 294
Aides. *See* Unlicensed assistive personnel (UAPs)
Alcohol–abusing employees, discipline of, 399
Alliances
  formation of, 162
  strategic, 103, 104
American Nurses Association (ANA)
  in collective bargaining, 334–335
  standards for nursing practice of, 351
Analytical thinking, 11–12
Androgogy, vs. pedagogy, 208t, 209t
Applicants, hiring of. *See* Interview(s); Recruitment; Selection
Arbitration, 331d, 398
Argument from analogy, 14
Argyris, Chris, 36
Assertive communication, 293–294, 295d

Assets, 98d
Assistants. *See* Subordinates; Unlicensed assistive personnel (UAPs)
Associate nurses, in primary nursing, 141, *141*
Audits, quality assurance, 351–352
Authoritarian leader, 39
Authority, 120
  delegation of, 274–286
  lines of, 116–118, *117, 119*
  vs. status, 118
Authority–power gap, 153–155
  bridging of, 154–155
Autonomy, 448–449
Average monthly patient days, 225d
Avoidance, in conflict resolution, 315

Baseline data, 98d
Behavioral theories, of leadership, 38–40
Behaviorism, 241
Beliefs. *See* Values
Benchmarking, 353
Beneficence, 449
Best practices research, 353
Bias, 432–433
Bill of Rights, patient, 430, 431d
Blake, R.R., 41
Blanchard, K., 41
Body language, 294–296
  cultural aspects of, 300
Bottom line, 319
Brainstorming, 13
Breach of duty, 428, 428t
Break–even point, 98d
Bridging, 317
Budget(s)
  analysis of, 97
  capital expenditure, 96
  continuous (perpetual), 97
  definition of, 95